FIRST AID FOR THE®

USMLE STEP 2 CS

Third Edition

TAO LE, MD, MHS
Assistant Clinical Professor of Medicine and Pediatrics
Chief, Section of Allergy and Immunology
Department of Medicine
University of Louisville

VIKAS BHUSHAN, MD
Diagnostic Radiologist

MAE SHEIKH-ALI, MD
Assistant Professor, Department of Medicine
Division of Endocrinology
University of Florida College of Medicine–Jacksonville

FADI ABU SHAHIN, MD
Fellow, Gynecologic Oncology
Cleveland Clinic

 Medical

New York / Chicago / San Francisco / Lisbon / London / Madrid / Mexico City
Milan / New Delhi / San Juan / Seoul / Singapore / Sydney / Toronto

First Aid for the® USMLE Step 2 CS, Third Edition

2 3 4 5 6 7 8 9 0   WDQ/WDQ   14 13 12 11 10

ISBN-13: 978-0-07-162425-1
MHID: 0-07-162425-2
ISSN: 1930-5354

NOTICE

This book was set in Electra LH by Rainbow Graphics.
The editor was Catherine A. Johnson.
The production supervisor was Phil Galea.
Production management was provided by Rainbow Graphics.
World Color Dubuque was printer and binder.

This book is printed on acid-free paper.

McGraw-Hill books are available at special quantity discounts to use as premiums and sales promotions, or for use in corporate training programs. To contact a representative please e-mail us at bulksales@mcgraw-hill.com.

DEDICATION

To the contributors of this and past editions, who took time to share their experience, advice, and humor for the benefit of future physicians.

and

To our families, friends, and loved ones, who supported us in the task of assembling this guide.

CONTENTS

SECTION V   TOP-RATED REVIEW RESOURCES   395

CONTRIBUTORS

David Beversluis
Case Western Reserve University School of Medicine
Class of 2010

Patrick Elliott
Case Western Reserve University School of Medicine
Class of 2010

Chad M. Fortun, MD
Resident, Orthopaedic Surgery
University Hospitals Case Medical Center

Mary Iruthayanathan, MBBS, PhD
Postdoctoral Scholar, Department of Internal Medicine
Division of Endocrinology and Metabolism
University of Iowa Carver College of Medicine

Neeraj Lalwani, MBBS, DMRD, MD
Fellow, Body Imaging
University of Texas, San Antonio

Shadi Mayasy, MD
Resident, Internal Medicine
Case Western Reserve University/St. Vincent Charity Hospital

FACULTY REVIEWERS

Kayla D. Chapman, MD
University of Kansas School of Medicine
Class of 2009

Roger Maalouf, MD
Assistant Professor of Medicine
Department of Medicine, Division of Hospital Medicine
University of Florida College of Medicine—Jacksonville

Senan Sultan, MD
Fellow
Department of Medicine, Divion of Endocrinology
University of Florida College of Medicine—Jacksonville

The USMLE Step 2 CS can be a source of stress and anxiety, especially among international medical graduates (IMGs), who find themselves at a disadvantage because of their non-U.S. training background. *First Aid for the USMLE Step 2 CS* is our "cure" for this exam. This book represents a virtual medicine bag of high-yield tools for students and IMGs, including:

- A thorough exam preparation guide for the new USMLE Step 2 CS. It includes proven study and exam strategies for the clinical encounters.
- Time management advice to maximize your clinical encounters.
- Step-by-step strategies for interacting with standardized patients, including "difficult" patients.
- Detailed descriptions of high-yield physical exam maneuvers that will win you points without costing time.
- A revised and expanded set of minicases representing common complaints designed to help you rapidly develop a working set of differential diagnoses.
- Forty-one full-length practice cases that allow you to simulate the real exam. They include all-new pediatric and telephone interviews as well as suggested "closing statements" for each case.

This book would not have been possible without the suggestions and feedback of medical students, IMGs, and faculty members. We invite you to share your thoughts and ideas to help us improve *First Aid for the USMLE Step 2 CS*. See How to Contribute, p. xv.

Louisville	Tao Le
Los Angeles	Vikas Bhushan
Jacksonville	Mae Sheikh-Ali
Cleveland	Fadi Abu Shahin

ACKNOWLEDGMENTS

We owe special thanks to the attendings, residents, and students who helped with this edition: Xiaotong Zhang, and Lin Wang; Attedings- From the University of Florida College of Medicine: Arshag D. Mooradian, M.D.; Malcom Foster, M.D.; Joe Chehade, M.D.; Kent Wehmeier, M.D.; Stanley JR. Nahman, M.D.; Aiham AlAshhab, M.D. From Mayo Clinic: Shon E. Meek, M.D. From University of Virginia Medical Center: Kurt P. Miceli, M.D. From Drexel University College of Medicine: Joseph M. Boselli, M.D.; Howard A. Miller, M.D. From Lankenau Hospital: Rita El-Hajj, M.D. Students, residents—Ruba Sheikh-Ali, M.D.; Andrew Darlington, M.D.; Ravindra Maharaj, M.D.; Karishma Ramsubeik, M.D.; Taren Ohman, M.D.; Amr El-Sergany, M.D. Special thanks for Nina Mirou for her help in editing.

Thanks to our editor, Catherine Johnson, for her enthusiasm, support, and commitment to the *First Aid* series. Thanks to Andi Fellows, our developmental editor, for her tireless dedication to our projects, and Selina Franklin and Louise Petersen for their organization and administrative assistance. Also, a special thanks to Rainbow Graphics, especially David Hommel and Susan Cooper, for remarkable editorial and production work. For support and encouragement throughout the process, we are grateful to Thao Pham and Jonathan Kirsch.

HOW TO CONTRIBUTE

First Aid for the USMLE Step 2 CS incorporates many contributions from students and faculty. We invite you to participate in this process. Please send us:

- Study and test-taking strategies for the Step 2 CS exam
- High-yield case topics that may appear on future Step 2 CS exams
- Personal comments on review books that you have examined

For each entry incorporated into the next edition, you will receive a $10 Amazon.com gift certificate and a personal acknowledgment in the next edition. Significant contributions will be compensated at the discretion of the authors. The preferred way to submit entries, suggestions, or corrections is via our blog:

www.firstaidteam.com

Otherwise, you can send entries, neatly written or typed or on disk (Microsoft Word), to:

First Aid Team
914 North Dixie Avenue, Suite 100
Elizabethtown, KY 42701
Attention: Step 2 CS

Contributions sent earlier will receive priority consideration for the next edition of *First Aid for the USMLE Step 2 CS.*

NOTE TO CONTRIBUTORS

All entries are subject to editing and reviewing. Please verify all data and spellings carefully. In the event that similar or duplicate entries are received, only the first entry received will be used. Please follow the style, punctuation, and format of this edition if possible. For additional space, use the back of this page. If you are submitting more than one entry, either photocopy this sheet before you write/type on it, or attach additional sheets.

INTERNSHIP OPPORTUNITIES

The author team of Le and Bhushan is pleased to offer part-time and full-time paid internships in medical education and publishing to motivated medical students and physicians. Internships may range from two to three months (e.g., a summer) up to a full year. Participants will have an opportunity to author, edit, and earn academic credit on a wide variety of projects, including the popular *First Aid* series. Writing/editing experience, familiarity with Microsoft Word, and Internet access are desired. For more information, e-mail a résumé or a short description of your experience along with a cover letter and writing sample to **firstaidteam@yahoo.com.**

Guide to the USMLE Step 2 CS

Since 1998, all international medical graduates (IMGs) have been required to pass a clinical skills exam known as the Clinical Skills Assessment, or CSA—a test involving clinical encounters with "standardized patients"—as a prerequisite to entering residency training in the United States. With the introduction of the USMLE Step 2 Clinical Skills (CS), however, U.S. and Canadian medical students as well as IMGs are now required to demonstrate basic clinical competencies in order to enter residency training and take the Step 3 exam.

Even if you are a seasoned pro at taking standardized exams such as the USMLE Step 1 and Step 2 Clinical Knowledge (CK), you may find it challenging to prepare for the USMLE Step 2 CS—which, like the CSA it has replaced, uses live patient actors to simulate clinical encounters. Common mistakes students and IMGs make in preparing for the Step 2 CS include the following:

- Panicking because of the unfamiliar format of the test
- Inadequate practice with mock patient scenarios prior to the actual exam
- Not developing a logical plan of attack based on patient "doorway information"
- Failing to understand the required objectives for each patient encounter
- Poor time management during patient encounters
- Becoming flustered by challenging questions or situations
- Taking unfocused histories and physical exams
- Failing to understand how to interact with a patient appropriately
- Neglecting to carry out easy but required patient interactions

This book will help guide you through the process of efficiently preparing for and taking the Step 2 CS with four organized sections:

- **Section I** introduces you to the USMLE Step 2 CS.
- **Section II** reviews critical, high-yield steps to take during the patient encounter.
- **Section III** provides high-yield minicases for common doorway chief complaints to help you rapidly develop focused differentials during the exam.
- **Section IV** has full-length practice cases to help you simulate the real thing.

What Is the USMLE Step 2 CS?

The United States Medical Licensing Examination (USMLE) Step 2 CS is a one-day exam whose objective is to ensure that all U.S. and Canadian medical students seeking to obtain their medical licenses—as well as all IMGs seeking to start their residencies in the United States—have the communication, interpersonal, and clinical skills necessary to achieve these goals. To pass the

test, all examinees must show that they can speak, understand, and communicate in English as well as take a history and perform a brief physical exam. Examinees are also required to exhibit competence in written English and to demonstrate critical clinical skills by writing a brief patient note (PN), some follow-up orders, and a differential diagnosis.

The Step 2 CS simulates clinical encounters that are commonly found in clinics, physicians' offices, and emergency departments. The test makes use of standardized patients, or SPs, all of whom are laypersons who have been extensively trained to simulate various clinical problems. SPs give the same responses to all candidates participating in the assessment. When you take the Step 2 CS, you will see 11–12 SPs, but cases will be mixed in terms of age, gender, ethnicity, organ system, and discipline. For quality assurance purposes, a video camera will record all clinical encounters, but the resulting videotapes will not be used for scoring. The cases used in the Step 2 CS represent the types of patients who would typically be encountered during core clerkships in the curricula of accredited U.S. medical schools. These clerkships are as follows:

- Internal medicine
- Surgery
- Obstetrics and gynecology
- Pediatrics
- Psychiatry
- Family medicine
- Emergency medicine

It should be noted that examinees do **not** interact with children during pediatric encounters. Instead, SPs assuming the role of pediatric patients' parents recount patients' histories, and no physical exam is required under such circumstances.

There is no physical exam in pediatric encounters and phone encounters.

How Is the Step 2 CS Structured?

Before entering a room to interact with an SP, you will be given an opportunity to review some preliminary information. This information, which is posted on the door of each room (and hence is often referred to as "doorway information"), includes the following:

- Patient characteristics (name, age, sex)
- Chief complaint and vitals (temperature, respiratory rate, pulse, blood pressure)

You will be given 15 minutes (with a warning bell sounded after 10 minutes) to perform the clinical encounter, which will include reading the doorway information, entering the room, introducing yourself, obtaining an appropriate history, conducting a focused physical exam, formulating a differential diagnosis, and planning a diagnostic workup. You will also be expected to answer any

Consider typing the PN if you are a slow or sloppy writer.

questions the SP might ask; to discuss the diagnoses being considered; and to advise the SP about follow-up plans. After leaving the room, you will have 10 minutes to write or type a PN.

How Is the Step 2 CS Scored?

Of your 11–12 patient encounters, 10 will be scored. Two people will score each encounter: the SP and a physician. The SP will evaluate you at the end of each encounter by filling out three checklists: one for the history, a second for the physical exam, and a third for communication skills. The physician will evaluate the PN you write after each encounter. Your overall score, which will be based on the clinical encounter as a whole and on your overall communication skills, will be determined by the following three components:

- **Integrated Clinical Encounter (ICE) score.** The skills you demonstrate in the clinical encounter are reflected in your ICE score. This score consists in turn of a **data-gathering (DG) score** and a **patient note (PN) score.**
  - **DG score.** To determine your DG score, SPs will document your ability to gather data pertinent to the clinical encounter. Specifically, SPs will note whether you asked the questions listed on their checklists, successfully obtained relevant information, and correctly conducted the physical exam (as indicated by your performance of the procedures on their checklists). Your final DG score will represent an average of your performance with all 10 SPs. If you asked questions or performed procedures that are not on an SP's checklist, you will not receive credit— but at the same time will not lose credit— for having done so.
  - **PN score.** A physician will score your PN according to predefined criteria, including organization, quality of information, data interpretation, legibility, and the absence of inappropriate or dangerous actions. Your final PN score will then represent the average of your individual PN scores over all 10 clinical encounters. Your ICE score will represent the sum of your DG and PN scores (ICE = DG + PN).
- **Communication and Interpersonal Skills (CIS) score.** In addition to assessing your data-gathering skills, SPs will evaluate your interpersonal skills (IPS). These include rapport, interviewing skills, personal manner, and counseling. Your overall CIS score will be the sum of your averaged IPS scores and your spoken English proficiency rating.
- **Spoken English Proficiency (SEP) score.** This component scores you on listening effort, pronunciation, and word choice.

You must pass all three components to pass the exam.

The grade you receive on the USMLE Step 2 CS will be either a "pass" or a "fail." In order to pass the Step 2 CS, candidates must pass all three components. Early results indicate that most U.S. and Canadian medical students are passing (see Table 1-1). The failure rate is higher among IMGs, with nearly 1 in 4 failing to pass.

TABLE 1-1. Step 2 CS Pass Rates

	THROUGH MARCH 2005		THROUGH JUNE 2007	
	NO. TESTED	PASSING	NO. TESTED	PASSING
U.S./Canadian	13,035	96%	17,284	97%
IMGs	10,225	83%	16,818	76%

In July 2007, the performance criteria for two subcomponents of the Step 2 CS—CIS and SEP—were raised by the USMLE Step 2 Committee. The committee anticipates an increase of about 8% in the failure rates of IMGs as a result of this change.

U.S. students rarely fail the SEP subcomponent. If they do fail, it is most likely because of poor ICE scores. Relatively few U.S. students fail both ICE and CIS. For IMGs, CIS is the most likely component to cause failure. SEP is more of a challenge but is still the least likely component to cause failure. Few IMGs fail all three subcomponents.

U.S. students are most likely to fail because of ICE. IMGs are most likely to fail because of CIS.

If you pass the Step 2 CS, your score report will not include any feedback with regard to your performance on any of the exam's subcomponents. If you fail the exam, however, your report will include a graphic representation of your strengths and weaknesses on the various subcomponents. Since October 2008, feedback on the CIS subcomponent of the exam has been further expanded to encompass three additional categories: questioning skills, information-sharing skills, and professional manners and rapport.

How Do I Register to Take the USMLE Step 2 CS?

As per the new rules and regulations, applicants can register directly for the Step 2 CS without having passed any other Step. Bear in mind, however, that registration information and procedures are constantly evolving. For the most current information on registering for the Step 2 CS, go to www.usmle.org or check with your dean's office. IMGs should also refer to the Web site of the Educational Commission for Foreign Medical Graduates (ECFMG) at www.ecfmg.org.

U.S. students must register using the National Board of Medical Examiners' (NBME's) interactive Web site for applicants and examinees (click the appropriate link at www.nbme.org). IMGs can either apply online using the ECFMG's Interactive Web Application (IWA) at http://iwa.ecfmg.org or download the paper application from the ECFMG Web site and mail it to the ECFMG along with the registration fee. Although there is no specific application deadline, you should apply early to ensure that you get your preferred test date and center.

Register as early as possible to get the best choice of dates and test centers!

After your application has been processed, you will receive a scheduling permit by e-mail as well as a CD containing an orientation manual and a video of sample encounters. This video is an excellent resource that you should find time to review before you take the test, as it shows exactly how the Step 2 CS is administered as well as how you should conduct yourself during the exam. Once you have received your scheduling permit, you will be eligible to take the Step 2 CS for one year, starting when you are entered into the scheduling system to take the exam. Your scheduling permit will list your eligibility period, scheduling instructions, and identification requirements for admission to the exam. You can schedule the test either through the NBME or ECFMG Web site or via telephone. Access information will be included with your registration materials. Note that test centers offer both morning and afternoon sessions. You may be offered an afternoon session if you select a date and center for which morning sessions are already filled. Try to select a date and center that will allow you to have a morning session (when you are fresher and more relaxed).

Apply early to get a first choice on test centers and morning-session dates.

Although you cannot extend your eligibility period for the Step 2 CS, you can cancel or reschedule your exam date. You will not be charged a fee if you cancel or reschedule 14 calendar days before your scheduled test date, not including the day of the test. However, a fee of $150 will be levied if you cancel or reschedule at any time during the 14-day period before (but not including) your scheduled test date. You will need to pay $400 if you miss an appointment without canceling or rescheduling.

Finally, a word of caution is in order with regard to the scheduling of test dates. Some applicants have been known to post requests on various online forums offering to exchange their appointments with other applicants. It should be noted that the Step 2 CS scheduling system does not allow anyone to schedule or reschedule an appointment on behalf of another applicant. In addition, the system works on a "first come, first served" basis—so if you cancel your appointment in anticipation of such an exchange, your test date might be claimed by someone else who happens to be logged onto the system at the same time. Applicants would therefore do well to avoid such temptations and opt for traditional routes in their efforts to reschedule their test dates.

Where Can I Take the Exam?

The Step 2 CS will be administered at five regional sites called Clinical Skills Evaluation Collaboration, or CSEC, centers (see Figure 1-1). Additional centers are currently under consideration.

For detailed information about cities, hotels, and transportation, please refer to the USMLE Web site (www.usmle.org), the ECFMG Web site (www.ecfmg.org), and the Section I Supplement (see p. 21).

FIGURE 1-1. Step 2 CS Test Centers

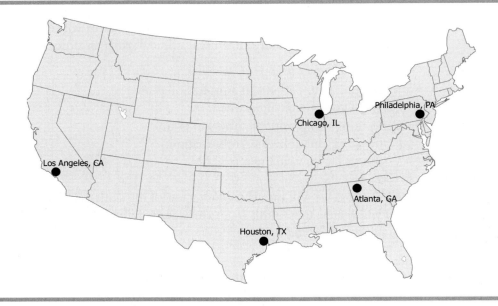

Philadelphia, PA

Chicago, IL

Los Angeles, CA

Atlanta, GA

Houston, TX

How Long Will I Wait to Get My Scores?

Step 2 CS results will be posted to your On-line Applicant Status and Information System (OASIS) account on the ECFMG/NBME Web site. An e-mail will be sent to you once your score report has been uploaded onto your account page. A fixed schedule of score-reporting periods will be published on the USMLE Web site well in advance of your test date. The vast majority of examinees who take the Step 2 CS will receive their scores on the first day of the corresponding reporting period, which is usually 1–3 months from the date of the test. If you do not receive your results within that time period, you must send a written request for a duplicate report to the NBME or the ECFMG. As mentioned above, the score report you receive will indicate only whether you passed or failed the exam. The numerical score you achieved will not be disclosed to you or to any of the programs to which you apply. Once you pass the Step 2 CS, your passing score will remain valid for the purpose of applying for residency training.

What If I Fail?

If you fail the Step 2 CS, you can retake it, but not more than three times within any 12-month period. In addition, each time you take the exam, you must submit a new application along with the appropriate fee.

If for some reason you feel that you unfairly received a failing score, you may be able to appeal and request a rescoring of your exam. However, doing so is unlikely to change your overall exam results. Check your orientation manual or the USMLE and/or ECFMG Web sites for the latest reexamination and appeal policies.

In preparing for the Step 2 CS, keep in mind that you will need to demonstrate certain fundamental but critical clinical skills in order to pass. These skills include:

- Interacting with patients in a professional way
- Taking a good medical history
- Performing an appropriate physical exam
- Counseling and delivering information
- Writing a logical and organized PN

In this section, we will briefly explore a few of the skills delineated above. Section II will review these skills in greater detail along with the mechanics of the clinical encounter and PN.

Ability to Interact with Patients in a Professional Way

There are several elements of the Communication and Interpersonal Skills (CIS) subcomponent that you must incorporate into each encounter. These are simple and easy to learn but require practice.

- **Introducing yourself to the patient.** When you first meet a patient, be sure to smile, address the patient by his or her last name (e.g., Mr. Jones), introduce yourself clearly, shake hands firmly, and establish good eye contact.
- **"Draping manners."** Always keep the patient well draped. You can cover the patient at any time before the physical exam, but it is better to do so at the beginning of the encounter. Don't expose large portions of the patient's body at the same time; instead, uncover only the parts that need to be examined, and only one at a time. Be sure to ask permission before you uncover any part of the body, and explain why you are doing so. You should also ask permission to untie the patient's gown and should tie the gown up again when you are done.
- **Appearance.** In your encounters, you should appear confident, calm, and friendly but at the same time serious and professional. You should also wear a clean white lab coat along with professional-looking but comfortable clothes. Do not wear shorts or jeans. Men should wear slacks, a shirt, and a tie. Women should consider slacks and low-heeled shoes and should avoid wearing skirts above the knee.
- **Appropriate use of body language.** During the clinical encounter, look the patient in the eye, smile when appropriate, and show compassion. You may place your hand on the patient's shoulder or arm but not on his leg or hand when you are trying to console him. Do not exaggerate your facial expressions in an effort to convince patients that you empathize with them. Never talk to a patient while standing somewhere he can't see you, especially during the history and closure.

- **Attitude toward the patient.** Always concentrate on your patient. Ask permission before you examine any part of his body, and provide explanations of what you intend to do. Pay attention to everything the patient says and does, because it is most likely purposeful. You can show concern by:
  - **Keeping the patient comfortable.** Help the patient sit up, lie down, and get onto and off the examination table. Do not repeat painful procedures.
  - **Showing compassion for the patient's pain.** If the patient does not allow you to touch his abdomen because of severe pain, say, "I know that you are in pain, and I want to help you, but I need to examine you to be able to locate the source of pain and give you the right treatment."
  - **Showing compassion for a patient's sadness.** To demonstrate empathy, you may take a brief moment of silence and place your hand lightly on the patient's shoulder or arm. You may then say something like "I know that you feel sad. Would you like to tell me about it?"
  - **Respecting the patient's beliefs.** Do not reject a patient's beliefs even if they sound incorrect to you. If a patient tells you, "I am sure that the pain I have is due to colon cancer," you may say something like "That may well be one possibility, but there are other possibilities that we need to consider as well."

Focus on communication and interpersonal skills if you are a foreign-born IMG.

Ability to Take a Good Medical History

The interviewing techniques you use should be effective enough to allow you to collect a thorough medical history. It is true that you can prepare a list of questions to use for every system or complaint. You should be aware, however, that you will not be able to cover everything. You should thus aim to choose only those questions that are most relevant to the case at hand so as to direct the interview toward exploring the chief complaint and uncovering any hidden complaints.

If you feel that a patient is not following with your line of questioning, be careful, as this may indicate that you are drifting away from the correct diagnosis. You should also bear in mind that physical findings may be feigned and may not look the same as real ones (e.g., feigning wheezing during chest auscultation). In such circumstances, you should pretend that the findings are real.

Do not be intimidated by angry patients. Remember that SPs are only actors, so stay calm, firm, and friendly. Ask about the reason for a patient's anger or complaint, and address it appropriately. Do not be defensive or hostile. If you do not understand what a patient has said or recognize a drug that has been prescribed, do not hesitate to ask, "Can you please repeat what you said?" or "What is the name of that drug again?"

The summary technique is an excellent patient communication strategy.

Finally, remember to use the **summary technique** at least once during the interview. This technique, which involves briefly summarizing what the patient has just told you, may be used either after you finish taking the history or fol-

lowing the physical exam. Doing so will help ensure that you remember the details of the history before you leave the room to write the PN.

Ability to Counsel and Deliver Information

At the end of each encounter, you will be expected to tell the patient about your findings, offer your medical opinion (including a concise differential diagnosis), describe the next step in diagnosis, and outline possible treatments. In doing so, you should always be clear and honest. Tell the patient only the things you know, and don't try to render a final diagnosis. Make sure the patient understands what you are saying, and avoid the use of complex medical terms. Before you leave, ask the patient if he still has any questions. After you respond, follow up by asking, "Did that answer your question?"

When counseling a patient, always be open. Tell him what you really think is wrong, and explain that the final diagnosis can be made only after some tests have been taken. You should also explain some of the tests you are planning to conduct. Address any concerns the patient may have in a realistic manner, and never offer false reassurances.

▶ TEST-DAY TIPS

The Step 2 CS is a one-day exam. You will be scheduled for either the morning or the afternoon session. The duration of the Step 2 CS, including orientation, testing, and breaks, is approximately eight hours. Once you have entered the secured area of the assessment center for orientation, you may not leave that area until the exam has been completed. During this time, the following conventions should be observed:

No watches of any kind, either analog or digital, are allowed in the test area.

- You may not use any watches (analog or digital), cell phones, or beepers at any time during the exam.
- The morning session starts at 8 A.M. and the afternoon session at 3 P.M. Test proctors will generally wait up to 30 minutes for latecomers, so the actual exam usually does not begin until 8:30 A.M. or 3:30 P.M. Nonetheless, you should plan to arrive 30 minutes before your session is scheduled to begin.
- Don't come to an afternoon session early in an attempt to meet candidates from the morning session, as they aren't allowed to leave until you are locked in.
- Bring a government-issued photo ID (e.g., a U.S. driver's license or a passport) that carries your signature.
- Be sure to bring your admission permit! You will not be admitted to the test center without it.

After the 30-minute waiting period has elapsed, the staff will give you a name tag, a numbered badge to be worn around your arm, a pen, and a clipboard. There is no need to bring a pen of your own, as you are not allowed to use anything other than the pen provided at the exam site.

Do not bring any of your luggage to the test site, as the staff will not store it for you. The staff will provide you with nothing more than a coat rack and a small storage locker for belongings that you are not allowed to carry during the encounter, such as watches, cell phones, purses, and handbags. If you are planning to travel immediately after the exam, you can keep your luggage at the front desk of the hotel where you stayed the night before.

Don't bring your luggage. Check it with the hotel front desk.

At the outset of your session, you will be asked to sign a confidentiality agreement. An orientation session will then be held to introduce you to all the equipment that you will find in the examination rooms. You are allowed to examine such equipment and to become familiar with it, especially the bed, foot extension, and head elevation. Do not hesitate to try every piece of equipment made available to you during this session.

You will be given two breaks during the exam. The first is for 30 minutes and takes place after the fourth encounter. During this break, the staff will serve you a meal. The second break is 15 minutes long and takes place after the eighth encounter. Use the bathroom during these breaks, as you will not have time to do so during the encounters. Finally, remember that smoking is strictly prohibited not only during the exam but also during breaks. You cannot leave the center during break periods.

In the break room, you will be assigned a seat and a desk. You can keep your food or drink on this desk so that it will be accessible during break time. Although the testing staff will provide you with one meal, you may want to bring some high-energy snacks for your breaks. Also remember that your personal belongings will not be accessible to you until the end of the exam—so if you do plan to bring some food along with you, keep it on your assigned desk, not in the storage area.

The Step 2 CS is not a social event, so when you meet with other candidates during breaks, do not mention anything about the cases you just encountered. Never speak with anyone in a language other than English, as this may be considered irregular behavior.

Finally, even though all your encounters are videotaped, it bears repeating that these tapes are not used for scoring purposes. To the contrary, they are used to ensure the safety of the SPs and candidates as well as to allow for quality monitoring. So don't worry about the camera, and don't try to look for it during the encounters. Instead, act as you would on a regular clinic day.

Some Final Words

The following general principles will also help you excel on the Step 2 CS:

- **"Don't think about the past; think about the present."** Clear your head when moving to the next encounter. Thinking about what you should

11

have done or should have asked will only distract you from your current encounter.

- **"Passing does not require perfection."** You need not be perfect. In fact, given the time constraints involved, the Step 2 CS rewards efficiency and relative completeness over perfection.

- **"There is a reason for everything you see."** If a patient is wearing a peculiar Mexican hat, inquire why this is the case. He might have been in Mexico, and the diarrhea he presents with may thus be a simple traveler's diarrhea.

▶ FIRST AID FOR THE IMG

If you are an IMG candidate seeking to pass the Step 2 CS, you must take a number of variables into account, from plotting a timetable to mastering logistical details to formulating a solid test preparation strategy.

Determining Eligibility

Before contacting the ECFMG for a Step 2 CS application, you must first take several preliminary steps. Begin by ascertaining whether you are eligible (see Table 1-2). Check the ECFMG Web site for the latest eligibility criteria.

Once you have established your eligibility to take the exam, you will also need to factor in the residency matching process. If you are planning to apply for a residency in the United States, your timetable should reflect that and should be carefully planned at least one year in advance.

Bear in mind that you are allowed to **register** (pay the fee) for the Match regardless of your ECFMG status. In order for you to **participate** in the Match, however, the National Residency Matching Program (NRMP) requires that you be ECFMG certified (or that you meet ECFMG requirements for certification even if you have not received your certificate) by the rank-order-list

TABLE 1-2. IMG Eligibility for the USMLE Step 2 CS[a]

MEDICAL STUDENTS	MEDICAL SCHOOL GRADUATES
You must be enrolled in a foreign medical school listed in the International Medical Education Directory (IMED, http://imed.ecfmg.org) both at the time you apply and at the time you take the assessment. You must also be within 12 months of graduation when you take the exam.	You must be a graduate of a medical school that was listed in the IMED at the time of your graduation.

[a] You do **not** have to have passed the English-language proficiency test or the Test of English as a Foreign Language (TOEFL) to be eligible for the Step 2 CS.

deadline (typically in February of each year). Otherwise, applicants will be automatically withdrawn from the Match. Therefore, you should take the Step 2 CS no later than October in the year before your target Match Day (see Figure 1-2).

There is a significant advantage to be gained by obtaining ECFMG certification by the time you submit your application for residency in the fall. Should you do so, programs are apt to consider you a ready applicant and may favor you over other candidates who have yet to take the Step 2 CS even if such candidates have more impressive applications. In addition, if you are certified early, you may be interested in taking Step 3 and getting your results back before the rank-order-list deadline. A good score on Step 3 can provide a perfect last-minute boost to your application and may also make you eligible for the H1B visa. In sum, you would be well advised to take the Step 2 CS as soon as you are eligible to do so (see Table 1-2). At the same time, of course, you should not take the Step 2 CS until you are confident that you are fully prepared to do so. Remember that in order to get ECFMG certification, you need to pass the Step 1, Step 2 CK, and Step 2 CS within a seven-year period.

Ideally, you should get your ECFMG certificate prior to submitting your residency applications.

USMLE exams need to be passed in a seven-year period for ECFMG certification.

FIGURE 1-2. Typical Step 2 CS Timeline for IMGs

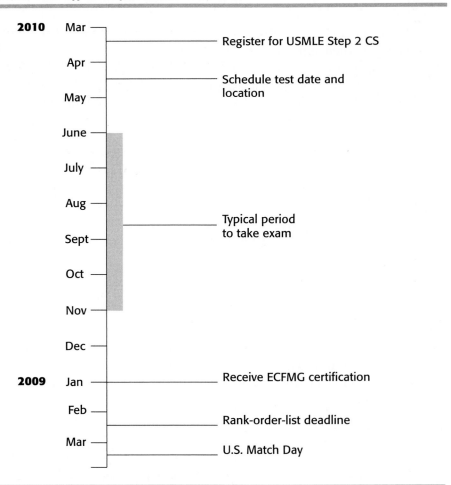

In deciding when to apply for the Step 2 CS, when to take it, and whether you are ready for it, you should keep the following points in mind:

- Scheduling your test date can be difficult during busy seasons. You should apply at least three months before your desired examination date. Ideally, you should aim to take the Step 2 CS in June or July in order to be certified when you apply for residency.
- You should schedule your exam on the date that you expect to be fully prepared for it. For IMGs, preparation for the exam typically requires anywhere between 1 and 12 weeks, factoring in your level of English proficiency as well as your medical knowledge and skills.
- If you choose to apply for the Step 2 CS using a paper application, it will take up to four weeks to receive your notification of registration—but it may take as few as 10 days to receive this information if you use the ECFMG's IWA.
- Don't be overly concerned if you are unable to meet these theoretically ideal deadlines. Most of the programs that would have invited you for an interview if you had received your Step 2 CS result will still invite you without it.

If you are an IMG living outside the United States, you must also factor in the time it may take to obtain a visa. You don't need a visa to come to the United States if you are a U.S. or Canadian citizen or a permanent resident. Citizens of countries participating in the Visa Waiver Program (such as European Union countries) may not need to obtain a visa either. You are responsible for determining whether you need a visa (usually B1 or B2) and, having done so, for obtaining that visa, regardless of how time-consuming and difficult this may be. Before you apply to take the Step 2 CS, you should therefore:

- Check with the U.S. embassy in your country to determine whether you need a visa.
- Determine how long it will take to get an appointment at the embassy.
- Find out how long it will take to get the visa and whether a clearance period is required.
- Check travel availability to the cities in which the exam centers are located.

As proof of the reason for your visit to the United States, the ECFMG will send you a letter that you can present to the U.S. consulate in your country. This letter will be sent to you only after you apply to take the Step 2 CS (i.e., after you have paid your fee) and will not guarantee that you will be granted a visa. For this reason, it would be wise not to schedule your actual exam day until you have arrived in the United States or have at least obtained your visa.

Application Tips

Once you have received an application form to take the Step 2 CS, be sure to read the form carefully before you start filling it out. You do not want to see your application returned to you—and thus squander valuable time—simply

because you forgot to answer one or more questions or made a careless mistake. Common errors that result in returned written applications include the following:

Use the ECFMG's Interactive Web Application to minimize delays and errors.

- Your application is not written in ink or is illegible.
- Your application is incomplete.
- You faxed your application or sent a photocopy rather than the original document.
- Your application contains a nonoriginal signature or photograph.
- Your photograph was taken more than six months before the date you submitted the application.
- The signature of the medical school official or the notary public is more than four months old.
- The medical school or notary public seal or stamp does not cover a portion of your photograph.
- You failed to explain why your application was signed by a notary public but not by your medical school official.
- Full payment was not included with the application.

Commonly encountered errors specific to IMGs include the following:

- You are a medical school graduate and you did not send the ECFMG a copy of your medical diploma with two full-face photographs.
- Your medical school diploma is not in English, and you did not send a translation along with it.
- The medical diploma and its translation are not stapled together, and the translator's stamp does not cover both of them together.

Once you have completed your application and have double-checked it for errors, you should make an effort to send it by express mail or courier service. To check the status of your application online, you can use OASIS (https://oasis2.ecfmg.org).

Improving Your English Proficiency

For many IMGs taking the Step 2 CS, a critical concern lies in the demonstration of proficiency in spoken English. In Step 2 CS terms, this refers to the ability to speak English clearly and comprehensibly and to understand English when the SP speaks to you.

You may not have a problem with English proficiency if you are a native English speaker, have studied in a U.S. or other English-speaking school, have learned medicine in English in your medical school, or have spent at least a few months or years of your life in an English-speaking country. English proficiency may, however, be the main obstacle facing IMGs at the other end of the spectrum. The good news is that most IMGs who have already passed the USMLE Step 1 have the basic English knowledge they need to pass the Step 2 CS. For such candidates, the key to passing the Step 2 CS lies in

organizing this knowledge and practicing. Your spoken English proficiency is based on the following skills:

- **The ability to speak in a manner that is easy for the SP to follow and understand.** Choose phrases that are simpler, more direct, and easier both for you to remember and for the SP to understand. Speaking slowly will also make it easier for SPs to understand you and will minimize the effect your accent has on your English.
- **The correct use of grammar.** The key to mastering this element is to be familiar with commonly used statements, transitions, and questions and to practice them as much as possible. This will minimize the probability that you will make significant grammatical errors.
- **Good pronunciation.** Again, the key to good pronunciation lies in practicing common statements and questions, repeating them to yourself aloud, and asking someone (preferably a native English speaker) to listen to you and correct your mistakes. The more you practice, the better your chances will be of reaching an acceptable and even a superior level of clear, comprehensible English.
- **The ability to correct and clarify your English if necessary.** You may find it difficult to practice for a situation in which an SP does not understand you and asks you for the meaning of something you have just said. Here again, however, you can avoid this situation by practicing common statements, questions, and transitions; speaking as slowly and clearly as possible; and using nontechnical words instead of complicated medical terminology. If an SP still cannot understand something you have said, simply repeat the phrase or question, or restate it in simple lay terms.

The key to better spoken English is to practice commonly used statements, transitions, and questions.

You should also make an effort to remain calm throughout your clinical encounters. If you are nervous, you may find that you mumble your words, making it difficult for the SP to understand what you are saying. So just relax and concentrate.

If you get nervous and start looking at the clock and rushing, you will further increase the likelihood of making mistakes. So remain calm and take your time. Fifteen minutes may seem like a short time to do and say all the things you think are necessary, but it will be more than enough if you follow an organized plan. In general, most of the things you have to say in the exam are the same in each encounter, so by thoroughly studying common cases and medical conditions (see Sections III and IV), you can go a long way toward overcoming this obstacle.

If you are still unsure about your mastery of English and would like to see if you have achieved the level of proficiency required to pass the Step 2 CS, the ECFMG suggests that you take the Test of Spoken English (TSE). If you score higher than 35 on this exam, you have probably attained the English proficiency level necessary for the Step 2 CS. In addition, you may consider taking TOEFL beforehand. However, doing so is no longer a prerequisite to

taking the Step 2 CS or to ECFMG certification. For more information about the TSE and the TOEFL, contact:

TOEFL/TSE Services
P.O. Box 6151
Princeton, NJ 08541-6151
(609) 771-7100
toefl@ets.org
www.toefl.org

Getting Observerships and Clinical Rotations

Many IMGs may also lack basic familiarity with the workings of U.S. medical schools. A clinical rotation or an observership in the United States can prepare IMGs for the Step 2 CS by introducing them to the U.S. system and, in the process, immersing them in the "American way" of taking a history, performing a physical exam, and writing PNs. Clinical rotations are also good to have on your curriculum vitae when you apply for residency programs. Furthermore, if you do a good job during your rotation, you can get strong letters of recommendation, which are the most important part of your application after your USMLE scores. The more time you spend in such a rotation, the better.

If you are still a **medical student,** it should not be difficult for you to find a clinical rotation. Check the Web sites of the universities in which you are interested, and send e-mails and letters to the program director and chairman of each. If you are already in the United States, call the relevant departments and make appointments to meet with those responsible for the rotations. Most of the time, such personnel will send you an application by mail. For the purposes of your residency application, however, it is highly recommended that you also do a rotation in the specialty in which you are interested.

If you are a **medical graduate,** your mission is more difficult but not impossible. You are no longer eligible for clinical rotations (clerkships), but you can still apply for observerships and externships.

The observership is perhaps the least active function you can fill in a hospital, but it can still be highly useful. Getting an observership is not an easy task because most hospitals do not have any such formal rotation or training program. Nonetheless, here is some advice that may help you:

- Prepare a list of hospitals in your area or any area in which you may reside. Include all types of teaching hospitals: university, community, and Veterans Administration medical centers.
- Contact people (attendings, senior residents, secretaries, administrators) whom you may know. Connections are an important way to uncover these unofficial rotations.

Internal medicine and emergency medicine are the best rotations for Step 2 CS preparation.

- Send e-mails and/or letters to the chairman and program director of each hospital.
- Call the office of the chairman or program director and try to set an appointment to meet them.
- Try to look for people (attendings, residents, secretaries, administrators) who are from your country and may be able to help you. Inform them that you would be willing to pay for your malpractice insurance if necessary.
- Talk to other physicians who are doing or have done observerships, and ask them where they did so and how to apply.

During your rotation, you will "officially" be an observer, which means that you cannot touch a patient or write on charts. The only things you are officially allowed to do are observe, do rounds with your team, answer an occasional question, present some topics, and attend conferences. On rare occasions, you may manage to examine some patients and write some notes. Here is some advice for making the most of your observership:

- Show a high level of enthusiasm.
- Come early and stay late (not very late, though).
- Follow up on patients your team is taking care of, and learn everything you can about them.
- Read about the cases your team is managing.
- Chat and spend time with the patients, but always let them know that you're an observer. This is the best way to practice taking histories and to improve your language skills.
- Write your own PNs and orders, ask your residents to correct them, and compare them to the official notes.
- Talk to the nurses, secretaries, and support staff. This will improve your communication skills.
- If you don't get a chance to examine patients, carefully observe the residents and medical students during the physical exam.
- Do as many presentations as you can.

Here is a brief and incomplete list of hospitals that have been known to offer observerships or externships:

- D.C. General Hospital, Washington, DC
- Emory University, Atlanta, GA
- Harbor Hospital, Baltimore, MD
- Providence Hospital, Washington, DC
- Veterans Administration Medical Center, Washington, DC
- University of Miami, Miami, FL
- Mayo Clinic, Rochester, MN (visiting physicians program)
- Mount Sinai Hospital, Miami, FL
- Hospital of St. Raphael, New Haven, CT
- Hahnemann Hospital, Philadelphia, PA
- Maricopa Medical Center, Phoenix, AZ

Some Final Tips

In addition to the above, there are a few final practical measures you can take to help ensure your success on the Step 2 CS exam:

- Check and recheck the ECFMG and USMLE Web sites for the latest information about the Step 2 CS. This will help you get a clear idea about regulations, requirements, registration, examination dates, and all other details concerning the Step 2 CS.
- Carefully prepare for the exam using the preparation materials included in this book.
- Check other Web sites and discussion forums. They can be a good source of information.
- Review the steps of history taking (see Section II). Choose and prepare common questions and cases (see Sections III and IV).
- Review the steps of the physical exam (see Section II). Practice the physical exam as if you were performing the real exam.
- Practice writing PNs (see Section IV).

The USMLE Step 2 CS Travel Guide

After you've worked hard to prepare for the Step 2 CS, the last thing you need is extra travel stress—or, worse still, potential problems on test day. The best way to ensure that everything works out well for you is to plan ahead. Getting all the details in place well in advance of your trip will help you focus on what's really important: doing a great job on the exam!

With this in mind, we've put together this quick guide as a tool that you can use both before and during your travels. For each of the five cities with a Step 2 CS testing center (called Clinical Skills Evaluation Collaboration, or CSEC centers), we've provided details on the best ways to get to your destination and the best things to do once you've arrived there. Since most of you will be flying, we've placed special emphasis on distances to the CSEC test sites and routes from the airports. Also listed are a number of nearby hotels, most of which are reasonably priced and within walking distance of the CSEC centers. As a cheaper option, we've included one youth hostel for each city. Finally, we have provided listings of a few well-known restaurants and tourist attractions for each destination. All five CSEC destinations are amazing cities, and we don't want you to miss out on what they have to offer. Although you shouldn't let sightseeing get in the way of your test, you might want to factor in at least a few hours to see the sights. Even better, think about leaving yourself an extra day or two so that you can relax and really enjoy yourself after you're done with the Step 2 CS exam.

It's important that you double-check the facts we've presented here before you leave for your destination of choice. We've put together a wealth of information for you, but by the time you get to your destination, some of the details may well have changed. There are other great sources of information you should look into as well, including the travel section on the USMLE Web site. Also note that the Association of American Medical Colleges (AAMC) has negotiated reduced hotel rates with many nearby hotels for the Step 2 CS exam. We've included many of these hotels here, but be sure to check the updated list online. Links to these sites are provided at the end of this section.

▶ TRAVELING TO THE UNITED STATES

We know that many of you who are planning on taking the Step 2 CS may be coming to the United States for the first time—so here are a few things you should keep in mind to ensure that your trip goes as smoothly as possible.

Arrange your documents. Generally, the most important document you'll need for the Step 2 CS is your **scheduling permit.** However, other documents may be required as well, especially if you're coming from another country. These may include the following:

- Your **passport**.
- A U.S. **tourist visa** (usually a B1/B2 visa; apply at the nearest U.S. embassy in your country).

- An **international driver's license** (consider getting one if you're planning to drive to your testing center).

Make sure your travel plans are in place. Be sure to make your reservations well in advance, and think about how you're going to get around in the test city. Once you've arrived at your destination, make sure you plan ahead and know how to get to the CSEC center on the morning of your test, especially if you're planning to stay a bit farther away.

Consider travel safety. When traveling abroad, particularly in major U.S. population centers, it's important to follow a few general guidelines for the sake of ensuring your safety. Here are some important points to bear in mind:

- In general, Americans are very kind and willing to help, but be aware that not everyone may have the best of intentions—particularly those who seem a bit too eager to go out of their way for you.
- Keep an eye on your baggage while traveling in a taxi, a train, or any form of public transportation. Pickpockets and petty thieves target visitors more often than they do the locals.
- Never carry anything in your baggage that doesn't belong to you. You will be responsible for the contents of your baggage, including anything illegal that might have been placed there by someone else.
- Dress like the locals.
- Avoid walking alone in deserted streets at night.

Pack appropriately. Packing before air travel requires a lot of preparation. Here are a few useful tips:

- There are many restrictions for carry-on luggage these days, particularly with regard to liquids. Check the U.S. Transportation Security Administration's Web site (www.tsa.gov) for the most up-to-date information available.
- Prepare for lost or delayed baggage. Do not keep your scheduling permit, lab coat, or stethoscope in your checked baggage. Also remember to put a copy of your itinerary in your baggage so that authorities can locate you in the event that your baggage gets lost.
- Using a mobile phone or a camera, take a photograph of your baggage to give to the authorities in the event that your baggage is delayed or lost.
- Tag your baggage with brightly colored tape or with a distinguishing mark so that you can easily identify it at baggage carousels.

Plan, plan, plan. Here are some guidelines for planning your visit and booking your hotel:

- Try to schedule your exam well in advance. Doing so will make it easier for you to get a good price on your tickets and accommodations.
- Before you book a hotel or a flight, always try to compare prices at multiple Web sites and at each organization's Web site (see "Useful Web sites" at the end of this chapter).

- Before you choose a hotel, be sure to factor in the distance to the testing center as well as the services each hotel offers—for example, whether it has a free airport shuttle, free breakfast, and access to Wi-Fi. Bear in mind that if you choose to stay in a youth hostel, you may well save money on hotel accommodations, but what you end up saving you're likely to pay for in travel time to the CSEC center on test day.

▶ ATLANTA ("THE BIG PEACH")

Clinical Skills Evaluation Collaboration Center
Two Crown Center
1745 Phoenix Boulevard, Suite 500
Atlanta, GA 30349-5585

The Atlanta metro area has a population of more than five million and is the capital city of the great state of Georgia. Throughout history, Atlanta has served as a main north-south and east-west railway hub; indeed, its name was derived from the Atlanta-Pacifica railway that ran through the town in the 1840s. Today, Atlanta is home to the Centers for Disease Control and Prevention as well as the headquarters of Coca-Cola. We know you'll enjoy your time in this diverse and thriving city!

Getting There

- **Air:** Atlanta's major airport is the Hartsfield-Jackson Atlanta International Airport (ATL), located about nine miles south of downtown and only a few blocks from the CSEC center.
- **Ground:**
  - Greyhound, 232 Forsyth Street Southwest (www.greyhound.com): The main bus terminal is located downtown, about 12 miles from the CSEC center.
  - Amtrak, 1688 Peachtree Street Northwest (www.amtrak.com): The main train station is also located downtown, about 16 miles from the testing center. Atlanta is on the Crescent Line, which runs between New Orleans and New York.

Getting Around When You Arrive

- **Shuttles:** Most hotels offer free shuttle service to and from the airport. There are also two airport shuttle services available from the airport. Both run into town on a regular basis; schedules are available online.
  - AAA Airport Express (www.aaaairportexpress.com).
  - Airport Metro Shuttle (www.airportmetro.com).
- **Taxis:** Taxis are available at the airport and at the bus/train terminals and cost $30–$35 from the airport to downtown. Local taxi companies include the following:

- Atlanta Checker Cab: 404-351-1111
- Yellow Cab: 404-521-0200
- National: 404-752-6834
- **Rental cars:** Automobile rentals are available at the airport from Alamo, Avis, Budget, Dollar, Enterprise, Hertz, and National, among others.
- **Public transportation:** Atlanta has a regional metro system called MARTA (Metropolitan Atlanta Rapid Transit Authority, www.itsmarta.com). The airport stop is at the south end of the main terminal; you will need to buy tokens to ride. A trip downtown will take approximately 15 minutes. For about $1.50, you can also get to the CSEC center from the airport on the southbound C-TRAN Route 503 bus. Board in the South Terminal ground transport area and expect a 10-minute ride.

CSEC Center Location

The Atlanta testing center is located a few minutes to the south of the Hartsfield-Jackson airport, about a quarter of a mile east of the intersection of West Fayetteville Road and Phoenix Boulevard. The V-shaped brown brick building that houses the CSEC center should be visible from the I-285 highway. The center is on the fifth floor, and plenty of free parking is available.

Where to Stay

The following are a few hotels located within walking distance of the test site. Most are just outside the airport, but there are some highways around, so plan your walk carefully. Remember to ask hotels about their USMLE deals, listed on the AAMC Web site.

- **Country Inn & Suites Atlanta Airport South:** 1808 Phoenix Boulevard, 770-991-1099, $85/night. Just around the corner from the CSEC center, making it very convenient (0.3 mile away).
- **Quality Hotel and Conference Center:** 1551 Phoenix Boulevard, 770-996-4321, $70/night. Also just down the street, and a good option (0.3 mile away).
- **Sheraton Gateway Atlanta Airport:** 1900 Sullivan Road, 770-997-1100, $100/night (approximately 2 miles away).
- **Best Western Hotel & Suites Airport South:** 1556 Phoenix Boulevard, 770-996-5800, $60/night (about 0.6 mile away).
- **Atlanta Youth Hostel:** 223 Ponce de Leon Avenue Northeast, 404-875-9449, $25/night in a dormitory. A cheaper option with plenty of nightlife. A bit farther away from the CSEC center (14 miles away), but a few blocks' walk from the MARTA North Avenue station.

Where to Eat and Play

Atlanta has amazing southern food. Take advantage of this and enjoy some of our favorites:

- **The Varsity ($):** 61 North Avenue Northwest, Downtown, 404-881-1706. The world's largest drive-in restaurant, the Varsity is an Atlanta icon that has been serving burgers and hot dogs since 1928.
- **Sweet Auburn Curb Market ($–$$):** 209 Edgewood Avenue Southeast, Downtown. A historic market with stalls that feature fresh produce and hot meals. Features many small ethnic restaurants as well.
- **Fat Matt's Rib Shack ($):** 1811 Piedmont Avenue Northeast, Midtown, 404-607-1622. An Atlanta hot spot serving up southern-style barbecue and live blues every night.

What to See

Atlanta has much to see and do. Here are just a few places to consider seeing while you're in town:

- **Georgia Aquarium:** The world's largest aquarium, with more that 1.8 million gallons of water and 100,000 species of sea life.
- **World of Coca-Cola:** Come and celebrate the original home of this sugary drink in historic Piedmont Park.
- **Underground Atlanta:** A mall located under the streets in the Five Points neighborhood.
- **Sweet Auburn District:** Home to the Martin Luther King, Jr. National Historic Site.

For more information, check out:

- www.lonelyplanet.com/worldguide/usa/atlanta/
- www.atlanta.net

▶ CHICAGO ("THE WINDY CITY")

Clinical Skills Evaluation Collaboration Center
8501 West Higgins Road, Suite 600
Chicago, IL 60631

Located on the shores of Lake Michigan, Chicago is the principal financial and cultural center of the Midwest and is currently the third largest city in the United States. Chicago is known for its gangster lore, blues clubs, and biting cold winters. With plenty of history, shopping, and culture, today's Windy City is bursting with life, so be sure to enjoy your stay!

Getting There

- **Air:** Chicago has two major airports. The larger is O'Hare International Airport (ORD), which is about 20 miles northwest of downtown and only five miles from the CSEC center. The other nearby destination is Chicago Midway Airport (MDW), located about 12 miles southwest of downtown

and roughly 20 miles from the testing center. If you can get a cheaper fare, it might be worth checking out Midway, but you probably won't save much on local transport costs. O'Hare is your best bet, as it serves a number of international destinations and is just down the road from the CSEC center.

- **Ground:**
  - Greyhound, 5800 North Cumberland Avenue (www.greyhound.com): The Chicago Cumberland Avenue Greyhound bus terminal is just a few blocks away from the CSEC center and is the closest of the six bus terminals in Chicago.
  - Amtrak, Canal Street between Adams and Jackson Boulevards (www.amtrak.com): The main train hub in Chicago is the downtown Union Station. This is a good choice, but you'll have to take public transportation or a taxi to get to the test site. The Chicago Transport Authority Blue Line runs to Cumberland Station from Union Station, taking you very close to the CSEC center.

Getting Around When You Arrive

- **Shuttles:** Most nearby hotels offer free shuttle service to and from the airport. You can also use either of the airport shuttle services. Schedules and up-to-date fares are available online.
  - Continental Airport Express: 1-888-284-3826 (www.airportexpress.com). A single one-way fare from O'Hare to downtown is approximately $27.
  - Omega Airport Shuttle: 773-734-6688 (www.omegashuttle.com). A regular shuttle service between O'Hare and Midway for approximately $16.
- **Taxis:** As in any big city, taxis are usually the most direct way to get around Chicago. They cost roughly $30–$40 from O'Hare to downtown and about $10 from O'Hare to the CSEC center.
  - Flash Cab: 773-561-4444
  - Yellow Cab: 312-225-7440
  - American United: 773-327-6161
- **Rental cars:** Rental cars are available at the airport from Alamo, Avis, Budget, Dollar, and Enterprise, among others.
- **Public transportation:** Ride the famous Chicago "L," an easy-to-use and cheap light-rail system, or take a Chicago Transit Authority bus! Both the CSEC center and O'Hare are on the "L" Blue Line, and both connect to downtown. For the CSEC center, you'll want Cumberland Station (5800 North Cumberland Avenue). Check out fares and schedules online at www.transitchicago.com.

CSEC Center Location

The exam center is located on the northwest side of Chicago, about 15 miles from downtown and just five miles east of O'Hare along I-90 (Kennedy

Expressway). From Cumberland Station, the CSEC center is a quick 0.8-mile walk or cab ride to the north over the highway. The CSEC center is located within the First Midwest Bank Building. There should be plenty of free parking at the site.

Where to Stay

The following are a few good hotel options near the testing center. Remember to ask hotels about their USMLE deals, listed on the AAMC Web site. If you have a car, you can also check out some of the hotels a bit farther west along I-90. You'll probably get a cheaper rate if you're willing to make a commute on the morning of the test.

- **Chicago Marriott O'Hare:** 8535 West Higgins Road, 773-693-4444, $95/night. Just next door to the testing center (0.1 mile away).
- **Chicago O'Hare Garden Hotel:** 8201 West Higgins Road, 773-693-2323, $80/night. A quick walk down the street (0.3 mile away).
- **Holiday Inn Chicago O'Hare:** 5615 North Cumberland Avenue, 773-693-5800, $89/night. Very close to the Cumberland Blue Line stop (0.7 mile away).
- **Hostelling International Chicago:** 24 East Congress Parkway, 312-360-0300, $30/ night in a dormitory. This large hostel is located downtown, about 15 miles from the testing center, so plan about at least an hour to make the trip on the Blue Line (15 miles away).

Where to Eat and Play

Chicago has hundreds of amazing restaurants of all varieties; here are just a few.

- **Giordano's World Famous Stuffed Pizza ($–$$):** 135 East Lake Street, 312-616-1200. Chicago is the town for pizza, and Giordano's delivers some of the best. There are branches all over the city, so find the one that works for you. This is likely to be the best and most filling meal you've had in a while.
- **Café Spiaggia ($$–$$$):** 980 North Michigan Avenue, 312-280-2750. Try lunch at the café. This relaxed restaurant is just next door to the world-famous Italian restaurant Spiaggia, which is known to be a favorite of the Obamas.
- **Blue Chicago ($$):** 736 North Clark Street, 312-642-6261. Check out one of Chicago's world-famous blues clubs, perhaps after you're done with the test.

What to See

Don't miss the sites of this amazing city by staying near the airport and the testing center. After you're done taking the exam, think about booking a late flight and jumping on the "L" for an afternoon downtown.

- **Sears Tower:** Visit the Skydeck for amazing views from the tallest building in North America.
- **Navy Pier:** Features museums, shops, restaurants, and even a Ferris wheel on the shore of Lake Michigan.
- **Magnificent Mile:** The heart of the city, with upscale shopping and fantastic restaurants running along Michigan Avenue.

For more information, check out:

- www.lonelyplanet.com/worldguide/usa/chicago/
- www.choosechicago.com
- www.cityofchicago.org/tourism

▶ HOUSTON ("SPACE CITY")

Clinical Skills Evaluation Collaboration Center
400 North Sam Houston Parkway, Suite 700
Houston, TX 77060

Houston was founded in 1836 on land near the Buffalo Bayou and was named after Sam Houston, then the president of the Republic of Texas. Today, Houston is one of the largest cities in the United States and is home to many major energy companies in addition to a substantial portion of the biomedical and aeronautical industries. It also boasts one of the best art festivals in the country, the Bayou City Art Festival, held here every spring and fall. Enjoy the show!

Getting There

- **Air:** Houston has two major airports: George Bush Intercontinental (IAH) and Hobby Airport (HOU). IAH is the larger of the two and is much closer to the CSEC center (8 miles); HOU is smaller and farther away (27 miles).
- **Ground:**
  - Greyhound, 2121 Main Street (www.greyhound.com): Houston has a terminal downtown. Outside of the station, there are plenty of taxis available. A ride to your hotel should take about 30 minutes.
  - Amtrak, 902 Washington Ave (www.amtrak.com): Houston is on the Sunset Limited line, which runs all the way from Louisiana to California.

Getting Around When You Arrive

- **Shuttles:** Most hotels around the CSEC center offer free shuttle service. If your hotel doesn't provide service, check out the following:
  - SuperShuttle: 713-523-8888, www.supershuttle.com, $19.

- **Taxis:** There are also a number of taxi companies that operate; below are just a few ($20–$40 to the CSEC center from the airport):
    - Square Deal Cab Company: 713-659-5105
    - Yellow Cab Company: 713-236-1111
    - Liberty Cab Company: 713-695-6700
- **Rental cars:** Multiple rental car companies are available in Houston. These include Alamo, Avis, Enterprise, Hertz, and National.
- **Public transportation:** If you're really adventurous, try Houston's Metro, which includes bus routes and light rail (www.ridemetro.org). Lines 102, 56, and 86 serve the area around the airport, the CSEC center, and hotels. Buses run every 10–45 minutes, depending on the route and time of day. The Web site has a trip planner to help you figure out the details.

CSEC Center Location

The CSEC center is located on the north side of Houston in a large office building at the intersection of Imperial Valley Drive and Beltway East Access Road. There is a parking garage with a large "400" on the side that is visible from the street. You'll see a McDonald's and an Arby's across the street. Free parking is available in the attached garage.

Where to Stay

The following are a few hotels around the test site. You can walk from most, although the sidewalks aren't great. Remember to ask hotels about their USMLE deals, listed on the AAMC Web site.

- **Crowne Plaza Houston North:** 425 North Sam Houston Parkway East, 866-573-4235, $231/night. The Crowne is clean, friendly, and quiet, but you pay for it (0.1 mile away).
- **Days Hotel Houston:** 500 North Sam Houston Parkway East, 866-678-6350, $99/night. The Days is cheap and close to the CSEC center (0.2 mile away).
- **Hyatt Place Houston:** 300 Ronan Park Place, 281-820-6060, $199/night. The Hyatt is a good deal, is close to the CSEC center, and is well recommended (0.7 mile away).
- **Baymont Inn & Suites Houston North:** 502 North Sam Houston Parkway East, 281-875-2000, $59/night. The Baymont gets high marks for cleanliness and service and is a great value (0.2 mile away).
- **Houston International Hostel:** 5302 Crawford Street, 713-523-1009, $15/night in a dormitory. The hostel is very cheap and is located about 30 minutes away from the CSEC center (18 miles away).

Where to Eat and Play

Houston has cuisine from all around the world but is especially well known for its Latin American fare. The restaurants we've listed aren't necessarily close to the test center, but we thought it might be fun for you to get out.

- **Americas ($$$):** 1800 Post Oak Boulevard, 713-961-1492. Americas serves Central and South American cuisine with flair.
- **Spanish Village Restaurant ($$):** 4720 Almeda Road, 713-523-2861. A restaurant that has been serving "Tex-Mex" food since 1953. Try their delicious margaritas.
- **Dry Creek Café ($):** 544 Yale Street, 713-426-2313. Relaxing and fun. Go for one of their "Bad Ass" burgers.

What to See

If your exam is over by early afternoon, you might have some extra time to enjoy the sights and sounds of Houston.

- **Theater district:** Located downtown with five great venues. Check out Bayou Place, with its many theaters, bars, and restaurants.
- **Museum district:** Located downtown near Rice University, with many museums and parks. It would be a shame to pass up the John C. Freeman Weather Museum.
- **Sports:** Check out an Astros (www.astros.com) or Rockets game (www.rockets.com) while you're there.

For more information, check out:

- www.houston-guide.com
- www.lonelyplanet.com/destinations/north_america/houston

▶ LOS ANGELES ("THE CITY OF ANGELS")

Clinical Skills Evaluation Collaboration Center
100 North Sepulveda Boulevard, 13th Floor
El Segundo, CA 90245

L.A. is one of the best-known cities in the United States and is rich in cultural and ethnic diversity. One of its most notable attractions, of course, is Hollywood, the hub of the U.S. motion picture industry. L.A. is also home to some amazing cultural sites, such as the Kodak Theatre, the Walt Disney Concert Hall, and all your favorite actors. Take in some stargazing while you're in town!

Getting There

- **Air:** Los Angeles is served by one major airport, Los Angeles International (LAX). It is one of the busiest airports in the world and is located only about three miles from the CSEC center.
- **Ground:**
  - Greyhound, 1716 East 7th Street (www.greyhound.com): L.A. has a terminal near downtown. Plenty of taxis are available outside the station. A ride to your hotel should take about 30 minutes.

- Amtrak, 800 North Alameda Street (www.amtrak.com): L.A. is on multiple rail routes that connect it to cities like New Orleans, Chicago, and Seattle. Take time to see the sights of the U.S. Southwest!

Getting Around When You Arrive

- **Shuttles:** Many hotels around the CSEC center offer free shuttle service from LAX. If your hotel doesn't provide such service, check out the following:
  - SuperShuttle: 800-258-3826, www.supershuttle.com, $15.
  - Prime Time Shuttle: 800-733-8267, www.primetimeshuttle.com, $10.
- **Taxis:** There are also a number of taxi companies that operate in L.A.; below are just a few ($10–$15 from airport to CSEC center):
  - City Cab: 818-780-1000
  - Yellow Cab: 310-851-5022
  - Independent Taxi: 213-666-0040
  - Checker Cab: 213-482-3456
- **Rental cars:** There are multiple rental car companies available in the area. These include Advantage, Alamo, Avis, Dollar, Enterprise, Hertz, and National.
- **Public transportation:** Despite its reputation, L.A. does have public transportation, and the CSEC center is not far away from both rail and bus stops. There is also a free shuttle from LAX to the Aviation station on the Green Line, a rail line that is just two stops away from the El Segundo/Nash station. The Green Line runs every 7–15 minute during rush hour. Get off at the El Segundo/Nash station, walk west on El Segundo Boulevard (0.5 mile) toward the park on the south side of El Segundo, and make a right on North Sepulveda Boulevard. The hotels listed are also generally within walking distance of the stop. You can find more information and use L.A.'s Metro trip planner on their Web site, www.metro.net.

CSEC Center Location

The CSEC center is located on the west side of L.A., only a few miles from LAX and about 20 miles from downtown. It is situated at the corner of North Sepulveda and El Segundo Boulevards. You'll see a series of large office towers; turn in the first driveway marked "Pacific Corporate Towers." Follow the signs to get to visitors' parking ($9/day).

Where to Stay

The following are a few hotels around the test site. You can walk from most, although not all have great walking routes. Remember to ask hotels about their USMLE deals, listed on the AAMC Web site.

- **Doubletree Hotel Los Angeles International Airport:** 1985 East Grand Avenue, 310-322-0999, $159/night. The Doubletree is routinely recommended by guests for its comfortable beds and clean rooms (0.6 mile away).
- **Residence Inn by Marriott El Segundo:** 2135 East El Segundo Boulevard, 310-333-0888, $199/night. Great, quiet rooms and a good complimentary breakfast (0.4 mile away).
- **Hacienda Hotel:** 525 North Sepulveda Boulevard, 310-615-0015, $78/night. A convenient 10-minute walk to the CSEC center. An older but decent choice. Just be ready for small elevators (0.4 mile away).
- **Travelodge Los Angeles Airport South:** 1804 East Sycamore Avenue, 310-615-1073, $72/night. An acceptable budget option, but service can be spotty (0.8 mile away).
- **USA Hostels Hollywood:** 1624 Schrader Boulevard, 323-462-3777, $30–$80/night. This hostel is very cheap and is about 30 minutes away from the center by car if traffic is normal. It's fun but loud, so if you plan on staying here, be sure to bring earplugs (24 miles away).

Where to Eat and Play

L.A. is one of the most ethnically diverse cities in the world, so you can find food for almost every taste. Here are just a few of our favorites:

- **Beachcomber Café ($$):** 23000 Pacific Coast Highway, Malibu, 310-456-9800. Situated on the historic Pacific Coast Highway about 40 minutes from El Segundo. Enjoy an amazing dinner on the beach in Malibu.
- **Pure Luck ($):** 707 North Heliotrope Drive, 323-660-5993. Located in Thai Town in East Hollywood, Pure Luck is a very popular vegetarian restaurant. Nothing on the menu costs more than $10.
- **WoodSpoon ($):** 107 West Ninth Street, 213-629-1765. Located downtown, this unassuming restaurant serves up Brazilian fare. Grilled plates come with rice, beans, plantains, and collard greens. Simple and delicious.
- **Medusa Lounge ($$$):** 3211 Beverly Boulevard, 213-382-5723. An exciting place to get dinner and enjoy the nightly DJs. Offers great beers, sushi, duck, and bratwurst. You'll have to see it to believe it.

What to See

Your exam might be over by early afternoon, so you might have some extra time to see the sights of L.A. Unfortunately, L.A.'s sights aren't always easy to reach without a car, but it's worth a try.

- **Hollywood:** Enjoy a stroll down Hollywood Boulevard and the Walk of Fame. If you don't have a car, you can ride the Metro Rail, but remember that this will take some time. Take the Green Line to the Blue Line and transfer to the Red Line. Exit at the Hollywood/Highland station.

- **Venice Beach:** Only 15 minutes away. Take in some of the uniqueness of L.A. with attractions like Muscle Beach and the area's renowned street performers!

For more information, check out: www.latourist.com

► PHILADELPHIA ("THE CITY OF BROTHERLY LOVE")

Clinical Skills Evaluation Collaboration Center
3624 Market Street, 3rd Floor
Philadelphia, PA 19104

Philadelphia is a great city that is steeped in U.S. history. It was a major hub of social and political activity during the American Revolution, and there is a wealth of places you can visit to soak it all up. Today, Philadelphia is thriving, boasting the fifth-largest metro area in the country. While you're in town, check out Independence Hall, where the Declaration of Independence was first signed on July 4, 1776. And be sure to eat a Philly cheesesteak!

Getting There

- **Air:** Philadelphia is served by one major airport, Philadelphia International Airport (PHL). It serves flights from all around the country and the world. PHL is located about 10 miles from the CSEC center.
- **Ground:**
    - Greyhound, 1001 Filbert Street (www.greyhound.com): The Greyhound terminal is located near the downtown area. Plenty of taxis are available outside the station. A ride to your hotel should take about 5 minutes.
    - Amtrak, 2955 Market Street (www.amtrak.com): Philadelphia is on multiple Amtrak lines, including the high-speed Acela line, which connects Boston, New York, Philadelphia, and Washington, D.C. Other lines connect Philadelphia to the South and the Midwest.

Getting Around When You Arrive

- **Shuttles:** There is limited shuttle service, but one does cover the area:
    - Lady Liberty Company: 215-724-8888, www.ladylibertyshuttle.com, $12.
- **Taxis:** There are also a number of taxi companies that operate in the city; below are just a few ($25 from the airport to the CSEC center):
    - Liberty Cab: 215-389-8000
    - Yellow Cab: 215-333-3333
    - Quaker City Cab: 215-728-8000

- **Rental cars:** There are multiple rental car companies available. These include Alamo, Avis, Dollar, Hertz, and National.
- **Public transportation:** Philadelphia has an extensive public transportation network, called SEPTA (www.septa.org). Both buses and a high-speed rail line connect to the airport. Although the rail line is more expensive ($7 one way), it is easier to use. The Airport rail line (R1) connects all the terminals to the 30th Street station, which is six blocks from the testing center—or you can transfer to the Market-Frankford line and take it to 34th and Market Street, which is just two blocks from the testing center. Fares for buses and the subway are $2 cash, or you can buy tokens for $1.45 that are good for one ride each.

CSEC Center Location

The CSEC center is located downtown, near the University of Pennsylvania campus. It can be found near the intersection of Market and 36th Streets. There is a parking lot right across the street ($14/day).

Where to Stay

The following are a few hotels within walking distance of the test site. Since the CSEC center is downtown, these hotels are fairly expensive. Remember to ask hotels about their USMLE deals, listed on the AAMC Web site.

- **Sheraton Philadelphia University City:** 36th and Chestnut Streets, 800-596-0369, $160/night. Well recommended, and one of the only moderately priced hotels close by (0.1 mile away).
- **Hilton Inn at Penn:** 3600 Sansom Street, 215-222-0200, $289/night. Located on the University of Pennsylvania's campus, this hotel is close but expensive (0.2 mile away).
- **Cornerstone Bed and Breakfast:** 3300 Baring Street, 215-387-6065, $150–$200/night. This B&B is a wonderful place to stay. The breakfasts are delicious (0.6 mile away).
- **Rodeway Inn Philadelphia:** 1208 Walnut Street, 215-546-7000, $136/night. An acceptable budget option, but not walkable. You can, however, ride the Market-Frankford line from City Hall to the 34th Street station (2.1 miles away).
- **Apple Hostels of Philadelphia:** 32 South Bank Street, 877-275-1971, $20–$80/night. This hostel offers both dorm-style and private rooms and is very well recommended. It is located just a block from the Market-Frankford line, so you can take the rail line to the 34th Street station and walk to the CSEC center (2.8 miles away).

Where to Eat and Play

Philadelphia is a great city with a variety of great restaurants. Here are a few of the best:

- **Geno's Steaks/Pat's King of Steaks ($):** 1219 South 9th Street, 215-389-0659/215-468-1547. The Philly cheesesteak (or "hoagie"), perhaps one of the best-known foods in the country, was born here. Just remember to drop the "Philly" while you're in town. Keys to a proper order: Cheese Whiz or provolone with or without fried onion rings.
- **Audrey Claire ($$):** 276 South 20th Street, 215-731-1222. One of the best restaurants in town, located in the heart of Rittenhouse Square.
- **Tangerine ($$$):** 232 Market Street, 215-627-5116. This is one of the tastiest experiences you'll ever have. There are too many great dishes to single out just one, but try the lobster risotto or the chicken tagine.

What to See

Your exam might be over by early afternoon, so you are likely to have some extra time to see the sights of Philadelphia. And since the CSEC center is downtown, you're already in the heart of it.

- **Independence Hall/Liberty Bell:** Located in the block between 5th and 6th Streets and Market and Chestnut Streets, Independence Hall and the Liberty Bell are two of the most iconic images in all of U.S. history. You may want to make a reservation beforehand (www.nps.gov/inde).
- **Museum District:** Close by and home of the Philadelphia Museum of Art, the Franklin Institute of Science, the Philadelphia Zoo, Fairmont Park, and Eastern State Penitentiary.

For more information, check out:

- www.philly.com
- www.lonelyplanet.com/destinations/north_america/philadelphia

► USEFUL WEB SITES

Here are a few other Web sites that you might find useful while you are planning your trip:

- **USMLE travel site:** www.usmle.org/Examinations/step2/cs/CSECAddresses.html
- **AAMC accommodations site:** www.aamc.org/meetings/clinicalskills/hotel rates
- **Travel and hotel sites:**
  - www.expedia.com
  - www.travelocity.com
  - www.orbitz.com
  - www.hotwire.com
  - www.hotels.com
  - www.priceline.com

- **Rental car sites:**
  - www.alamo.com
  - www.avis.com
  - www.budget.com
  - www.dollar.com
  - www.hertz.com
  - www.nationalcar.com
  - www.enterprise.com
  - www.thrifty.com
  - www.paylesscarrental.com
  - www.arac.com

The Patient Encounter

As previously described in Section I, the Clinical Skills (CS) exam consists of 10–12 clinical encounters with trained "standardized patients" (SPs), with each encounter designed to replicate situations commonly seen in clinics, doctors' offices, and emergency departments.

Each encounter in the Step 2 CS is 15 minutes long. You will be given a warning when five minutes remain in the session. The 15-minute period allotted for each of your interviews includes meeting the patient, taking the history, performing the physical exam, discussing your findings and plans, and answering any questions the patient might have. After that, you will have 10 minutes to summarize the patient history and physical exam and to formulate your differential diagnosis and workup plan. All this may seem overwhelming, but it need not be. This chapter will guide you through the process step by step.

Any time saved from the patient encounter can be used to write the patient note.

Fifteen minutes should be adequate for most patient encounters as long as you budget your time wisely. The most common reasons for running out of time are as follows:

- Taking an overly detailed history
- Conducting an unnecessarily detailed physical exam
- Carrying out the encounter in a slow or disorganized fashion
- Allowing the patient to stray away from relevant topics
- Failing to adequately control challenging (e.g., unresponsive, angry, crying) patients

To best manage your encounter, it is recommended that you distribute your time in the following way:

- **Doorway information** (assessing preliminary information posted on the door of each room): 10–20 seconds
- **History:** 7–8 minutes
- **Physical exam:** 3–5 minutes
- **Closure:** 2–3 minutes

Of course, this is only an approximation of how you should divide your time during your 15-minute encounter. In reality, each encounter is different, so some will require more time for taking the history or doing the physical exam, while others will demand that more time be spent on closure and patient counseling. You should thus tailor your time to fit each case. Here are some additional time management tips:

- Do not waste valuable time looking at the clock on the wall. We recommend using the official announcement that five minutes remain in the encounter as your only time indicator. If you have not begun to perform the physical exam by that point, you should do so.

- An organized and well-planned history is key. Stay focused on asking questions that are pertinent to the chief complaint.
- A brief and focused physical exam is also critical. There is no need to conduct a comprehensive physical exam during encounters.
- Never try to save time by ignoring the patient's questions, requests, or emotional status.
- Practice is the best way to improve your performance, efficiency, and sense of timing.

Figure 2-1 further describes the key components and desired outcomes of the clinical encounter. The sections that follow will guide you through each of these components.

FIGURE 2-1. Overview of the Clinical Encounter

Doorway Information
Must get: Chief complaint, age, sex, and abnormal vital signs.
Leads to: Forming a hypothesis (broad differential, relevant points that should be elicited in the history, systems to examine).

History
Must get: Details of the chief complaint, associated symptoms, and any other relevant information that will help rule in or rule out each item in the differential.
Leads to: A more well-defined differential diagnosis, which will help narrow down the procedures that should be performed and the systems that should be examined in the physical exam.

Physical Exam
Must get: Evaluation of the appropriate systems to help rule in or rule out each item in the differential; any additional information on the patient's history if required.
Leads to: A final differential and an appropriate workup plan.

Closure
Explaining the findings, differential, and workup plan to the patient.
Answering the patient's questions and addressing his concerns.

As has previously been described, you will be given a chance to review some preliminary patient information, known as "doorway information," at the outset of each encounter. This information, which is posted on the door of the examination room, includes the patient's name, age, and gender; the reason for the visit; the patient's vital signs (pulse, blood pressure, temperature in both centigrade and Fahrenheit, and respiratory rate); and the task you will be called on to perform.

You should begin by reading the doorway information carefully, checking the chief complaint, and trying to organize in your mind the questions you will need to ask and the systems you will have to examine. Toward this goal, you should look for abnormalities in vital signs without trying to memorize actual numbers. Assume that these vital signs are accurate.

At this time, you should remain calm and confident by reminding yourself that what you are about to encounter is a common medical case. You should also bear in mind that SPs are easier to deal with than real patients in that they are more predictable and already know what you are expected to do. Remember that a second copy of the doorway information sheet will be available on the other side of the door, so you can review that information at the end of each encounter. Note, however, that the time you spend reading the doorway information is included in the 15-minute time limitation.

Address the patient by his or her name when you enter the room.

Your entrance into the examination room is also a critical part of the encounter as a whole. So before you enter the room, be sure to read and commit to memory the patient's last name. Then knock on the door and, once you have entered the examination room, ask the patient if he or she is the person identified on the door ("Mr. Smith?"). You will receive credit for having done so and will not have to worry about remembering the patient's name for the remainder of the encounter. If the patient does not respond to your query, consider the possibility that there may be a change in mental status and that the SP might have been instructed not to respond to his or her name.

After your initial entrance, you should shake hands with the patient and introduce yourself in a confident yet friendly manner (e.g., "Hi, I am Dr. Morton. Nice to meet you."). You may also add something like "I would like to ask you some questions and do a physical exam." You should make an effort to establish eye contact with the patient during this initial period.

▶ TAKING THE HISTORY

Your ability to take a detailed yet focused history is essential to the formulation of a differential diagnosis and workup plan. The discussion that follows will help guide you through this process in a manner that will maximize your chances of success.

Guidelines

You may take the history while either standing in front of the patient or sitting on the stool that is usually located near the bed. You will find a sheet placed on this stool. Begin by removing the sheet and draping the patient. Doing so prior to taking the history is a good idea to guarantee your credit for that early on.

Don't cross your arms in front of your chest when talking to the patient, especially with the clipboard in your hands. It's best to sit down on the stool, relax, and keep the clipboard on your lap. If you decide to stand, maintain a distance of approximately two feet between yourself and the patient.

As previously described, the interview as a whole should take no more than 7–8 minutes. You can start your interview by asking the patient an open-ended question such as "So what brought you to the hospital/clinic today?" or "How can I help you today?" See Figure 2-2 to get an overview of the process.

FIGURE 2-2. History-Taking Overview

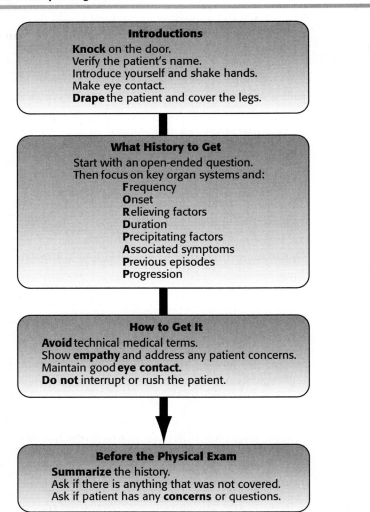

Introductions
Knock on the door.
Verify the patient's name.
Introduce yourself and shake hands.
Make eye contact.
Drape the patient and cover the legs.

What History to Get
Start with an open-ended question.
Then focus on key organ systems and:
      Frequency
      Onset
      Relieving factors
      Duration
      Precipitating factors
      Associated symptoms
      Previous episodes
      Progression

How to Get It
Avoid technical medical terms.
Show **empathy** and address any patient concerns.
Maintain good **eye contact.**
Do not interrupt or rush the patient.

Before the Physical Exam
Summarize the history.
Ask if there is anything that was not covered.
Ask if patient has any **concerns** or questions.

Use simple, nontechnical terminology when speaking to the patient.

Additional Tips

Once the interview has begun, be sure to maintain a professional yet friendly demeanor. You should speak clearly and slowly, and your questions should be short, well phrased, and simple. Toward that end, avoid the use of medical terms; instead, use simple words that a layperson can understand. For example, don't use the term *renal calculus*; use *kidney stone* instead. If you find yourself obliged to use a medical term that the patient may not understand, try to offer a quick explanation. Don't wait for the patient to ask you for the meaning of a term, or you may lose credit.

If you don't understand something the patient has said, you may ask him either to explain his statement or to repeat it: "Can you please explain what you mean by that?" or "Can you please repeat what you have just said?" At the same time, do not rush the patient. Instead, give him the time he needs to respond. In interacting with the patient, you should always remember to ask questions in a neutral and nonjudgmental way.

You should also remember not to interrupt the patient unless it is absolutely necessary. If the patient starts telling lengthy stories that are irrelevant to the chief complaint, you can interrupt him politely but firmly by saying something like "Excuse me, Mr. Johnson. I understand how important those issues are for you, but I'd like to ask you some additional questions about your current problem." You can also redirect the conversation by summarizing what the patient has told you thus far and then moving to the next step. For example, you can say, "So as I understand it, your abdominal pains are infrequent, last a short time, and are always in the middle of your belly. Now tell me about. . . ."

Summarizing key facts for the patient will earn you credit.

It is critical to summarize what the patient has told you, not only to verify that you have understood him but also to ensure that you receive credit. You need to use this summary technique no more than once during the encounter in order to get credit, but you may use it more often should you consider it necessary. It is recommended, however, that you give a summary (1) after you have finished taking the history and before you start examining the patient, or (2) just after you have finished examining the patient and before you give him your medical opinion. In either case, your summary should include only the points that are relevant to the patient's chief complaint.

Minor transitions may also be used during the history. For example, when you want to move from the history of present illness (HPI) to the patient's past medical history or social and sexual history, you can say something like "I need to ask you some questions about your health in the past," or "I'd like to ask you a few questions about your lifestyle and personal habits."

To ensure that you stay on track in gathering information, you will also need to watch the patient carefully, paying attention to his every word, move, or sign. Remember that clinical encounters are staged, so it is uncommon for

something to occur for no reason. Although accidents do happen (e.g., an SP once started to hiccup inadvertently), an SP will most likely cough in an encounter because he is intending to convey that he has bronchitis, not because he "feels like" doing so.

By the same logic, you should address every sign you see in the patient (e.g., "You look sad; do you know the reason?" or "You look concerned; is there anything that is making you worry?"). If your patient is coughing, ask him about his cough even if he didn't cite it as the reason for his visit. If he is using a tissue, ask to see it in order to check the color of the sputum. A spot of blood on the tissue may take you by surprise!

Look for nonverbal clues.

Finally, take brief notes throughout the interview, mainly to record relevant yet easy-to-forget pieces of information such as the duration of the chief complaint or the number of years the patient smoked. To facilitate this note taking, you will be given a clipboard with 12 blank blue sheets, one for each encounter. The extent of your note taking inside the encounter will depend on how much you trust your memory. Before you finish your interview and move to the physical exam, you may ask the patient something like "Is there anything else you would like to tell me about?" or "Is there anything else you forgot to tell me about?"

Common Questions to Ask the Patient

In this section, we will cover a wide spectrum of questions that you may need to pose in the course of each of your patient interviews. This is not meant to be a complete list. You do not have to use all of the questions outlined below. Instead, be selective in choosing the questions you ask in your efforts to obtain a concise, relevant history. You should also be sure to ask only one question at a time. If you ask complex questions (e.g., "Is there any redness or swelling?"), the SP will likely answer only the last question you posed. Instead, you should slow down and ask about one symptom at a time.

Opening of the encounter:
- "Mr. Jones, hello; I am Dr. Singh. It's nice to meet you. I'd like to ask you some questions and examine you today."
- "How can I help you today?"
- "What brought you to the hospital/clinic today?"
- "What made you come in today?"

Pain:
- "Do you have pain?"
- "When did it start?"
- "How long have you had this pain?"
- "How long does it last?"
- "How often does it come on?"
- "Where do you feel the pain?"
- "Can you show me exactly where it is?"

45

- "Does the pain travel anywhere?"
- "What is the pain like?"
- "Can you describe it for me?"
- "Is it sharp, dull, burning, pulsating, cramping, or pressure-like?"
- "Is it constant, or does it come and go?"
- "On a scale of 1 to 10, with 10 being the worst pain of your life, how would you rate your pain?"
- "What brings the pain on?"
- "Do you know what causes the pain to start?"
- "Does anything make the pain better?"
- "Does anything make it worse?"
- "Have you had similar pain before?"

Nausea:
- "Do you feel nauseated?"
- "Do you feel sick to your stomach?"

Vomiting:
- "Did you vomit?"
- "Did you throw up?"
- "What color was the vomit?"
- "Did you see any blood in it?"

Cough:
- "Do you have a cough?"
- "When did it start?"
- "How often do you cough?"
- "Do you bring up any phlegm with your cough, or is it dry?"
- "Does anything come up when you cough?"
- "What color is it?"
- "Is there any blood in it?"
- "Can you estimate the amount of the phlegm? A teaspoon? A tablespoon? A cupful?"
- "Does anything make it better?"
- "Does anything make it worse?"

Headache:
- "Do you get headaches?"
- "Tell me about your headaches."
- "Tell me what happens before/during/after your headaches."
- "When do your headaches start?"
- "How often do you get them?"
- "When your headache starts, how long does it last?"
- "Can you show me exactly where you feel the headache?"
- "What causes the headache to start?"
- "Do you have headaches at certain times of the day?"
- "Do your headaches wake you up at night?"

- "What makes the headache worse?"
- "What makes it better?"
- "Can you describe the headache for me, please? Is it sharp, dull, pulsating, pounding, or pressure-like?"
- "Do you notice any change in your vision before/during/after the headaches?"
- "Do you notice any numbness or weakness before/during/after the headaches?"
- "Do you feel nauseated? Do you vomit?"
- "Do you notice any fever or stiff neck with your headaches?"

Fever:
- "Do you have a fever?"
- "Do you have chills?"
- "Do you have night sweats?"
- "Do you sweat during the night?"
- "How high is your fever?"

Shortness of breath:
- "Do you get short of breath?"
- "Do you get short of breath when you're climbing stairs?"
- "How many steps can you climb before you get short of breath?"
- "When did it start?"
- "When do you feel short of breath?"
- "What makes it worse?"
- "What makes it better?"
- "Do you wake up at night short of breath?"
- "Do you have to prop yourself up on pillows in order to sleep at night? How many?"
- "Have you been wheezing?"
- "How far do you walk on level ground before you have shortness of breath?"
- "Have you noticed any fluid retention around your ankles?"

Urinary symptoms:
- "Has there been any change in your urinary habits?"
- "Do you have any pain or burning during urination?"
- "Have you noticed any change in the color of your urine?"
- "How often do you have to urinate?"
- "Do you have to wake up at night to urinate?"
- "Do you have any difficulty urinating?"
- "Do you feel that you haven't completely emptied your bladder after urination?"
- "Do you need to strain/push during urination?"
- "Have you noticed any weakness in your stream? Any dribbling of urine?"
- "Have you noticed any blood in your urine?"
- "Do you feel as though you need to urinate but then very little urine comes out?"

- "Do you feel as though you have to urinate all the time?"
- "Do you feel as though you have very little time to make it to the bathroom once you feel the urge to urinate?"

Bowel symptoms:
- "Has there been any change in your bowel movements?"
- "Do you have diarrhea?"
- "Are you constipated?"
- "How long have you had diarrhea/constipation?"
- "How many bowel movements do you have per day/week?"
- "What does your stool look like?"
- "What color is your stool?"
- "Is there any mucus or blood in it?"
- "Do you feel any pain when you have a bowel movement?"
- "Did you travel recently?"
- "Do you feel as though you strain to go to the bathroom and then very little feces or none at all come out?"
- "Have you lost control of your bowels?"
- "Do you feel as though you have very little time to make it to the bathroom once you have the urge to have a bowel movement?"

Weight:
- "Have you noticed any change in your weight?"
- "How many pounds did you gain/lose?"
- "Over what period of time did it happen?"
- "Was the weight gain/loss intentional?"

Appetite:
- "How is your appetite?"
- "Has there been any change in your appetite?"

Diet:
- "Has there been any change in your eating habits?"
- "What do you usually eat?"
- "Did you eat anything unusual lately?"
- "What did you eat before the symptoms started?"
- "Is there any kind of special diet that you are following?"

Sleep:
- "Do you have any problems falling asleep?"
- "Do you have any problems staying asleep?"
- "Do you have any problems waking up?"
- "Do you feel refreshed when you wake up?"
- "Do you snore?"
- "Do you feel sleepy during the day?"
- "How many hours do you sleep?"
- "Do you take any pills to help you go to sleep?"

Dizziness:
- "Do you ever feel dizzy?"
- "Tell me exactly what you mean by dizziness."
- "Did you feel the room spinning around you, or did you feel lightheaded as if you were going to pass out?"
- "Did you black out?"
- "Did you lose consciousness?"
- "Did you notice any change in your hearing?"
- "Do your ears ring?"
- "Do you feel nauseated? Do you vomit?"
- "What causes this dizziness to happen?"
- "What makes you feel better?"

Joint pain:
- "Do you have any painful joints in your body?"
- "Do you have pain in any of your joints?"
- "Have you noticed any rash with your joint pain?"
- "Is there any redness or swelling of the joint?"

Travel history:
- "Have you traveled recently?"

Past medical history:
- "Have you had this problem or anything similar before?"
- "Have you had any other major illnesses before?"
- "Do you have any other medical problems?"
- "Have you been hospitalized before?"
- "Have you had any surgeries before?"
- "Have you had any accidents or injuries before?"
- "Are you taking any medications?"
- "Are you taking any over-the-counter drugs, vitamins, or herbs?"
- "Do you have any allergies?"

Family history:
- "Does anyone in your family have the same problem or anything similar?"
- "Are your parents alive?"
- "Are they in good health?"
- "What did your mother/father die of?"
- "Are your brothers or sisters alive?"
- "Are they in good health?"

Social history:
- "Do you smoke?"
- "How many packs a day?"
- "How long have you smoked?"
- "Do you drink alcohol?"
- "What do you drink?"
- "How much do you drink per week?"

- "Do you use any recreational drugs such as marijuana or cocaine?"
- "Which ones do you use?"
- "How often do you use them?"
- "Do you smoke or inject them?"
- "What type of work do you do?"
- "Where do you live? With whom?"
- "Tell me about your life at home."
- "Are you married?"
- "Do you have children?"
- "Do you have a lot of stressful situations on your job?"
- "Are you exposed to environmental hazards on your job?"

Alcohol history:
- "How much alcohol do you drink?"
- "Tell me about your use of alcohol."
- "Have you ever had a drinking problem?"
- "When was your last drink?"
- Administer the CAGE questionnaire:
  - "Have you ever felt a need to **cut down** on drinking?"
  - "Have you ever felt **annoyed** by criticism of your drinking?"
  - "Have you ever had **guilty** feelings about drinking?"
  - "Have you ever had a drink first thing in the morning ('**eye opener**') to steady your nerves or get rid of a hangover?"

Sexual history:
- "I would like to ask you some questions about your sexual health and practice."
- "Are you sexually active?"
- "Do you use condoms? Always? Other contraceptives?"
- "Are you sexually active? With men, women, or both?"
- "Tell me about your sexual partner or partners."
- "How many sexual partners have you had in the past year?"
- "Do you currently have one partner or more than one?"
- "Have you ever had a sexually transmitted disease?"
- "Do you have any problems with sexual function?"
- "Do you have any problems with erections?"
- "Do you use any contraception?"
- "Have you ever been tested for HIV?"

Gynecologic/obstetric history:
- "At what age did you have your first menstrual period?"
- "How often do you get your menstrual period?"
- "How long does it last?"
- "When was the first day of your last menstrual period?"
- "Have you noticed any change in your periods?"
- "Do you have cramps?"
- "How many pads or tampons do you use per day?"

- "Have you noticed any spotting between periods?"
- "Have you ever been pregnant?"
- "How many times?"
- "How many children do you have?"
- "Have you ever had a miscarriage or an abortion?"
- "In what trimester?"
- "Do you have pain during intercourse?"
- "Do you have any vaginal discharge?"
- "Do you have any problems controlling your bladder?"
- "Have you had a Pap smear before?"

Pediatric history:
- "Was your pregnancy full term (40 weeks or 9 months)?"
- "Did you have routine checkups during your pregnancy? How often?"
- "Did you have any complications during your pregnancy/during your delivery/after delivery?"
- "Was an ultrasound performed during your pregnancy?"
- "Did you smoke, drink, or use drugs during your pregnancy?"
- "Was it a vaginal delivery or a C-section?"
- "Did your child have any medical problems after birth?"
- "When did your child have his first bowel movement?"

Growth and development:
- "When did your child first smile?"
- "When did your child first sit up?"
- "When did your child start crawling?"
- "When did your child start talking?"
- "When did your child start walking?"
- "When did your child learn to dress himself?"
- "When did your child learn to tie his shoes?"
- "When did your child start using short sentences?"
- "When did your child start putting things in his mouth?"

Feeding history:
- "Did you breast-feed your child?"
- "When did your child start eating solid food?"
- "How is your child's appetite?"
- "Does your child have any allergies?"
- "Is your child's formula fortified with iron?"
- "Are you giving your child pediatric multivitamins?"

Routine care:
- "Are your child's immunizations up to date?"
- "When was the date of your child's last routine checkup?"
- "Has your child had any serious illnesses?"
- "Is your child taking any medications?"
- "Has your child ever been hospitalized?"

Psychiatric history:

- "Tell me about yourself and your future goals."
- "How long have you been feeling unhappy/sad/anxious/confused?"
- "Do you have any idea what might be causing this?"
- "Would you like to share with me what made you feel this way?"
- "Do you have any friends or family members you can talk to?"
- "Has your appetite changed lately?"
- "Has your weight changed recently?"
- "Tell me how you spend your time/day."
- "Do you have any problems falling asleep/staying asleep/waking up?"
- "Has there been any change in your sleeping habits lately?"
- "What interests/hobbies do you have? Do you enjoy them?"
- "Do you take interest or pleasure in your daily activities?"
- "Do you have any memory problems?"
- "Do you have difficulty concentrating?"
- "Do you have hope for the future?"
- "Have you ever thought about hurting yourself or ending your life?"
- "Do you think of killing yourself/putting an end to your own life?"
- "Do you have a plan to end your life?"
- "Would you mind telling me about it?"
- "Do you feel that you want to hurt other people? Have you ever done so?"
- "Do you ever see or hear things that others can't see or hear?"
- "Do you hold beliefs about yourself or the world that other people would find odd?"
- "Do you feel as if other people are trying to harm or control you?"
- "Has anyone in your family ever experienced depression?"
- "Has anyone in your family ever been diagnosed with a mental illness?"
- "Would you like to meet with a counselor to help you with your problem?"
- "Would you like to join a support group?"
- "What do you think makes you feel this way?"
- "Can you tell me more about it?"
- "Have you lost any interest in your social activities and relationships?"
- "Do you feel hopeless?"
- "Do you feel guilty about anything?"
- "How is your energy level?"
- "Can you still perform your daily functions or activities?"
- "Do you have any thoughts of harming yourself?"
- "Do you have any thoughts of harming others?"
- "Whom do you live with?"
- "How do they react to your behavior?"
- "Do you have any problems in your job?"
- "How is your performance on your job?"
- "Have you had any recent emotional or financial problems?"
- "Have you had any recent traumatic event in your family?"
- "Does anyone support you?"

Daily activities (for dementia patients):

- "Tell me about your day yesterday."
- "Do you need any help bathing?"
- "Do you need any help getting dressed?"
- "What do you need help with when you are getting dressed?"
- "Do you need any help going to the toilet?"
- "Do you need any help transferring from your bed to the chair?"
- "Do you ever have accidents with your urine or bowel movements?"
- "Do you ever not make it to the toilet on time?"
- "Do you need any help feeding yourself?"
- "What do you need help with when you eat?"
- "Do you need any help taking your medications/using the telephone/shopping/ preparing food/cleaning your house/doing laundry/getting from place to place/ managing money?"

Abuse:

- "Are you safe at home?"
- "Is there any threat to your personal safety at home or anywhere else?"
- "Does anyone (your husband/wife/parents/boyfriend) treat you in a way that hurts you or threatens to hurt you?"
- "Can you tell me about the bruises on your arm?"

▶ THE PHYSICAL EXAM

Guidelines

In this section, we will suggest a systematic way to perform the physical exam. You can use this method or any other system with which you feel comfortable. Regardless of the method you choose, however, it is essential that you practice until you can perform the physical exam without mistakes or hesitation.

The key is a focused physical exam.

As described earlier, the physical exam can take up to five minutes. Given that the history portion of the encounter is estimated to take 7–8 minutes, you should already have started the physical exam by the time you hear the announcement that you have five minutes remaining in the encounter. Bear in mind that there is no time for a complete physical exam. Instead, you should aim at conducting a focused exam to look for physical findings that can support the differential diagnosis you made after taking the history. See Figure 2-3 for an overview of the process.

Before you begin, you should announce to the patient the need for the physical exam. Then, don't forget to wash your hands with soap and water and dry them carefully. (You can wear gloves instead if you so choose.) While you are washing your hands, use the time to think about what you should examine and whether there is anything you neglected to ask the patient. You should then drape the patient if you have not yet done so. The drape will be on the stool; unfold it and cover the patient from the waist down.

FIGURE 2-3. Physical Exam Overview

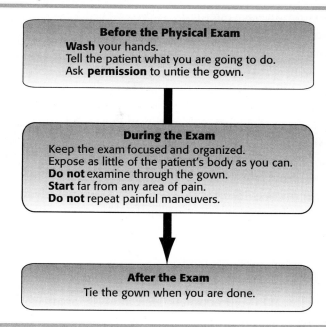

Before the Physical Exam
Wash your hands.
Tell the patient what you are going to do.
Ask **permission** to untie the gown.

During the Exam
Keep the exam focused and organized.
Expose as little of the patient's body as you can.
Do not examine through the gown.
Start far from any area of pain.
Do not repeat painful maneuvers.

After the Exam
Tie the gown when you are done.

Before you touch the patient, make sure your hands are warm (rub your hands together if they are cold). In a similar manner, rub the diaphragm of your stethoscope to warm it up before you use it. Do not auscultate or palpate through the patient's gown.

Ask permission before touching or uncovering the patient.

As you proceed, be sure to ask the patient's permission before you uncover any part of his body (e.g., "Is it okay if I untie your gown in order to examine your chest?" or "Can I move down the sheet to examine your belly?"). You may also ask the patient to uncover himself. You should expose only the area you need to examine. Do not expose large areas of the patient's body at once. After you have examined a given area, cover it immediately.

During the physical exam, you will be scored both for performing a given procedure and for doing so correctly. You will not get credit for conducting an extra maneuver or for examining a nonrequired system, but failure to perform a required procedure will cost you a check mark on your list. You should also bear in mind that you are not allowed to perform a corneal reflex, breast, rectal, pelvic, or genital exam. If you think any of the above-mentioned exams is indicated, you should tell the patient that you will need to do the specific exam later and then remember to add the exam to your orders on your patient note (PN). When you have concluded a given procedure, remember to say "thank you." Then explain the next step, and ask the patient for his permission to proceed. The patient should always be made to feel that he is in control of his body.

In the course of the physical exam, you may ask the patient any additional questions that you feel may be pertinent to the history. It is recommended,

however, that you stop the physical exam while doing so in order to reestablish eye contact. After the patient has answered your questions, you may resume the exam.

Finally, you should remain alert to special situations that may not unfold as would an ordinary physical exam. When you enter the examination room, for example, the patient may hand you an insurance form requesting that only certain systems be examined. In such cases, the patient will usually tell you that you do not need to take a history. Should this occur, simply introduce yourself, proceed to examine the systems listed, and then leave the room. No PN is required under such circumstances; instead, you are required only to fill out the form the patient gave you with the appropriate findings. In such encounters, the emphasis will be on the correct performance of the physical exam maneuvers and on professional and appropriate interaction with the patient.

Be alert to special situations that may occur during a patient encounter.

Physical Exam Review

The following is a review of the steps involved in the examination of each of the body's main systems. Included are samples of statements that can be used during the physical exam. Remember that it is crucial to keep the patient informed of what is going on as well as to ask his consent before each step.

1. **HEENT exam:**
    -   **What to say to the patient before and during the exam:**
        -   "I need to examine your sinuses, so I am going to press on your forehead and cheeks. Please tell me if you feel pain anywhere."
        -   "I would like to examine your eyes now."
        -   "I am going to shine this light in your eyes. Can you please look at the clock on the wall?"
        -   "I need to examine your ears now."
        -   "Can you please open your mouth? I need to check the inside of your mouth and your throat."
    -   **What to perform during the HEENT exam:**
        -   Head:
            1. Inspect the head for signs of trauma and scars.
            2. Palpate the head for tenderness or abnormalities.
        -   Eyes:
            1. Inspect the sclerae and conjunctivae for color and irritation.
            2. Check the pupils for symmetry and reactivity to light.
            3. Check the extraocular movements of the eyes.
            4. Check visual acuity with the Snellen eye chart.
            5. Perform a funduscopic exam. Remember the rule "right-right-right" (ophthalmoscope in examiner's right hand—patient's right eye—examiner's right eye) and the rule "left-left-left" (ophthalmoscope in examiner's left hand—patient's left eye—examiner's left eye).

- Ears:
    1. Conduct an external ear inspection for discharge, skin changes, or masses.
    2. Palpate the external ear for pain (otitis externa); do the same for the mastoid.
    3. Examine the ear canal and the tympanic membrane using an otoscope. (Don't forget to use a new speculum for the patient.)
    4. Conduct the Rinne and Weber tests.
- Nose:
    1. Inspect the nose.
    2. Palpate the nose and sinuses.
    3. Inspect the nasal turbinates and the nasal septum with a light source.
- Mouth and throat:
    1. Inspect with a light.
    2. Tooth tapping may be performed if needed.

2. **Cardiovascular exam:**
   - **What to say to the patient before and during the exam:**
     - "I need to listen to your heart."
     - "Can you hold your breath, please?"
     - "Can you sit, please?"
     - "Can you turn to your left side, please?"
     - "I am going to examine your legs to check for fluid retention. Is that okay with you?"
     - "I need to check the pulse in your arms and legs now."
   - **What to perform during the cardiovascular exam:**
     - When examining the heart, do not lift up the patient's gown. Rather, pull the gown down the shoulder, exposing only the area to be examined.
     - Listen to the carotids for bruits (use the diaphragm of the stethoscope).
     - Look for JVD.
     - Palpate the chest for the PMI, retrosternal heave, and thrills.
     - Listen to at least two of the four cardiac areas. (Listen to the mitral area with the patient on his left side.)
     - Listen to the base of the heart with the patient leaning forward.
     - Check for pedal edema.
     - Check the peripheral pulses.

3. **Pulmonary exam:**
   - **What to say to the patient before and during the exam:**
     - "I need to listen to your lungs now."
     - "Can you take a deep breath for me, please?"
     - "Can you say '99' for me, please?"
     - "I am going to tap on your back to check your lungs. Is that okay with you?"
   - **What to perform during the pulmonary exam:**
     - Examine both the front and the back of the chest.
     - Don't percuss or auscultate through the patient's gown.

- Don't percuss or auscultate over the scapula.
- Allow a full inspiration and expiration in each area of the chest.
- Inspect: The shape of the chest, respiratory pattern, deformities.
- Palpate: Tenderness, tactile fremitus.
- Percuss.
- Auscultate, egophony.

4. **Abdominal exam:**
   - **What to say to the patient before and during the exam:**
     - "I need to examine your belly/stomach now."
     - "I am going to listen to your belly now."
     - "I am going to press on your belly. Tell me if you feel any pain or discomfort."
     - "Now I need to tap on your belly."
     - "Do you feel any pain when I press in or when I let go? Which hurts more?"
   - **What to perform during the abdominal exam:**
     - Inspect.
     - Auscultate (always auscultate before you palpate the abdomen).
     - Percuss.
     - Palpate: Start from the point that is farthest from the pain; be gentle on the painful area, and don't try to reelicit the pain. Check for rebound tenderness, CVA tenderness, obturator sign, psoas sign, and Murphy's sign.
     - Check the liver span.

5. **Neurologic exam:**
   - **What to say to the patient before and during the exam—mini-mental status exam questions:**
     - "I would like to ask you some questions to test your orientation."
     - "I would like to check your memory and concentration by asking you some questions."
     - "Can you tell me your name and age?"
     - "Do you know where are you now?"
     - "Do you know the date today?"
     - Show the patient your pen and ask him, "Do you know what this is?"
     - "Now I would like to ask you some questions to check your memory."
     - "I will name three objects for you, and I want you to repeat them immediately, okay? Chair, bed, and pen." (Tests immediate memory.)
     - "I will ask you to repeat the names of these three objects after a few minutes." (Tests short-term memory.)
     - "Do you remember what you had for lunch yesterday?" (Tests recent memory.)
     - "When did you get married?" (Tests distant memory.)
     - "Now, can you repeat for me the names of the three objects that I mentioned to you?" (Tests short-term memory.)
     - "Are you left-handed or right-handed?"

- "I will give you a piece of paper. I want you to take the paper in your right hand, fold the paper in half, and put it on the floor." (Three-step command.)
- "Now I want you to write your name on the paper."
- "I want you to count backward starting with the number 100," or "Take 7 away from 100 and tell me what number you get; then keep taking 7 away until I tell you to stop." (Tests concentration.)
- "Spell 'world' forward and backward." (Tests concentration.)
- "What would you do if you saw a fire coming out of a paper basket?" (Tests judgment.)

- **What to say to the patient before and during the exam—neurologic exam questions:**
  - "I am going to check your reflexes now."
  - "I am going to test the strength of your muscles now."
  - "This is up, and this is down. Tell me which direction I am moving your big toe."
  - "Can you walk across the room for me, please?"

- **What to perform during the neurologic exam:**
  - Mental status examination: Orientation, memory, concentration.
  - Cranial nerves:
    1. II: Vision.
    2. III, IV, VI: Extraocular movements.
    3. V: Facial sensation, muscles of mastication.
    4. VII: Smile, lifting of brows, close your eyes and don't let me open them.
    5. IX, X: Symmetrical palate movement, gag reflex.
    6. XI: "Shrug your shoulders."
    7. XII: "Stick out your tongue."
  - Motor system:
    1. Passive motion.
    2. Active motion: Arms—flexion ("pull in"), extension ("push out"); wrists—flexion ("push down"), extension ("pull up").
    3. Hands: "Spread your fingers apart; close your fist."
    4. Legs: Knee extension ("kick out"), knee flexion ("pull in").
    5. Ankles: "Push on the gas pedal."
  - Reflexes: Biceps, triceps, brachioradialis, patellar, Achilles, Babinski.
  - Sensory system: Sharp (pin)/dull (cotton swab), vibration, position sense.
  - Cerebellum: Finger-to-nose, heel-to-shin, rapid alternating movements, Romberg sign, gait.
  - Meningeal signs: Neck stiffness, Kernig, Brudzinski.

6. **Joint exam:**
   - **What to say to the patient before and during the exam:**
     - "Tell me if you feel pain anywhere."
     - "I am going to examine your knee/ankle now."
   - **What to perform during the joint exam:**
     - Inspect and compare joint with the opposite side.
     - Palpate.

- Check for joint effusion.
- Check for crepitus.
- Check the joint range of motion.
- **Useful scales:**
  - Reflexes (0–4), with 0 being completely areflexic:
    - **1:** Hyporeflexia.
    - **2:** Normal reflexes.
    - **3:** Hyperreflexia.
    - **4:** Hyperreflexia plus clonus (test the ankle and the knee).
  - Strength (0–5), with 0 representing an inability to move the limb:
    - **1:** Can move limb (wiggle toes).
    - **2:** Can lift limb against gravity.
    - **3:** Can lift limb with one-finger resistance from the examiner.
    - **4:** Can lift limb with two-finger resistance from the examiner.
    - **5:** Has full strength.
  - Pulses (0–4), with 0 representing pulselessness:
    - **1:** Weak pulse.
    - **2:** Regular pulse.
    - **3:** Increased pulse.
    - **4:** Pounding pulse.

Special Challenges During the Physical Exam

During the course of the physical exam, you may encounter any number of special problems. The following are examples of such challenges along with potential responses to them.

- **Listening to the heart in a female patient:** You can place the stethoscope anywhere around the patient's bra and between the breasts. To auscultate or palpate the PMI, if necessary, ask the patient, "Can you please lift up your breast?"
- **Examining a patient who is in severe pain:** A patient in severe pain may initially seem unapproachable, refuse the physical exam, and insist that you give him something to stop his pain. In such cases, you should first ask the patient's permission to perform the physical exam. If he refuses, gently say, "I understand that you are in severe pain, and I want to help you. The physical exam that I want to do is very important to help determine what is causing your pain. I will be as quick and gentle as possible, and once I find the reason for your pain, I should be able to give you something to make you more comfortable."
- **Examining lesions:** If you see a scar, a mole (nevus), a psoriatic lesion, or any other skin lesion during the exam, you should mention it and ask the patient about it even if it is not related to the patient's complaint.
- **Examining bruising:** Inquire about any bruises you see on the patient's body, and think about abuse as a possible cause.
- **Running out of time:** If you don't have time for a full mini-mental status exam, at least ask patients if they know their name, where they are, and what day it is.

SP Simulation of Physical Exam Findings

It bears repeating that during the physical exam, it is necessary to remain cautious and attentive, as the symptoms patients exhibit during the encounter are seldom accidental and are usually reproducible. So when you notice any positive sign, take it seriously. The following are some physical signs that may be simulated by the SP:

1. **Abdomen:**
   - Abdominal tenderness: The patient feels pain when you press on his abdomen. Remember that the patient is an actor. When you palpate the area, he will feel pain where he is supposed to feel pain regardless of the amount of pressure you exert. So don't try to palpate the same area again; instead, move on, and consider the pain on palpation a positive sign.
   - Abdominal rigidity: The patient will contract his abdominal muscles when you try to palpate the abdomen.
   - Rebound tenderness of the abdomen.
   - CVA tenderness.

2. **Chest:**
   - Shortness of breath.
   - Wheezing: This may often sound strange, as if the patient were whistling from his mouth.
   - Decreased respiratory sounds: The patient will move his chest without really inhaling any air so that you do not hear any respiratory sounds.
   - Increased fremitus: The patient will say "99" in a coarse voice, creating more fremitus than usual.

3. **Nervous system:**
   - Confusion.
   - Dementia.
   - Extensor plantar response (Babinski's sign).
   - Absent or hyperactive tendon reflexes (stroke, diabetes mellitus): Eliciting the reflex in the SP is not like doing so in a real patient, where you must try more than once to ensure that you have not missed the tendon and that your strike is strong enough. In a clinical encounter, try the reflex only once; if you don't see it, it is not there. If the patient wants to show you hyperactive DTRs, he will make sure to respond with an exaggerated jerk even to the lightest and most awkward hammer hit.
   - Facial paralysis.
   - Hemiparesis.
   - Gait abnormalities.
   - Ataxia.
   - Chorea.
   - Hearing loss.
   - Tinel's sign.
   - Phalen's sign.
   - Nuchal rigidity.
   - Kernig's sign.
   - Brudzinski's sign.

4. **Eyes:**
   - Visual loss (central, peripheral): In a young patient, this may be multiple sclerosis.
   - Photophobia: The patient will say, "I hate the light" or "I don't feel comfortable in bright light." Dim the light to make the patient feel more comfortable.
   - Lid lag.
   - Nystagmus.
5. **Muscles and joints:**
   - Muscle weakness.
   - Rigidity.
   - Spasticity.
   - Parkinsonism: Shuffling gait (difficulty initiating and stopping ambulation, small steps, no swinging of the arms), resting tremor, masked facies, rare blinking, and cogwheel rigidity.
   - Restricted range of motion of joints.
6. **Bruits and murmurs:**
   - Renal artery stenosis: A patient with hypertension who is not responding to multiple antihypertensive medications. Do not be surprised if you hear an abdominal bruit.
   - Thyroid bruit.
   - Carotid bruit: The patient says "Hush, hush" when you place the stethoscope over his neck.
   - Heart murmur: Once you place the stethoscope on the patient's heart, you will hear him saying "Hush, hush."
7. **Skin:**
   - Skin lesions: You may see artificial skin discoloration (e.g., painful red spots on the shin for erythema nodosum in a patient with sarcoidosis; redness over an inflamed joint in a patient with arthritis).
8. **Real physical exam findings:**
   - You may see real C-section, appendectomy, cholecystectomy, or other scars. Don't overlook them. Always inquire about any scar you see.
   - You may see a real nevus (mole). Ask the patient about it and advise him to check it routinely and report any change in it.
   - You may see real skin lesions, such as pityriasis rosea in a Christmas tree pattern, seborrheic dermatitis of the scalp, or acne vulgaris.
   - When you listen to a patient's heart, don't be surprised to hear a real heart murmur.
   - A patient with a sore throat may present with real enlarged tonsils.

▶ CLOSURE

Finishing the history and the physical exam does not mean that the encounter is over. To the contrary, closure is a critical part of the encounter. See Figure 2-4 for an overview of the process. During closure, you are expected to do several things:

FIGURE 2-4. Closure Overview

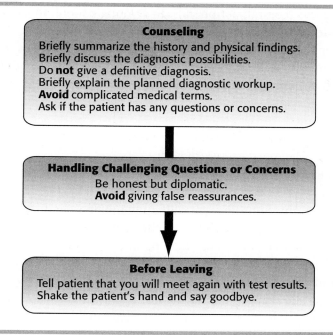

Counseling
Briefly summarize the history and physical findings.
Briefly discuss the diagnostic possibilities.
Do **not** give a definitive diagnosis.
Briefly explain the planned diagnostic workup.
Avoid complicated medical terms.
Ask if the patient has any questions or concerns.

Handling Challenging Questions or Concerns
Be honest but diplomatic.
Avoid giving false reassurances.

Before Leaving
Tell patient that you will meet again with test results.
Shake the patient's hand and say goodbye.

Leave a few minutes for closure. Don't rush it.

- Make a transition to mark the end of your encounter.
- Summarize the chief complaint and the HPI if you have not already done so before the physical exam.
- Summarize your findings from the physical exam.
- Give your impression of the patient's clinical condition and most likely diagnosis.
- Suggest a diagnostic workup.
- Answer any questions the patient might have.
- Address the patient's concerns.
- Check to see if the patient has any more questions.
- Leave the room.

To transition into the closure, you should begin by saying something like "Thank you for letting me examine you, Mrs. Jones. Now I would like to sit down with you and give you my impression." You should then tell the patient about the possible differential diagnoses (keep to a maximum of three) and explain the meaning of any complicated medical terms you might use. You might also point out the organ or system that you think is involved and explain a simple mechanism of the disease. You should not, however, give the patient a definitive diagnosis at this time. Instead, tell him that you still need to run some tests in order to establish the final diagnosis. In some cases there will actually be no final diagnosis; instead, the case will be constructed in such a way as to be a mixture of signs and symptoms that can be construed to indicate any number of diseases.

During closure, almost every patient will have at least one challenging question to which you must respond (e.g., "Do you think I have cancer, doctor?"

or "Am I going to get better?"). In answering these questions, be honest yet diplomatic. Essentially, being honest with the patient means not giving false reassurances such as "I am sure you will be cured after a week of antibiotics," or "Don't worry, I am sure that it is not cancer." What you might say instead is, "Well, I cannot exclude the possibility of cancer at this point. We need to do additional testing. Regardless of the final diagnosis, however, I want you to be assured that I will be available for any support you need."

If you do not know the answer to a patient's question, you should state as much. See the end of this chapter for examples of challenging questions patients might pose along with potential responses to them.

During closure, you should also explain to the patient the diagnostic tests you are planning to order. In doing so, you should again use nontechnical terms— for example, "We need to run some blood tests to check the function of your liver and kidneys," or "You need to have a chest x-ray and a CT scan of the head." You may further explain the latter by saying, "The CT scan is a type of x-ray imaging that gives us clear images of sections of the body." You should then add, "After we get the results of those tests, we will meet again to discuss them in detail along with the final diagnosis and the treatment plan." Finally, you should conclude by asking the patient if he still has any questions.

If you find you are running out of time, do not compromise the closure. If time constraints dictate that you choose between a thorough physical exam and an appropriate closure, give priority to the execution of a proper closure.

Before you leave the room, you can finish your encounter by looking the patient in the eye and saying something like "Okay, Mr. Jones, I'll contact you when I have your test results. It was nice meeting you." You may then shake the patient's hand and leave the room. You are allowed to leave the room as soon as you think you have completed the encounter. Once you have left the encounter room, you will not be allowed to go back inside.

You cannot reenter the examination room once you leave.

▶ HOW TO INTERACT WITH SPECIAL PATIENTS

The following are guidelines for dealing with atypical or uncommon patients or encounters.

- **The anxious patient:** Encourage the patient to talk about his feelings. Ask him about the things that are causing him to feel anxious. Give him reasonable reassurance.
- **The angry patient:** Stay calm and don't be scared. Remember that the patient is not really angry; he is just acting angry to test your response. Let him express his feelings, and ask about the reason for his anger. You should also address the patient's anger in a reasonable way. For example, if the patient is complaining that he has been waiting for a long time, tell him you understand. Explain that the clinic is crowded, and there were many

patients who had appointments prior to his. Reassure the patient that now that it is his turn, you will focus on his case and take care of him.

- **The crying patient:** Allow the crying patient to express his feelings, and wait in silence for him to finish. Offer him a tissue, and show him empathy in your facial expressions. You may also place your hand lightly on the patient's shoulder or arm and say something like "I know that you feel sad. Would you like to tell me about it?" Don't worry about time constraints in such cases. Remember that the patient is an actor and that his crying is timed. He will allow you to continue the encounter in peace if you respond correctly.

- **The patient who is in pain:** Show compassion for the patient's pain. Say something like "I know that you are in pain." Offer help by asking, "Is there anything I can do for you to help you feel more comfortable?" Do not repeat painful maneuvers. If the patient does not allow you to touch his abdomen because of the severe pain he is experiencing, tell him, "I know that you are in pain, and I want to help you. I need to examine you, though, to be able to locate the source of pain and give you the right treatment." Reassure the patient by saying, "I will be as quick and gentle as possible."

- **The patient who can't pay for the tests or for treatment:** Reassure the patient by saying, "Not having enough money doesn't mean you can't get treatment." You might also add, "We will refer you to a social worker who can help you find resources."

- **The patient who refuses to answer your question or let you examine him:** Explain to the patient why the question or the physical exam is important. Tell him that they are necessary to allow you to understand the problem and arrive at a diagnosis. If the patient still refuses to cooperate, skip the question or the maneuver and document his refusal and your counseling in the PN.

- **The hard-of-hearing patient:** Face the patient directly to allow him to read your lips. Speak slowly, and do not cover your mouth. Use gestures to reinforce your words. If the patient has unilateral hearing loss, sit close to the hearing side.

- **The patient who doesn't know the names of his medications or is taking medications whose names *you* don't recognize:** Ask the patient if he has a prescription or a written list of the medications he is currently taking.

- **The phone encounter:** The Step 2 CS exam may include a telephone encounter. As with other encounters, patient information will be posted on the door before you enter the examination room. Once you are inside, sit in front of the desk with the telephone, and push the speaker button by the yellow dot to be connected to the patient. Do not dial any numbers or touch any other buttons. You are permitted to call the SP only once. Treat this like a normal encounter and gather all the necessary information. To end the call, press the speaker button above the yellow dot. As in the pediatric encounter, there is no physical exam, so leave this portion of the PN blank.

During your encounters, every patient will ask you one or more challenging questions. Your reactions and answers to these questions will be scored. Such questions may be explicit ones that you are expected to answer directly, or they may take the form of indirect comments or statements that must be properly addressed in order to reveal an underlying concern. When answering the challenging questions, try to remember the following guidelines:

- Be honest and diplomatic.
- Before addressing the patient's issue, you might restate the issue back to the patient to let him know that you understand.
- Don't give the patient a final diagnosis. Instead, tell the patient about your initial impressions and about the workup you have in mind to reach a conclusive diagnosis.
- Do not give false reassurances.
- If you do not know the answer to the patient's question, just tell him so.

Do not give the patient a definitive diagnosis.

The following are examples of challenging questions:

Confidentiality/Ethical Issues

Challenging Question	Possible Response
A patient who needs emergent surgery says, "I can't afford the cost of staying in the hospital. I have no insurance. Just give me something to relieve the pain, and I will leave."	"I know that you are concerned about medical costs, but your life will be in danger if you don't have surgery. Let our social workers help you with the cost issues."
"Should I tell my sexual partner about my venereal disease?"	"Yes. There is a chance that you have already transmitted the disease to your partner, or he/she may be the source of your infection. The important step is to have you both evaluated and appropriately treated."
An anxious patient who you suspect has been abused asks, "Why are you asking me these questions?"	"I am concerned that domestic abuse may be involved. My goal is to make sure that you are in a safe environment and that you are not a victim of abuse."
A patient recently diagnosed with HIV asks, "Do I have to tell my wife?"	"I know that it's difficult, but doing so will allow you and your wife to take the appropriate precautions to treat and prevent the transmission of the disease."

Patient Belief/Behavioral Issues

Challenging Question	Possible Response
An elderly patient says, "I think that it is normal at my age to have this problem" (impotence), or "I am just getting old."	"Age may play a role in the change you are experiencing in your sexual function, but your problem may have other causes that we should rule out, such as certain diseases (hypertension, diabetes) or certain medications. We also have medications that may improve your sexual function."
"I read in a journal that the treatment of this disease is herbal compounds."	"Herbal medicines have been suggested for many diseases. However, their safety and efficacy may not always be clear-cut. Let me know the name of the herbal medicine and I will check into its potential treatment role for this disease."
"I am afraid of surgery."	"I understand your feelings. It is normal and very common to have these feelings before surgery. Is there anything specific that you are concerned about?"
A patient who has a serious problem (unstable angina, colon cancer) asks, "I want to go on a trip with my wife. Can we do the tests after I come back?"	"I know that you don't want to put off your trip, but you may have a serious problem that may benefit from early diagnosis and management."
"I did not understand your question, doctor. Could you repeat it, please?"	Repeat the question again slowly. If the patient still doesn't comprehend the question, ask if there is any specific word he didn't understand and try to explain it or use a simpler one.
"What is a bronchoscopy?" (MRI, CT, x-ray, colonoscopy)	Explain the meaning using simple words. For example, "Bronchoscopy is using a thin tube connected to a camera to look into your respiratory airways and parts of your lungs," or "An MRI is a machine that uses a big magnet to obtain detailed pictures of your brain or body."

Challenging Question	Possible Response
"What do you mean by 'workup'?"	"It means all the tests that we are going to do to help us make the final diagnosis."
A patient who is late in seeking medical advice asks, "Do you think it is too late for recovery?"	"I am glad that you came for help. We will do our best and hope for the best."
A patient with pleuritic chest pain asks, "Is this a heart attack? Am I going to die?"	"Given your current presentation, my suspicion for a heart attack is low. It is more likely that inflammation of the membranes surrounding your lungs is causing your pain, and this is usually not a life-threatening condition. However, we still need to do some tests to confirm the diagnosis and rule out heart problems."
"Do you think I have colon cancer?" "Do you think I have a brain tumor?" "Do I have endometrial cancer?"	"That is one of the possibilities, but there are other explanations for your symptoms that we should rule out before making a diagnosis."
"My friend told me that you are a very fine doctor. That's why I came to you to refill my prescription."	"I am flattered, but since this is your first visit, I can't give you a refill without reviewing your history to better understand your need for this medication. I will also need to do a physical exam and perhaps order some tests."
"Will my insurance cover the expenses of this test?"	"I'm not sure, but I can refer you to a social worker who does have that information. If necessary, I can write a note to your insurance company indicating the importance of this test."
A person who wants to return to work at a job that can negatively affect his health asks, "Can I go back to work?"	"Unfortunately, work may actually worsen your condition. Therefore, I would prefer that you stay at home for now. I can write a letter to your employer explaining your situation."
"Do you think that this tumor I have could become malignant?"	"We really won't know until we remove the mass and get a pathology report on it."

Challenging Question	Possible Response
"Since I stopped smoking, I have gained weight. I want to go back to smoking in order to lose weight."	"There are healthier ways to lose weight than smoking, such as exercise and diet. Smoking will increase your risk of cancer, heart problems, and lung disease."
A patient with a shoulder injury says, "I am afraid of losing my job if my shoulder doesn't get better."	"We will do our best to help you recover from your shoulder injury. With your permission, I will communicate the situation to your employer."
"Will I ever feel better, doctor?"	The answer differs depending on the prognosis of the disease and can vary from "Yes, most people with this disease are completely cured" to "Complete cure may be difficult at this advanced stage, but we have a lot to offer in terms of controlling the symptoms and improving your quality of life."
A person who has a broken arm asks, "Doctor, do you think I will be able to move my arm again like before?"	"It is hard to tell right now, but those fractures usually heal well, and with physical therapy you should regain the normal range of motion of your arm."
"I think that life is full of misery. Why do we have to live?"	"Life can be challenging. Is there something in particular that is bothering you? Have you thought of ending your life?" You can then continue screening for depression.
A young man with multiple sexual partners and a recent-onset skin rash says, "I am afraid that I might have AIDS."	"Having multiple sexual partners does put you at risk for HIV infection, but this rash may be due to many other causes. I agree that we should do an HIV test on you in addition to a few other tests."
A patient who needs hospitalization says, "My child is at home alone. I have to leave now."	"I understand your concern about your child, but right now staying in the hospital is in your best interest. One of our social workers can make some phone calls to arrange for child care."

Challenging Question	Possible Response
"Do you have anything that will make me feel better? Please, doctor, I am in pain."	"I know that you're in pain, but I need to know what's causing your pain in order to give you the appropriate treatment. After I am done with my evaluation, we can decide on the best way to help manage your pain."
A patient you believe is pretending (malingering) says, "Please, doctor, I need a week off from work. The pain in my back is terrible."	"I know that you are uncomfortable, but after examining you, I don't find disability significant enough to keep you out of work. I plan to prescribe pain medication and exercises, but a big part of your recovery will be continuing your normal daily activities."
"Stop asking me all these stupid questions and just give me something for this pain."	"I know that you're in pain, but I need to determine the cause of the pain in order to give you the right treatment. After I am done with my evaluation, we will give you the appropriate treatment."
"So what's the plan, doctor?"	"After we get the results of your tests, we will meet again. At that time, I will try to answer any questions you may have."
"Do you think I will need surgery?"	"I will try to manage your problem medically, but if that doesn't work, you may need surgery. We can see how things go and then try to make that decision together in the future."
A female patient has only one sexual partner, and she is diagnosed with an STD. She asks you, "Could he possibly be cheating on me?"	"You most likely contracted this infection from your partner. It would be best to talk to your partner about this to clear things up. He needs to be tested and treated, or else you risk becoming reinfected."
A patient is shouting angrily, "Where have you been, doctor? I have been waiting here for the whole day."	"I am sorry you had to wait so long. We had some unexpected delays with a few of the earlier patients this morning. But I'm here now, and I will focus on you and your concerns."

Disease-Related Issues

Challenging Question	Possible Response
An educated 58-year-old woman asks, "I read in a scientific journal that hormonal replacement therapy causes breast cancer. What do you think of that, doctor?"	"It appears to be true. Studies show a slight increase in the risk of developing breast cancer after four years of combination estrogen and progesterone use for hormonal replacement therapy. The current recommendations are to use hormonal replacement therapy solely for the relief of hot flashes, and only for a limited period of time."
"Did I have a stroke?"	"We don't know yet. Your symptoms could be explained by a small stroke, but we need to wait for the results of your MRI."
"Do I have lung cancer?"	"We don't know at this point. It is a possibility, but we still need to do additional tests."
An African-American man with sickle cell anemia presents with back and chest pain and says, "Please, doctor, I need some Demerol now or I will die from pain."	"I know that you are in pain, but I need to ask you a few questions first to better understand your pain. Then we will get you medicines for your pain."
A patient with symptoms of a common cold says, "I think I need antibiotics, doctor."	"It appears that you have a viral common cold. Antibiotics do not treat viruses, and they have adverse effects that could even make you feel worse. We should focus on treating your symptoms."
"My mother had breast cancer. What is the possibility that I will have breast cancer, too?"	"You are at increased risk, but it doesn't mean that you will get it. There are other risk factors that need to be considered, and regular screening tests will be very important."
A 55-year-old man says, "I had a colonoscopy six years ago, and they removed a polyp. Do you think that I have to repeat the colonoscopy?"	"Yes, it should be repeated. We need to screen for more polyps, and in this way we hope to prevent the development of colon cancer."

Challenging Question	Possible Response
A patient with headache or confusion asks, "Do you think I have Alzheimer's disease?"	"I don't know. Alzheimer's is one of several possible causes that we will investigate."
"Can I get pregnant even though my tubes are tied?"	"There is no single contraceptive method that is 100% effective. The risk of pregnancy after tubal ligation is less than 1%, but it is a real risk."
A woman who is in her first trimester of pregnancy with vaginal bleeding asks, "Do you think I am losing my pregnancy?"	"Bleeding early in pregnancy increases your risk of losing the pregnancy, but at the same time, most women who have bleeding carry the pregnancy to term without problems."
"My brother has colon cancer. What are the chances that I will have colon cancer as well?"	"Some types of colon cancer are hereditary, and you may be at increased risk, but it doesn't mean that you will get colon cancer for sure. I need to get more information about your personal and family history to determine your level of risk."
A patient with palpitations says, "My mother had a thyroid problem; do you think it is my thyroid?"	"It's possible. We always check a thyroid blood test, but we will also consider many other possible causes of palpitations."
"Obesity runs in my family. Do you think that this is why I am overweight?"	"Genes play an important role in obesity, but lifestyle, diet, and daily habits are also major factors influencing weight. These factors can be used in a way that can help you lose weight."
A young man with dysuria asks, "Do you think I have an STD?"	"That is one of the possibilities. We will do some cultures to find out for sure, and we will also check a urine sample, since your symptoms may be due to a urinary tract infection."
"I am drinking a lot of water, doctor. What do you think the reason is?"	"This may simply be due to dehydration, or it may be a sign of a disease such as diabetes. We need to do some tests to determine the cause."

Challenging Question	Possible Response
A patient with COPD asks, "Will I get better if I stop smoking?"	"Most patients with your condition who stop smoking will experience a gradual improvement in their symptoms, in addition to a significantly decreased risk of lung cancer in the future."
A patient with possible appendicitis is asking for a cup of water to drink.	"I am sorry, but I can't give you anything to eat or drink right now. You may need emergent surgery, and anesthesia is much safer if your stomach is completely empty."
A patient with infectious mononucleosis asks, "Can I go back to school, doctor?"	"Now that you have recovered from the acute stage of the disease, you can go back to school, but I want you to stay away from any strenuous exercise or contact sports, as you may rupture your spleen."

▶ COUNSELING

During at least one of your encounters, you are likely to find a patient who smokes, drinks, or has another habit that may adversely affect his health. Although these behaviors may or may not be relevant to your primary diagnosis, it is important that they be addressed in a rapid yet caring manner. Here are some examples of conversations you might have with your patient. Try to practice saying some of these aloud, making sure to change them to fit your personality and style.

*The **5 A's** are recommended guidelines to help patients quit smoking.*

*1. **A**sk the patient about tobacco use.*

*2. **A**dvise him or her to quit.*

*3. **A**ssess the patient's willingness to make an attempt to quit.*

*4. **A**ssist in the quit attempt.*

*5. **A**rrange for follow-up.*

The Smoker

Examinee: Do you smoke cigarettes?

SP: Yes, I have smoked one pack a day for 20 years.

Examinee: Have you ever tried to quit?

SP: Of course, but it never works.

Examinee: Well, I strongly recommend that you quit smoking. Smoking is a major cause of cancer and heart disease. Are you interested in trying to quit now?

SP1: Yes. (If the answer is "no," see below.)

Examinee: I would be happy to help you quit smoking. We have many tools to help you do that, and I will be with you every step of the way. Let's set up an appointment for two weeks from today, and we can get started on it then. Is that okay with you?

SP2: No, I don't want to quit.

Examinee: I understand that you aren't ready to quit smoking yet, but I want to assure you that whenever you are ready, I will be here to help you.

The Alcoholic

Examinee: How many drinks do you have in a week?

SP: It is hard to say. Too many.

Examinee: How many drinks do you have per day?

SP: Oh, maybe five or so.

Examinee: Have you ever felt the need to **cut down** on your drinking? Have you ever felt **annoyed** by criticism of your drinking? Have you ever felt **guilty** about drinking? Have you ever had to take a morning **eye opener**? (A "yes" answer to any one of the questions in the CAGE questionnaire should raise suspicion and prompt further questioning.)

SP: All of these things apply.

Examinee: I am concerned about your drinking. It can lead to liver disease, cause problems with bleeding, or even predispose you to early dementia. Are you interested in cutting down or quitting?

SP1: Yes. (If the answer is "no," see below.)

Examinee: I am glad you want to quit. A variety of resources are available to help you quit drinking, and I would like to discuss them with you. Let's make an appointment later this week to talk about your options. In the meantime, I have printed up a list of resources, and my office assistant will bring it to you.

SP2: No, I am not ready to quit.

Examinee: I realize that you are not ready to quit drinking, but I want to assure you that if you do decide to try, I will be here for you. Okay?

The Patient with Uncontrolled Diabetes

Examinee: Apparently, your diabetes is not adequately controlled according to your blood glucose readings. How often do you forget to take your medication? (Check for noncompliance.)

SP1: Taking all these medications just gets so confusing. I can never remember when to take them.

Examinee: Diabetes can certainly be a challenge to manage. Do you have someone who could help you take your medications? If not, we have a social worker who might be able to arrange for a nurse to come to your home. Are you interested in that?

SP2: I have been taking my medications exactly as they were prescribed to me.

Examinee: Tell me about your diet. (Check for dietary management.)

SP2: I eat regular meals, but I really like to drink soda. Diet soda tastes awful!

Examinee: You must be very careful about your sugar consumption. It is prudent to keep your blood sugar within normal limits. Persistently high blood sugar can cause damage to your eyes, kidneys, and nerves. Also, you will be at

higher risk for developing infections, heart attacks, and strokes. Fortunately, we have a diabetes educator who may be able to help you. Are you interested in meeting with him?

The Sexually Promiscuous Patient

Examinee: Are you currently in a sexual relationship?
SP: Yes.
Examinee: Can you tell me about your partner or partners?
SP: I have a girlfriend, but I also see a couple of other women on the side.
Examinee: Are you using any type of protection with these partners?
SP: My girlfriend is on the pill, but I don't use anything with the other women I see.
Examinee: Condoms reduce the risk of sexually transmitted infections. Do you think you could try to use condoms?
SP: I tried them, but I just don't like them.
Examinee: I understand that you may not like to use condoms, but I am concerned that you may be putting yourself at risk for STDs. You could contract HIV, herpes, chlamydia, or any of a number of other STDs. The complications of these diseases include infertility, painful infections, or even death. If anyone with whom you have sexual contact has an STD, you could share it among all of them, including your girlfriend. I hope you will consider using a condom in the future. Do you have any questions for me?

The Depressed Patient

Examinee: Do you have problems **sleeping**? Have you lost **interest** in things that used to interest you? Do you feel **guilty**? Do you lack your usual **energy**? Has it been difficult for you to **concentrate**? Has your **appetite** changed? Do you feel as though you want to hurt yourself or someone else or commit **suicide**? (If you suspect depression, ask the questions posed in the mnemonic **SIG E CAPS.**)
SP: (Answers affirmatively to many of these questions.)
Examinee: You answered "yes" to many of my questions. I believe that you might have the diagnosis of depression. Depression is a common disease; it is due to a chemical imbalance in the brain that causes many of the symptoms you have described to me. Fortunately, we have medications that can help; however, these medications work best when they are combined with counseling. I can write you a prescription and also give you a referral to see a therapist. Is this something you are interested in?

The Patient with an STD (Trichomoniasis)

Examinee: Your symptoms are due to an infection called trichomoniasis, a sexually transmitted infection that has been given to you by one of your sexual partners. This infection responds well to treatment with antibiotics and is curable. You will also need to be tested for all other STDs. Your sexual partner needs to be treated as well; otherwise, you will be at risk of contracting the infection again. You should avoid sexual intercourse (unless you use condoms) until you finish the course of antibiotics and your partner gets treated.

▶ THE PATIENT NOTE

Once you have completed an encounter, your final task will be to compose a PN. (See Figure 2-5 for a detailed overview of the clinical encounter and PN.) Toward this goal, you will find a desk with a sheet of paper on it immediately outside the encounter room. You will be given 10 minutes to write the PN and will be notified when two minutes remain. If you leave the encounter room before the end of the 15-minute period allotted for your patient encounter, you can devote the extra time you have to writing the PN. You are allowed to review the doorway information while you are writing the PN.

The PN sheet located outside the encounter room will have your name, the number of the encounter, and a bar code printed on it. You will not be provided with additional paper, so use the space wisely. You should also take care not to write outside the frame of the sheet, because the paper will be scanned and nothing outside the frame will be read. Be sure to use the pen provided by the examination center, as you are not allowed to use your own pens.

Before you start writing the PN, take a few seconds to review the history, including the chief complaint, how it started, its progression, and the main symptoms. Then take a deep breath and try to relax. If you get nervous and try to rush, your thoughts may become garbled, and you will risk losing the point of your story. As you begin to write, also remember that your handwriting must be legible in order for your PN to be properly scored.

As mentioned previously, you have the option of typing your PNs instead of writing them. Typing is a good choice if you are fast with the keyboard or have bad handwriting. Make a decision about which method you prefer and practice it beforehand. Note that you will not be able to render diagrams such as the neurology stick figure for reflexes. You can simulate typing the PN online at the USMLE Web site. Whether you choose to type or write, you will have to do the same for all PNs.

FIGURE 2-5. Summary Overview of the Patient Encounter

First announcement:
"Examinees, you may enter the room."

10–20 SECONDS

DOORWAY
Read the doorway information and note the **vital signs/age/chief complaint.**
Note the encounter objectives: history and physical exam vs. just history.
Develop a list of likely differential diagnoses.

KNOCK on the door and enter the room.

7–8 MINUTES

HISTORY
Greet the patient/shake hands/introduce yourself.
Make **eye** contact; maintain a **proper posture.**
Put the drape on the patient and cover the legs.
Start with an **open**-ended question.
Avoid technical terms.
Show **empathy** and address the patient's concern and expressions.
Do not interrupt/rush the patient.
Obtain past medical, surgical, medication, family, social, sexual, and allergy history.

WASH your hands.

3–5 MINUTES

PHYSICAL EXAM
Tell the patient what you are going to do.
Ask **permission** to start the physical exam.
Never examine through the gown.
Use a respectful draping technique.

Second announcement:
"Examinees, you have **five minutes left** for this encounter."
By this time you should be **halfway** through your exam.

Writing the Patient Note

You will be required to fill out four main sections in your PN: the history, physical exam, differential diagnosis, and initial diagnostic workup.

Decide first if you will type or handwrite the PNs.

Summarizing the history. In writing the history, be clear, direct, and concise, and avoid long and complex phrases. Make sure the history flows in a logical sequence. Also bear in mind that it is not necessary to write a detailed, all-inclusive history. The components that should be included are as follows:

- Chief complaint (CC)
- History of present illness (HPI)
- Review of systems (ROS)
- Past medical history (PMH)

FIGURE 2-5. **Summary Overview of the Patient Encounter** *(continued)*

2–3 MINUTES

CLOSURE
Explain your diagnostic possibilities/workups.
Avoid complicated medical terms.
Ask if the patient has any concerns.
Be prepared to handle **challenging questions.**
Avoid giving false reassurances.
Do the **counseling.**
Say goodbye, thank the patient, and leave the encounter.

Third announcement:
*"This encounter is now **finished.**"*

10 MINUTES

WRITTEN PATIENT NOTE
Document **key** CC, HPI, PMH, meds, SH, ROS.
Document **key** physical findings.
Include **pertinent positives** and **negatives.**
Give a maximum of **five** diagnostic possibilities.
Order maximum of **five** diagnostic tests.
Do **not** consult, hospitalize, or treat the patient.
Order **rectal, pelvic, genital,** or **breast** exams if needed.

Fourth announcement:
"You have two minutes left."

Fifth announcement:
"Your time is now finished."

- Past surgical history (PSH)
- Social history (SH)
- Family history (FH)

When you are summarizing the history, you should be prudent in using the space assigned to you for that purpose. Many examinees run out of space while writing this section. One way to save both time and space is to make ample use of abbreviations. Train yourself to use the abbreviations that are listed in the USMLE Step 2 CS exam orientation materials. (Please see inside back cover.) You will find a copy of this list on each desk. You are allowed to use any abbreviations that are commonly used in U.S. hospitals. If you are unsure of the correct abbreviation, it is better to spell out the word or phrase.

In general, many different styles of writing are acceptable as long as your history is both comprehensive and legible. Two examples can be found in the candidate orientation manual.

Outlining the physical exam. To summarize the physical exam, write a list of the systems that you examined, outlining all the relevant positive and negative findings. If you did not perform a maneuver that you think was necessary, it is better not to lie and pretend that you did. Be honest and list only the items you examined. For example, do not claim that you saw diabetic retinopathy in a patient with diabetes mellitus if you did not even get to see the eye fundus. See Figure 2-6 for some examples of how to document physical exam findings.

Developing a differential. In writing the differential, you should list a maximum of five diagnoses. You are not required to list that many if three or four diagnoses suffice. The diagnoses should be directly related to the history and physical exam, and it is preferable that they be listed in order of probability, from the most to the least probable.

Specifying the initial diagnostic workup. In summarizing your workup, list a maximum of five tests. It is best to start with the "forbidden physical exam maneuvers" (e.g., rectal exam, pelvic exam) if you feel such procedures are indicated. Then state the required laboratory and radiologic tests, starting with the most simple and straightforward tests and ending with the most complex. Do not include referrals, treatments, hospitalizations, or consults, as these will not be scored.

Be specific in your orders. Instead of "chem 7," "thyroid panel," or "liver function tests," you should specify "Na, K," "TSH and total T_4," and "AST and ALT." You may, however, order electrolytes. Each group of related tests (blood tests, x-rays) should be listed together.

Tests in the diagnostic workup should be specific.

Scoring the Patient Note

The PN will be scored by a physician on the basis of its organization, quality of information, interpretation of data, and legibility. The final score will represent the average PN score of all 10 scored encounters.

How to Prepare

The cardinal rule for preparing to write a PN is to practice, practice, and practice. Imagine that you are in the actual exam, and try to write the PN within 10 minutes. You should also practice writing the note so that it will fit in the allotted space. When using the cases presented in this book, try to write your PN and then compare your note with ours. The main things you should look for are the following:

- Is your history complete?
- Does it make sense?

FIGURE 2-6. Examples of How to Document Physical Exam Findings

- **HEENT:**
  - Head: Atraumatic, normocephalic.
  - Eyes: EOMI, PERRLA, normal eye fundus.
  - Nose: No nasal congestion.
  - Throat: No tonsillar erythema, exudates, or enlargement.
  - Mouth: Moist mucous membranes, good dentition, no lesions.

- **Neck:** Supple, no JVD, normal thyroid, no cervical LAD.

- **Nervous System:**
  - Mental status: Alert and oriented x 3, good concentration.
  - Cranial nerves II–XII grossly intact.
  - Motor: Strength 5/5 in all muscle groups.
  - DTRs: 2+ intact and symmetric, Babinski ⊖.
  - Sensation: Intact to sharp and dull.
  - Cerebellum: ⊖ Romberg sign, intact finger to nose.

- **Chest/Lung:**
  - Clear to percussion bilaterally.
  - No rales, rhonchi, wheezing, or rubs.
  - No tenderness to palpation.
  - Tactile fremitus WNL.

- **Heart:**
  - PMI not displaced.
  - Regular rate and rhythm.
  - Normal S1, S2.
  - No murmurs, rubs, or gallops.

- **Abdomen:**
  - Soft, nontender, nondistended, BS ⊕, no hepatosplenomegaly.

- **Extremities:**
  - No clubbing, cyanosis, or edema.

- **Mental Status Exam:**
  - Patient speaks slowly.
  - No hostile behavior toward the interviewer.
  - Blunt affect with poor eye contact.
  - Inattentive to interviewer.
  - 3/3 registration, 3/3 recall at 3 times.
  - Distant memories are impaired.
  - Oriented to person, date, and place.
  - Completed three-step command.
  - Right-handed.
  - 1/5 on serial 7s.
  - Poor judgment.

- Are the physical exam results complete?
- Is your differential diagnosis correct?
- Are your tests correct and in the right order?

There are several styles you can use both to document the physical exam and to compose the PN. So choose a method, memorize it, and stick with it. Note, however, that in this book we used only one method to write PNs.

If you are running out of time, start from the bottom of the PN. Write down the differential diagnosis, the tests conducted, the physical exam, and then the history and the review of systems (listing only the positives first).

SECTION III

Minicases

In this chapter, we will attempt to cover most of the clinical cases that you are likely to encounter in the Step 2 CS. The main title of each case represents a chief complaint that you may see on the doorway information sheet before you enter the examination room. After each chief complaint, key points pertinent to the history and physical exam are reviewed. Each clinical case consists of three components:

- **Presentation:** A brief clinical case with some pertinent positives and negatives.
- **Differential:** An appropriate differential diagnosis, with the most likely diagnosis appearing in boldface.
- **Workup:** The main diagnostic tests that should be considered for each disease. Note that the diagnostic tests in the third column are generally listed in order of priority. In clinical practice, many tests may be performed at the same time or not at all.

The sum of the **Differential** column will give you a wide differential diagnosis for the chief complaint, while the sum of the **Workup** column will give you a pool of tests from which to choose in the exam.

If you are studying by yourself, we suggest that you start by reading the vignette and then try to figure out the diagnosis and the workup.

If you are studying with a partner or in a group, we suggest that you read a vignette aloud and have others develop the differential diagnosis and workup.

Key History

Location (especially unilateral vs. bilateral), quality, intensity, duration, timing (does it disturb sleep?); presence of associated neurologic symptoms (paresthesias, visual stigmata, weakness, numbness, ataxia, photophobia, dizziness, auras, neck stiffness); nausea/vomiting; jaw claudication; recent trauma, dental surgery, sinusitis symptoms; exacerbating (stress, fatigue, menses, exercise, certain foods) and alleviating factors (rest, medications); past history of headache; family history of migraines.

Key Physical Exam

Vital signs; inspection and palpation of entire head; ENT inspection; complete neurologic exam, including funduscopic exam.

Presentation	Differential	Workup
▪ 21 yo F presents with several episodes of throbbing left temporal pain that lasts for 2–3 hours. Prior to its onset, she sees flashes of light in her right visual field and feels weakness and numbness on the right side of her body for a few minutes. Headaches are often associated with nausea and vomiting. She has a family history of migraine.	**Migraine (complicated)** Tension headache Cluster headache Pseudotumor cerebri Trigeminal neuralgia CNS vasculitis Partial seizure Intracranial neoplasm	CBC ESR CT—head MRI—brain LP
▪ 26 yo M presents with severe right temporal headaches associated with ipsilateral rhinorrhea, eye tearing, and redness. Episodes have occurred at the same time every night for the past week and last for 45 minutes.	**Cluster headache** Migraine Tension headache Sinusitis Pseudotumor cerebri Trigeminal neuralgia Intracranial neoplasm	CBC ESR CT—head MRI—brain LP
▪ 65 yo F presents with severe, intermittent right temporal headache, fever, blurred vision in her right eye, and pain in her jaw when chewing.	**Temporal arteritis (giant cell arteritis)** Migraine Cluster headache Tension headache Meningitis Carotid artery dissection Pseudotumor cerebri Trigeminal neuralgia Intracranial neoplasm	CBC ESR CRP Temporal artery biopsy Doppler U/S—carotid MRI—brain

Presentation	Differential	Workup
30 yo F presents with frontal headache, fever, and nasal discharge. There is pain on palpation of the frontal and maxillary sinuses. She has a history of sinusitis.	**Sinusitis** Migraine Tension headache Meningitis Intracranial neoplasm	CBC XR—sinus CT—sinus LP
50 yo F presents with recurrent episodes of bilateral squeezing headaches that occur 3–4 times a week, typically toward the end of her work day. She is experiencing significant stress in her life.	**Tension headache** Migraine Depression Caffeine or analgesic withdrawal Hypertension Cluster headache Pseudotumor cerebri Intracranial neoplasm	CBC Electrolytes ESR CT—head LP
35 yo M presents with sudden severe headache, vomiting, confusion, left hemiplegia, and nuchal rigidity.	**Subarachnoid hemorrhage** Migraine Meningitis/encephalitis Intracranial hemorrhage Vertebral artery dissection Intracranial venous thrombosis Acute hypertension Intracranial neoplasm	CT without contrast—head LP CBC PT/PTT MRI/MRA—brain
25 yo M presents with high fever, severe headache, confusion, photophobia, and nuchal rigidity. Kernig's and Brudzinski's signs are positive.	**Meningitis** Migraine Subarachnoid hemorrhage Sinusitis/encephalitis Intracranial or epidural abscess	CBC CT—head MRI—brain LP—CSF analysis (cell count, protein, glucose, Gram stain, PCR for antigens, culture)
18 yo obese F presents with a pulsatile headache, vomiting, and blurred vision for the past 2–3 weeks. She is taking OCPs.	**Pseudotumor cerebri** Tension headache Migraine Cluster headache Meningitis Intracranial venous thrombosis Intracranial neoplasm	Urine hCG CBC CT—head LP—opening pressure and CSF analysis

Presentation	Differential	Workup
■ 57 yo M c/o daily pain in the right cheek over the past month. The pain is electric and stabbing in character and occurs while he is shaving. Each episode lasts 2–4 minutes.	**Trigeminal neuralgia** Tension headache Migraine Cluster headache TMJ dysfunction Intracranial neoplasm	CBC ESR MRI—brain

► CONFUSION/MEMORY LOSS

Key History

Must include history from family members/caregivers. Detailed time course of cognitive deficits (acute vs. chronic/gradual onset), associated symptoms (constitutional, incontinence, ataxia, hypothyroid symptoms, depression); screen for delirium (waxing/waning level of alertness); falls, medications (and recent medication changes); history of stroke or other atherosclerotic vascular disease, syphilis, HIV risk factors, alcohol use, or vitamin B_{12} deficiency; family history of Alzheimer's disease.

Key Physical Exam

Vital signs; complete neurologic exam, including mini-mental status exam and gait; general physical exam, including ENT, heart, lungs, abdomen, and extremities.

Presentation	Differential	Workup
■ 81 yo M presents with progressive confusion over the past several years together with forgetfulness and clumsiness. He has a history of hypertension, diabetes mellitus, and two strokes with residual left hemiparesis. His mental status has clearly worsened after each stroke (stepwise decline in cognitive function).	**Vascular ("multi-infarct")** **dementia** Alzheimer's disease Normal pressure hydrocephalus Chronic subdural hematoma Intracranial tumor Depression B_{12} deficiency Neurosyphilis Hypothyroidism	CBC VDRL/RPR Serum B_{12} TSH MRI—brain CT—head LP—CSF analysis (rare)

Presentation	Differential	Workup
84 yo F brought by her son c/o forgetfulness (e.g., forgets phone numbers, loses her way back home) along with difficulty performing some of her daily activities (e.g., bathing, dressing, managing money, using the phone). The problem has gradually progressed over the past few years.	**Alzheimer's disease** Vascular dementia Depression Hypothyroidism Chronic subdural hematoma Normal pressure hydrocephalus Intracranial neoplasm B_{12} deficiency Neurosyphilis	CBC VDRL/RPR Serum B_{12} TSH MRI—brain (preferred) CT—head LP—CSF analysis (rare)
72 yo M presents with memory loss, gait disturbance, and urinary incontinence for the past six months.	**Normal pressure hydrocephalus** Alzheimer's disease Vascular dementia Chronic subdural hematoma Intracranial neoplasm Depression B_{12} deficiency Neurosyphilis Hypothyroidism	CT—head LP—opening pressure and CSF analysis Serum B_{12} VDRL/RPR TSH
55 yo M presents with a rapidly progressive change in mental status, inability to concentrate, and memory impairment for the past two months. His symptoms are associated with myoclonus and ataxia.	**Creutzfeldt-Jakob disease** Vascular dementia Lewy body dementia Wernicke's encephalopathy Normal pressure hydrocephalus Chronic subdural hematoma Intracranial neoplasm Depression Delirium B_{12} deficiency Neurosyphilis	CBC, electrolytes, calcium Serum B_{12} VDRL/RPR MRI—brain (preferred) CT—head EEG LP—CSF analysis Brain biopsy
70 yo insulin-dependent diabetic M presents with episodes of confusion, dizziness, palpitation, diaphoresis, and weakness.	**Hypoglycemia** Transient ischemic attack Arrhythmia Delirium Angina	Glucose CBC, electrolytes Echocardiography ECG MRI—brain Doppler U/S—carotid
55 yo F presents with gradual altered mental status and headache. Two weeks ago she slipped, hit her head on the ground, and lost consciousness for two minutes.	**Subdural hematoma** SIADH (causing hyponatremia) Creutzfeldt-Jakob disease Intracranial neoplasm	Electrolytes CT—head MRI—brain LP

Key History

Onset, duration; sleep patterns; appetite and weight change; drug and alcohol use; life stresses, excessive guilt, suicidality, social function, decreased interest (anhedonia), decreased energy, decreased concentration, psychomotor agitation or retardation; family history of mood disorders; prior episodes; medications.

Key Physical Exam

Vital signs; head and neck exam; neurologic exam; mental status exam, including documentation of appearance, behavior, speech, mood, affect, thought process, thought content, cognition (measured by the 30-point mini-mental status exam), insight, and judgment.

Presentation	Differential	Workup
68 yo M presents with a two-month history of crying spells, excessive sleep, poor hygiene, and a 7-kg weight loss, all following his wife's death. He cannot enjoy time with his grandchildren and reluctantly admits to thinking he has seen his dead wife in line at the supermarket or standing in the kitchen making dinner.	**Normal bereavement** Adjustment disorder with depressed mood Major depressive disorder with psychotic features Schizoaffective disorder Depressive disorder not otherwise specified (NOS)	Physical exam Mental status exam TSH CBC Urine toxicology
42 yo F presents with a four-week history of excessive fatigue, insomnia, and anhedonia. She states that she thinks constantly about death. She has suffered five similar episodes in the past, the first in her 20s, and has made two previous suicide attempts. She further admits to increased alcohol use in the past month.	**Major depressive disorder** Substance-induced mood disorder Dysthymic disorder	Physical exam Mental status exam Blood alcohol level TSH CBC Urine toxicology
26 yo F presents with a 3-kg weight loss over the past two months, accompanied by early-morning awakening, excessive guilt, and psychomotor retardation. She does not identify a trigger for the depressive episode but reports several weeks of increased energy, sexual promiscuity, irresponsible spending, and racing thoughts approximately six months before her presentation.	**Bipolar I disorder** Bipolar II disorder Cyclothymic disorder Major depressive disorder Schizoaffective disorder	Physical exam Mental status exam Urine toxicology

Key History

Positive symptoms (delusions, hallucinations, disorganized thoughts, disorganized or catatonic behavior), negative symptoms (blunted affect, social withdrawal, decreased motivation, decreased speech/thought), cognitive symptoms (disorganized speech or thought patterns, paranoia); age of first symptoms and/or hospitalization; previous psychiatric medications; alcohol and substance use.

Key Physical Exam

Vital signs; mental status exam.

Presentation	Differential	Workup
19 yo M c/o receiving messages from his television set. He reports that he did not have many friends in high school. In college, he started to suspect his roommate of bugging the phone. In the same time frame, he stopped going to classes because he felt that his professors were saying horrible things about him that no one else noticed. He rarely showered or left his room and has recently been hearing a voice from his television set telling him to "guard against the evil empire."	**Schizophrenia** Schizoid or schizotypal personality disorder Schizophreniform disorder Psychotic disorder due to a general medical condition Substance-induced psychosis Depression with psychotic features	Mental status exam Urine toxicology TSH CBC Electrolytes
28 yo F c/o seeing bugs crawling on her bed over the past two days and reports hearing loud voices when she is alone in her room. She has never experienced symptoms such as these in the past. She recently ingested an unknown substance.	**Substance-induced psychosis** Brief psychotic disorder Schizophreniform disorder Schizophrenia Psychotic disorder due to a general medical condition	Urine toxicology Mental status exam TSH CBC Electrolytes, BUN/Cr, AST/ALT
48 yo F presents with a one-week history of auditory hallucinations, stating, "I am worthless" and "I should kill myself." She also reports a two-week history of weight loss, early-morning awakening, decreased motivation, and overwhelming feelings of guilt.	**Schizoaffective disorder** Mood disorder with psychotic features Schizophrenia Schizophreniform disorder Psychotic disorder due to a general medical condition	Mental status exam Beck Depression Inventory TSH CBC Electrolytes

Key History

Lightheadedness vs. vertigo, ± auditory symptoms (hearing loss, tinnitus), duration of episodes, context (occurs with positioning, following head trauma), other associated symptoms (visual disturbance, URI, nausea); neck pain or injury; medications; history of atherosclerotic vascular disease.

Key Physical Exam

Vital signs; complete neurologic exam, including Romberg test, nystagmus, tilt test (e.g., Dix-Hallpike maneuver), gait, hearing, and Weber and Rinne tests; head and neck exam; cardiovascular exam.

Presentation	Differential	Workup
35 yo F presents with intermittent episodes of vertigo, tinnitus, nausea, and hearing loss over the past week.	**Ménière's disease** Vestibular neuronitis Labyrinthitis Benign positional vertigo Acoustic neuroma	CBC VDRL/RPR (syphilis is a cause of Ménière's disease) MRI—brain
55 yo F c/o dizziness for the past day. She feels faint and has severe diarrhea that started two days ago. She takes furosemide for her hypertension.	**Orthostatic hypotension due to dehydration** (diarrhea, diuretic use) Vestibular neuronitis Labyrinthitis Benign positional vertigo Vertebrobasilar insufficiency	Orthostatic vital signs CBC Electrolytes Stool exam (occult blood, fecal leukocytes)
65 yo M presents with postural dizziness and unsteadiness. He has hypertension and was started on hydrochlorothiazide two days ago.	**Drug-induced orthostatic hypotension** Vestibular neuronitis Labyrinthitis Benign positional vertigo Brain stem or cerebellar tumor Acute renal failure	Orthostatic vital signs CBC Electrolytes BUN/Cr MRI—brain
44 yo F c/o dizziness on moving her head to the left. She feels that the room is spinning around her head. Tilt test results in nystagmus and nausea.	**Benign positional vertigo** Vestibular neuronitis Labyrinthitis Ménière's disease	MRI—brain Audiogram

Presentation	Differential	Workup
■ 55 yo F c/o dizziness that started this morning. She is nauseated and has vomited once in the past day. She had a URI two days ago and has experienced no hearing loss.	**Vestibular neuronitis** Labyrinthitis Ménière's disease Benign positional vertigo Vertigo associated with cervical spine disease/injury Vertebrobasilar insufficiency	CBC Electrolytes Electronystagmography MRI/MRA—brain
■ 55 yo F c/o dizziness that started this morning and of "not hearing well." She feels nauseated and has vomited once in the past day. She had a URI two days ago.	**Labyrinthitis** Vestibular neuronitis Ménière's disease Acoustic neuroma Vertebrobasilar insufficiency	Audiogram Electronystagmography MRI/MRA—brain

► LOSS OF CONSCIOUSNESS (LOC)

Key History

Presence or absence of preceding symptoms (nausea, diaphoresis, palpitation, pallor, lightheadedness), context (exertional, postural, traumatic; stressful, painful, or claustrophobic experience; dehydration); associated tongue biting, incontinence, tonic-clonic movements, prolonged confusion; dyspnea or pulmonary embolism risk factors; history of heart disease, arrhythmia, hypertension, or diabetes; alcohol and drug use.

Key Physical Exam

Vital signs, including orthostatics; complete neurologic exam; carotid and cardiac exam; lung exam; exam of the lower extremities.

Presentation	Differential	Workup
■ 26 yo M presents after falling and losing consciousness at work. He had rhythmic movements of the limbs, bit his tongue, and lost control of his bladder. He was subsequently confused (as witnessed by his colleagues).	**Seizure, grand mal** (now called complex tonic-clonic seizure) Convulsive syncope Substance abuse/overdose Malingering Hypoglycemia	CBC, electrolytes, glucose Urine toxicology EEG MRI—brain CT—head LP—CSF analysis ECG

Presentation	Differential	Workup
▪ 55 yo M c/o falling after feeling dizzy and unsteady. He experienced transient LOC. He has hypertension and is on numerous antihypertensive drugs.	**Drug-induced orthostatic hypotension (causing syncope)** Cardiac arrhythmia Syncope (vasovagal, other causes) Stroke MI Pulmonary embolism	Orthostatic vital signs CBC Electrolytes CT—head ECG V/Q scan CT—chest with IV contrast
▪ 65 yo M presents after falling and losing consciousness for a few seconds. He had no warning prior to passing out but recently had palpitations. His past history includes coronary artery bypass grafting (CABG).	**Cardiac arrhythmia (causing syncope)** Severe aortic stenosis Syncope (other causes) Seizure Pulmonary embolism	ECG Holter monitoring CBC, electrolytes Glucose Echocardiography CT—head

▶ NUMBNESS/WEAKNESS

Key History

Distribution (unilateral, bilateral, proximal, distal), duration, ± progressive, pain (especially headache, neck or back pain); constitutional symptoms, other neurologic symptoms; history of diabetes, alcoholism, atherosclerotic vascular disease.

Key Physical Exam

Vital signs; neurologic and musculoskeletal exams; relevant vascular exam.

Presentation	Differential	Workup
▪ 68 yo M presents following a 20-minute episode of slurred speech, right facial drooping and numbness, and right hand weakness. His symptoms had totally resolved by the time he got to the ER. He has a history of hypertension, diabetes mellitus, and heavy smoking.	**Transient ischemic attack (TIA)** Hypoglycemia Seizure Stroke Facial nerve palsy	CBC Glucose Electrolytes ECG CT—head MRI—brain Doppler U/S—carotid Echocardiography EEG

Presentation	Differential	Workup
68 yo M presents with slurred speech, right facial drooping and numbness, and right hand weakness. Babinski's sign is present on the right. He has a history of hypertension, diabetes mellitus, and heavy smoking.	**Stroke** TIA Seizure Intracranial neoplasm Subdural or epidural hematoma	CBC, electrolytes PT/PTT CT—head MRI—brain (preferred) Doppler U/S—carotid Echocardiography
33 yo F presents with ascending loss of strength in her lower legs over the past two weeks. She had a recent URI.	**Guillain-Barré syndrome** Multiple sclerosis Polymyositis Myasthenia gravis Peripheral neuropathy Tumor in the vertebral canal	CBC, electrolytes CPK LP—CSF analysis MRI—spine EMG/nerve conduction study Tensilon test Serum B_{12}
30 yo F presents with weakness, loss of sensation, and tingling in her left leg that started this morning. She is also experiencing right eye pain, decreased vision, and double vision. She reports feeling "electric shocks" down her spine upon flexing her head.	**Multiple sclerosis** Stroke Conversion disorder Malingering CNS tumor Neurosyphilis Syringomyelia CNS vasculitis	CBC, ESR VDRL/RPR MRI—brain LP—CSF analysis Retinal evoked potentials
55 yo M presents with tingling and numbness in the hands and feet (glove-and-stocking distribution) over the past two months. He has a history of diabetes mellitus, hypertension, and alcoholism. There is decreased soft touch, vibratory, and position sense in the feet.	**Diabetic peripheral neuropathy** Alcoholic peripheral neuropathy B_{12} deficiency Hypocalcemia Hyperventilation Paraproteinemia/myeloma	HbA_{1c} ESR Calcium Serum B_{12} Serum and urine protein electrophoresis
40 yo F presents with occasional double vision and droopy eyelids at night with normalization by morning.	**Myasthenia gravis** Horner's syndrome Multiple sclerosis Intracranial tumor compressing CN III, IV, or VI Amyotrophic lateral sclerosis	Tensilon test ACh receptor antibodies (in serum) CXR CT—chest MRI—brain EMG
25 yo M presents with hemiparesis (after a tonic-clonic seizure) that resolves over a few hours.	**Todd's paralysis** TIA Stroke Complicated migraine Malingering	CBC, electrolytes EEG MRI—brain Doppler U/S—carotid

Key History

Duration; sleep hygiene, snoring, waking up choking/gasping, witnessed apnea; overexertion; stress, depression, or other emotional problems; lifestyle changes, shift changes at work; diet, weight changes; other constitutional symptoms; symptoms of thyroid disease; history of bleeding or anemia; medications; alcohol and drug use.

Key Physical Exam

Vital signs; head and neck exam (conjunctival pallor, oropharynx/palate, lymphadenopathy, thyroid exam); heart, lung, abdominal, and neurologic exams; consider rectal exam and occult blood testing.

Presentation	Differential	Workup
40 yo F c/o feeling tired, hopeless, and worthless and of having suicidal thoughts. She recently discovered that her husband is homosexual.	**Depression** Adjustment disorder Hypothyroidism Anemia	CBC TSH HIV/STD testing (given husband's possible risk factors)
44 yo M presents with fatigue, insomnia, and nightmares about a murder that he witnessed in a mall one year ago. Since then, he has avoided that mall and has not gone out at night.	**Post-traumatic stress disorder (PTSD)** Depression Generalized anxiety disorder Psychotic or delusional disorder Hypothyroidism	CBC TSH Calcium Urine toxicology
55 yo M presents with fatigue, weight loss, and constipation. He has a family history of colon cancer.	**Colon cancer** Hypothyroidism Renal failure Hypercalcemia Depression	Rectal exam, stool for occult blood CBC, electrolytes, calcium, BUN/Cr, AST/ALT, TSH Colonoscopy Barium enema
40 yo F presents with fatigue, weight gain, sleepiness, cold intolerance, constipation, and dry skin.	**Hypothyroidism** Depression Diabetes Anemia	TSH, FT_3, FT_4 CBC Glucose, HbA_{1c}
50 yo obese F presents with fatigue and daytime sleepiness. She snores heavily and naps 3–4 times per day but never feels refreshed. She also has hypertension.	**Obstructive sleep apnea** Hypothyroidism Chronic fatigue syndrome Narcolepsy	CBC TSH Nocturnal pulse oximetry Polysomnography ECG

Presentation	Differential	Workup
■ 20 yo M presents with fatigue, thirst, increased appetite, and polyuria.	**Diabetes mellitus** Atypical depression Primary polydipsia Diabetes insipidus	Glucose tolerance test, HbA_{1c} UA CBC, electrolytes, glucose BUN/Cr
■ 35 yo M policeman c/o feeling tired and sleepy during the day. He changed to the night shift last week.	**Sleep deprivation** Sleep apnea Depression Anemia	CBC Nocturnal pulse oximetry Polysomnography

Key History

Onset, duration, severity, frequency, timing, patterns; recent URIs, associated cough, hemoptysis, pleuritic chest pain; lymphadenopathy, fever, rash, malaise, weight loss, itching; diarrhea, nausea/vomiting, early satiety, anorexia; alcohol history, sexual exposure, sick contacts, exposure to high-risk populations; menstrual history, perimenopause.

Key Physical Exam

Vital signs; HEENT exam, including throat inspection for lymphadenopathy; heart and lung exam; abdominal exam for hepatosplenomegaly; skin exam; musculoskeletal exam for joint pain.

Presentation	Differential	Workup
■ 30 yo M presents with night sweats, cough, and swollen glands of one month's duration.	**Tuberculosis** Acute HIV infection Lymphoma Leukemia Hyperthyroidism	PPD CBC CXR Sputum Gram stain, acid-fast stain, and culture HIV antibody TSH, FT_4

Key History

Primary vs. secondary, duration, description (trouble falling asleep vs. multiple awakenings vs. early-morning awakening); daytime sleepiness; other medical problems keeping patient awake at night, such as arthritis (pain) or diabetes (polyuria); associated symptoms, including loud snoring, nightmares, and depression; caffeine use, recreational drug use; work or lifestyle (jet lag or shift work), stressors, sleep hygiene.

Key Physical Exam

Vital signs; mental status exam.

Presentation	Differential	Workup
25 yo F presents with a three-week history of difficulty falling asleep. She sleeps seven hours per night without nightmares or snoring. She recently began college and is having trouble with her boyfriend. She drinks 3–4 cups of coffee a day.	**Stress-induced insomnia** Caffeine-induced insomnia Insomnia with circadian rhythm sleep disorder Insomnia related to major depressive disorder	Polysomnography Mental status exam Urine toxicology CBC TSH
55 yo obese M presents with several months of poor sleep and daytime fatigue. His wife reports that he snores loudly.	**Obstructive sleep apnea** Daytime fatigue in primary hypersomnia Insomnia with circadian rhythm sleep disorder Insomnia related to major depressive disorder	CBC TSH Polysomnography ECG
33 yo F c/o three weeks of fatigue and trouble sleeping. She states that she falls asleep easily but wakes up at 3 A.M. and cannot return to sleep. She also reports an unintentional weight loss of 3.5 kg along with an inability to enjoy the things she once liked to do.	**Insomnia related to major depressive disorder** Primary hypersomnia Insomnia with circadian rhythm sleep disorder	Mental status exam TSH CBC Polysomnography

Key History

Duration, fever, other ENT symptoms (ear pain, URI), odynophagia, swollen glands, ± cough, rash; sick contacts, HIV risk factors.

Key Physical Exam

Vital signs; ENT exam, including oral thrush, tonsillar exudate, and lymphadenopathy; lung, abdominal, and skin exams.

Presentation	Differential	Workup
26 yo F presents with sore throat, fever, severe fatigue, and loss of appetite for the past week. She also reports epigastric and LUQ discomfort. She has cervical lymphadenopathy and a rash. Her boyfriend recently experienced similar symptoms.	**Infectious mononucleosis** Hepatitis Viral or bacterial pharyngitis Acute HIV infection Secondary syphilis	CBC, peripheral smear Monospot test Throat culture AST/ALT/bilirubin/alkaline phosphatase HIV antibody and viral load Anti-EBV antibodies VDRL/RPR
26 yo M presents with sore throat, fever, rash, and weight loss. He has a history of IV drug abuse and sharing needles.	**HIV, acute retroviral syndrome** Infectious mononucleosis Hepatitis Viral pharyngitis Streptococcal tonsillitis/ scarlet fever Secondary syphilis	CBC Peripheral smear HIV antibody and viral load CD4 count Monospot test Throat culture VDRL/RPR AST/ALT/bilirubin/alkaline phosphatase
46 yo F presents with fever and sore throat.	**Pharyngitis (bacterial or viral)** *Mycoplasma* pneumonia Acute HIV infection Infectious mononucleosis	Throat swab for culture and rapid streptococcal antigen Monospot test CBC HIV antibody and viral load

Key History

Acute vs. chronic; presence/description of sputum; associated symptoms (constitutional, URI, postnasal drip, dyspnea, wheezing, chest pain, heartburn, other), exacerbating and alleviating factors, timing, exposures; smoking history; history of lung disease; allergies; medications (especially ACE inhibitors).

Key Physical Exam

Vital signs ± pulse oximetry; exam of nasal mucosa, oropharynx, heart, lungs, lymph nodes, and extremities (clubbing, cyanosis, edema).

Presentation	Differential	Workup
30 yo M presents with shortness of breath, cough, and wheezing that worsen in cold air. He has had several such episodes over the past four months.	**Asthma** GERD Bronchitis Pneumonitis Foreign body	CBC CXR Peak flow measurement PFTs Methacholine challenge test
56 yo F presents with shortness of breath as well as with a productive cough that has occurred over the past two years for at least three months each year. She is a heavy smoker.	**COPD—chronic bronchitis** Bronchiectasis Lung cancer Tuberculosis	CBC Sputum Gram stain and culture CXR PFTs CT—chest PPD
58 yo M presents with pleuritic chest pain, fever, chills, and cough with purulent yellow sputum. He is a heavy smoker with COPD.	**Pneumonia** Bronchitis Lung abscess Lung cancer Tuberculosis Pericarditis	CBC Sputum Gram stain and culture CXR CT—chest ECG PPD
25 yo F presents with two weeks of a nonproductive cough. Three weeks ago she had a sore throat and a runny nose.	**Atypical pneumonia** Reactive airway disease URI-associated ("postinfectious") Postnasal drip GERD	CBC Induced sputum Gram stain and culture CXR IgM detection for *Mycoplasma pneumoniae* Urine *Legionella* antigen

Presentation	Differential	Workup
65 yo M presents with worsening cough over the past six months together with hemoptysis, dyspnea, weakness, and weight loss. He is a heavy smoker.	**Lung cancer** Tuberculosis Lung abscess COPD Vasculitis (i.e., Wegener's) Interstitial lung disease CHF	CBC Sputum Gram stain, culture, and cytology CXR CT—chest PPD Bronchoscopy
55 yo M presents with increased dyspnea and sputum production over the past three days. He has COPD and stopped using his inhalers last week. He also stopped smoking two days ago.	**COPD exacerbation (bronchitis)** Lung cancer Pneumonia URI CHF	CBC CXR PFTs Sputum Gram stain and culture CT—chest
34 yo F nurse presents with worsening cough of six weeks' duration together with weight loss, fatigue, night sweats, and fever. She has a history of contact with tuberculosis patients at work.	**Tuberculosis** Pneumonia Lung abscess Vasculitis Lymphoma Metastatic cancer HIV/AIDS Sarcoidosis	CBC PPD Sputum Gram stain, acid-fast stain, and culture CXR CT—chest Bronchoscopy HIV antibody
35 yo M presents with shortness of breath and cough. He has had unprotected sex with multiple sexual partners and was recently exposed to a patient with active tuberculosis.	**Tuberculosis** Pneumonia (including *Pneumocystis jiroveci*) Bronchitis CHF (cardiomyopathy) Asthma Acute HIV infection	CBC PPD Sputum Gram stain, acid-fast stain, silver stain, and culture CXR HIV antibody
50 yo M presents with a cough that is exacerbated by lying down at night and improved by propping up on three pillows. He also reports exertional dyspnea.	**CHF** Cardiac valvular disease GERD Pulmonary fibrosis COPD Postnasal drip	CBC CXR ECG Echocardiography PFTs BNP

Key History

Location, quality, severity, radiation, duration, context (exertional, postprandial, positional, cocaine use, trauma), associated symptoms (sweating, nausea, dyspnea, palpitation, sense of doom), exacerbating and alleviating factors (especially medications); prior history of similar symptoms; known heart or lung disease or history of diagnostic testing; cardiac risk factors (hypertension, hyperlipidemia, smoking, family history of early MI); pulmonary embolism risk factors (history of DVT, coagulopathy, malignancy, recent immobilization).

Key Physical Exam

Vital signs ± BP in both arms; complete cardiovascular exam (JVD, PMI, chest wall tenderness, heart sounds, pulses, edema); lung and abdominal exams.

Presentation	Differential	Workup
60 yo M presents with sudden onset of substernal heavy chest pain that has lasted for 30 minutes and radiates to the left arm. The pain is accompanied by dyspnea, diaphoresis, and nausea. He has a history of hypertension, hyperlipidemia, and smoking.	**Myocardial infarction (MI)** GERD Angina Costochondritis Aortic dissection Pericarditis Pulmonary embolism Pneumothorax	ECG CPK-MB, troponin CXR CBC, electrolytes Echocardiography Cardiac catheterization
20 yo African-American F presents with acute onset of severe chest pain. She has a history of sickle cell disease and multiple previous hospitalizations for pain and anemia management.	**Sickle cell disease—pulmonary infarction** Pneumonia Pulmonary embolism MI Pneumothorax Aortic dissection	CBC, reticulocyte count, LDH, peripheral smear ABG CXR CPK-MB, troponin ECG CT—chest with IV contrast
45 yo F presents with a retrosternal burning sensation that occurs after heavy meals and when lying down. Her symptoms are relieved by antacids.	**GERD** Esophagitis Peptic ulcer disease Esophageal spasm MI Angina	ECG Barium swallow Upper endoscopy Esophageal pH monitoring

Presentation	*Differential*	*Workup*
▪ 55 yo M presents with retrosternal squeezing pain that lasts for two minutes and occurs with exercise. It is relieved by rest and is not related to food intake.	**Angina** Esophageal spasm Esophagitis	ECG CPK-MB, troponin CXR CBC, electrolytes Exercise stress test Upper endoscopy/pH monitor Cardiac catheterization
▪ 34 yo F presents with retrosternal stabbing chest pain that improves when she leans forward and worsens with deep inspiration. She had a URI one week ago.	**Pericarditis** Aortic dissection MI Costochondritis GERD Esophageal rupture	ECG CPK-MB, troponin CXR Echocardiography CBC Upper endoscopy
▪ 34 yo F presents with stabbing chest pain that worsens with deep inspiration and is relieved by aspirin. She had a URI one week ago. Chest wall tenderness is noted.	**Costochondritis** Pneumonia MI Pulmonary embolism Pericarditis Muscle strain	ECG CPK-MB, troponin CXR CBC
▪ 70 yo F presents with acute onset of shortness of breath at rest and pleuritic chest pain. She also presents with tachycardia, hypotension, tachypnea, and mild fever. She is recovering from hip replacement surgery.	**Pulmonary embolism** Pneumonia Costochondritis MI CHF Aortic dissection	ECG CXR ABG CPK-MB, troponin CBC, electrolytes CT—chest with IV contrast Doppler U/S—legs D-dimer

▪ 55 yo M presents with sudden onset of severe chest pain that radiates to the back. He has a history of uncontrolled hypertension.	**Aortic dissection**
	MI
	Pericarditis
	Esophageal rupture
	Esophageal spasm
	GERD
	Pancreatitis
	Fat embolism
		ECG, CPK-MB, troponin
		CXR
		CBC, amylase, lipase
		Transesophageal
		   echocardiography (TEE),
		   MRI/MRA—aorta
		Aortic angiography
		Upper endoscopy

Key History

Gradual vs. acute onset/offset, context (exertion, caffeine, anxiety), associated symptoms (lightheadedness, chest pain, dyspnea); hyperthyroid symptoms; history of bleeding or anemia; history of heart disease.

Key Physical Exam

Vital signs; endocrine/thyroid exam, including exophthalmos, lid retraction, lid lag, gland size, bruit, and tremor; complete cardiovascular exam.

Presentation	Differential	Workup
■ 70 yo diabetic M presents with episodes of palpitations and diaphoresis. He is on insulin.	**Hypoglycemia** Cardiac arrhythmias Angina Hyperthyroidism Hyperventilation episodes Panic attacks Pheochromocytoma Carcinoid	Glucose CBC, electrolytes TSH BUN/Cr ECG Holter monitor

Key History

Amount, duration, ± intentional; diet history, body image, anxiety or depression; other constitutional symptoms; palpitation, tremor, diarrhea, family history of thyroid disease; HIV risk factors; alcohol and drug use; medications; history of cancer.

Key Physical Exam

Vital signs; complete physical.

Presentation	Differential	Workup
■ 42 yo F presents with a 7-kg weight loss over the past two months. She has a fine tremor, and her pulse is 112.	**Hyperthyroidism** Cancer HIV infection Dieting/diet drugs Anorexia nervosa Malabsorption	TSH, FT_4 CBC, electrolytes HIV antibody Urine toxicology

Key History

Amount, duration, timing (relation to medication changes, smoking cessation, depression); diet history; hypothyroid symptoms (fatigue, constipation, skin/hair/nail changes); menstrual irregularity; past medical history; alcohol and drug use.

Key Physical Exam

Vital signs; complete exam, including signs of Cushing's syndrome (hypertension, central obesity, moon face, buffalo hump, supraclavicular fat pads, purple abdominal striae).

Presentation	Differential	Workup
■ 44 yo F presents with a weight gain of > 11 kg over the past two months. She quit smoking three months ago and is on amitriptyline for depression. She also reports cold intolerance and constipation.	**Smoking cessation** Drug side effect Hypothyroidism Cushing's syndrome Polycystic ovary syndrome Diabetes mellitus Atypical depression	CBC, electrolytes, glucose TSH 24-hour urine free cortisol Dexamethasone suppression test

Key History

Solids vs. both solids and liquids, ± progressive, constitutional symptoms (especially weight loss), drooling, regurgitation, odynophagia, GERD symptoms; medications; HIV risk factors, history of smoking, history of Raynaud's phenomenon.

Key Physical Exam

Vital signs; head and neck exam; heart, lung, and abdominal exams; skin exam (for signs of scleroderma/CREST).

Presentation	Differential	Workup
■ 75 yo M presents with dysphagia that started with solids and progressed to liquids. He is an alcoholic and a heavy smoker. He has had an unintentional weight loss of 7 kg over the past four months.	**Esophageal cancer** Achalasia Esophagitis Systemic sclerosis Esophageal stricture Amyotrophic lateral sclerosis	CBC CXR Endoscopy with biopsy Barium swallow CT—chest

Presentation	Differential	Workup
■ 45 yo F presents with dysphagia for two weeks together with fatigue and a craving for ice and clay.	**Plummer-Vinson syndrome** Esophageal cancer Esophagitis Achalasia Systemic sclerosis Mitral valve stenosis	CBC Serum iron, ferritin, TIBC Barium swallow Endoscopy
■ 48 yo F presents with dysphagia for both solid and liquid foods that has slowly progressed in severity over the past year. It is associated with regurgitation of undigested food, especially at night.	**Achalasia** Plummer-Vinson syndrome Esophageal cancer Esophagitis Systemic sclerosis Mitral valve stenosis Esophageal stricture Zenker's diverticulum	CXR Endoscopy Barium swallow Esophageal manometry
■ 38 yo M presents with dysphagia and pain on swallowing solids more than liquids. Exam reveals oral thrush.	**Esophagitis** (CMV, HSV, pill-induced) Systemic sclerosis GERD Esophageal stricture Zenker's diverticulum	CBC Endoscopy Barium swallow HIV antibody CD4 count

► **NAUSEA/VOMITING**

Key History

Acuity of onset, ± abdominal pain, relation to meals, sick contacts, possible food poisoning, possible pregnancy; neurologic symptoms (headache, stiff neck, vertigo, focal numbness or weakness), other associated symptoms (GI, chest pain), exacerbating and alleviating factors; medications.

Key Physical Exam

Vital signs; ENT; consider funduscopic exam (increased intracranial pressure); complete abdominal exam; consider heart, lung, and rectal exams.

Presentation	Differential	Workup
■ 20 yo F presents with nausea, vomiting (especially in the morning), fatigue, and polyuria. Her last menstrual period was six weeks ago, and her breasts are full and tender. She is sexually active with her boyfriend, and they use condoms for contraception.	**Pregnancy** Gastritis Hypercalcemia Diabetes mellitus UTI Depression	Urine hCG Pelvic exam U/S—pelvis CBC, electrolytes, calcium, glucose UA, urine culture Baseline Pap smear, cervical cultures, rubella antibody, HIV antibody, hepatitis B surface antigen, and VDRL/RPR

► ABDOMINAL PAIN

Key History

Location, quality, intensity, duration, radiation, timing (relation to meals), associated symptoms (constitutional, GI, cardiac, pulmonary, renal, pelvic, other), exacerbating and alleviating factors; prior history of similar symptoms; history of abdominal surgeries, gallstones, renal stones, atherosclerotic vascular disease; medications; alcohol and drug use; domestic violence.

Key Physical Exam

Vital signs; heart and lung exams; abdominal exam, including guarding, rebound, Murphy's sign, and CVA palpation; rectal exam; pelvic exam (women).

Presentation	Differential	Workup
■ 45 yo M presents with sudden onset of colicky right-sided flank pain that radiates to the testicles, accompanied by nausea, vomiting, hematuria, and CVA tenderness.	**Nephrolithiasis** Renal cell carcinoma Pyelonephritis GI etiology (e.g., appendicitis)	Rectal exam UA Urine culture and sensitivity BUN/Cr CT—abdomen U/S—renal IVP

Presentation	Differential	Workup
◼ 60 yo M presents with dull epigastric pain that radiates to the back, together with weight loss, dark urine, and clay-colored stool. He is a heavy drinker and smoker.	**Pancreatic cancer** Acute viral hepatitis Chronic pancreatitis Cholecystitis/choledocholithiasis Abdominal aortic aneurysm Peptic ulcer disease	Rectal exam CBC, electrolytes Amylase and lipase AST/ALT/bilirubin/alkaline phosphatase U/S—abdomen CT—abdomen
◼ 56 yo M presents with severe midepigastric abdominal pain that radiates to the back and improves when he leans forward. He also reports anorexia, nausea, and vomiting. He is an alcoholic and has spent the past three days binge drinking.	**Acute pancreatitis** Peptic ulcer disease Cholecystitis/choledocholithiasis Gastritis Abdominal aortic aneurysm Mesenteric ischemia Alcoholic hepatitis Mallory-Weiss tear	Rectal exam CBC, electrolytes, BUN/Cr, amylase, lipase, AST/ALT/ bilirubin/alkaline phosphatase U/S—abdomen CT—abdomen Upper endoscopy ECG
◼ 41 yo obese F presents with RUQ abdominal pain that radiates to the right scapula and is associated with nausea, vomiting, and a fever of 101.5°F. The pain started after she had eaten fatty food. She has had similar but less intense episodes that lasted a few hours. Exam reveals positive Murphy's sign.	**Acute cholecystitis** Hepatitis Choledocholithiasis Ascending cholangitis Peptic ulcer disease Fitz-Hugh–Curtis syndrome	Rectal exam CBC AST/ALT/bilirubin/alkaline phosphatase U/S—abdomen HIDA scan
◼ 43 yo obese F presents with RUQ abdominal pain, fever, and jaundice. She was diagnosed with asymptomatic gallstones one year ago.	**Ascending cholangitis** Acute cholecystitis Hepatitis Choledocholithiasis Sclerosing cholangitis Fitz-Hugh–Curtis syndrome	Rectal exam CBC AST/ALT/bilirubin/alkaline phosphatase Viral hepatitis serologies U/S—abdomen MRCP ERCP
◼ 25 yo M presents with RUQ pain, fever, anorexia, nausea, and vomiting. He has dark urine and clay-colored stool.	**Acute hepatitis** Acute cholecystitis Ascending cholangitis Choledocholithiasis Pancreatitis Acute glomerulonephritis	Rectal exam CBC, amylase, lipase AST/ALT/bilirubin/alkaline phosphatase UA Viral hepatitis serologies U/S—abdomen

Presentation	Differential	Workup
35 yo M presents with burning epigastric pain that starts 2–3 hours after meals. The pain is relieved by food and antacids.	**Peptic ulcer disease** Gastritis GERD Cholecystitis Chronic pancreatitis Mesenteric ischemia	Rectal exam Amylase, lipase, lactate AST/ALT/bilirubin/alkaline phosphatase Endoscopy (including *H. pylori* testing) Upper GI series
37 yo M presents with severe epigastric pain, nausea, vomiting, and mild fever. He appears toxic. He has a history of intermittent epigastric pain that is relieved by food and antacids. He also smokes heavily and takes aspirin on a regular basis.	**Peptic ulcer perforation** Acute pancreatitis Hepatitis Cholecystitis Choledocholithiasis Mesenteric ischemia	Rectal exam CBC, electrolytes, amylase, lipase, lactate AST/ALT/bilirubin/alkaline phosphatase AXR Upright CXR Endoscopy (including *H. pylori* testing)
18 yo M boxer presents with severe LUQ abdominal pain that radiates to the left scapula. He had infectious mononucleosis three weeks ago.	**Splenic rupture** Kidney stone Rib fracture Pneumonia Perforated peptic ulcer Splenic infarct	Rectal exam CBC, electrolytes CXR CT—abdomen U/S—abdomen
40 yo M presents with crampy abdominal pain, vomiting, abdominal distention, and inability to pass flatus or stool. He has a history of multiple abdominal surgeries.	**Intestinal obstruction** Small bowel or colon cancer Volvulus of the bowel Gastroenteritis Food poisoning Ileus Hernia	Rectal exam CBC, electrolytes AXR CT—abdomen/pelvis CXR
70 yo F presents with acute onset of severe, crampy abdominal pain. She recently vomited and had a massive dark bowel movement. She has a history of CHF and atrial fibrillation, for which she has received digitalis. Her pain is out of proportion to the exam.	**Mesenteric ischemia/infarction** Diverticulitis Peptic ulcer disease Gastroenteritis Acute pancreatitis Cholecystitis/choledocholithiasis MI	Rectal exam CBC, amylase, lipase, lactate ECG, CPK-MB, troponin AXR CT—abdomen Mesenteric angiography Barium enema

Presentation	Differential	Workup
21 yo F presents with acute onset of severe RLQ pain, nausea, and vomiting. She has no fever, urinary symptoms, or vaginal bleeding and has never taken OCPs. Her last menstrual period was regular, and she has no history of STDs.	**Ovarian torsion** Appendicitis Nephrolithiasis Ectopic pregnancy Ruptured ovarian cyst PID Bowel infarction or perforation	Pelvic exam Rectal exam Urine hCG UA CBC Doppler U/S—pelvis CT—abdomen Laparoscopy
68 yo M presents with LLQ abdominal pain, fever, and chills for the past three days. He also reports recent onset of alternating diarrhea and constipation. He consumes a low-fiber, high-fat diet.	**Diverticulitis** Crohn's disease Ulcerative colitis Gastroenteritis Abscess	Rectal exam CBC, electrolytes CXR AXR CT—abdomen
20 yo M presents with severe RLQ abdominal pain, nausea, and vomiting. His discomfort started yesterday as a vague pain around the umbilicus. As the pain worsened, it became sharp and migrated to the RLQ. McBurney's and psoas signs are positive.	**Acute appendicitis** Gastroenteritis Diverticulitis Crohn's disease Nephrolithiasis Volvulus or other intestinal obstruction/perforation	Rectal exam CBC, electrolytes AXR CT—abdomen U/S—abdomen
30 yo F presents with periumbilical pain for six months. The pain never awakens her from sleep. It is relieved by defecation and worsens when she is upset. She has alternating constipation and diarrhea but no nausea, vomiting, weight loss, or anorexia.	**Irritable bowel syndrome** Crohn's disease Celiac disease Chronic pancreatitis GI parasitic infection (amebiasis, giardiasis) Endometriosis	Rectal exam, stool for occult blood Pelvic exam Urine hCG CBC Electrolytes CT—abdomen/pelvis Stool for ova and parasitology, *Entamoeba histolytica* antigen
24 yo F presents with bilateral lower abdominal pain that started with the first day of her menstrual period. The pain is associated with fever and a thick, greenish-yellow vaginal discharge. She has had unprotected sex with multiple sexual partners.	**PID** Endometriosis Dysmenorrhea Vaginitis Cystitis Spontaneous abortion Pyelonephritis	Pelvic exam Rectal exam Urine hCG Cervical cultures CBC/ESR UA, urine culture U/S—pelvis

Key History

Frequency and volume of stools, duration of change in bowel habits, associated symptoms (constitutional, abdominal pain, bloating, sense of incomplete evacuation, melena or hematochezia); thyroid disease symptoms; diet (especially fiber and fluid intake); medications (including recent antibiotics); sick contacts, travel, camping, HIV risk factors; history of abdominal surgeries, diabetes, pancreatitis; alcohol and drug use; family history of colon cancer.

Key Physical Exam

Vital signs; relevant thyroid/endocrine exam; abdominal and rectal exams; ± female pelvic exam.

Presentation	Differential	Workup
67 yo M presents with alternating diarrhea and constipation, decreased stool caliber, and blood in the stool for the past eight months. He also reports unintentional weight loss. He is on a low-fiber diet and has a family history of colon cancer.	**Colorectal cancer** Irritable bowel syndrome Diverticulosis GI parasitic infection (ascariasis, giardiasis) Inflammatory bowel disease Angiodysplasia	Rectal exam CBC AST/ALT/bilirubin/alkaline phosphatase Colonoscopy Barium enema CT—abdomen/pelvis
28 yo M presents with constipation (very hard stool) for the last three weeks. Since his mother died two months ago, he and his father have eaten only junk food.	**Low-fiber diet** Irritable bowel syndrome Substance abuse (e.g., heroin) Depression Hypothyroidism	Rectal exam TSH Electrolytes Urine toxicology
30 yo F presents with alternating constipation and diarrhea and abdominal pain that is relieved by defecation. She has no nausea, vomiting, weight loss, or blood in her stool.	**Irritable bowel syndrome** Inflammatory bowel disease Celiac disease Chronic pancreatitis GI parasitic infection (ascariasis, giardiasis) Lactose intolerance	Rectal exam, stool for occult blood CBC Electrolytes Stool for ova and parasitology AXR CT—abdomen/pelvis

Presentation	Differential	Workup
33 yo M presents with watery diarrhea, vomiting, and diffuse abdominal pain that began yesterday. He also reports feeling hot. Several of his coworkers are also ill.	**Infectious diarrhea (gastroenteritis)**—bacterial, viral, parasitic, protozoal Food poisoning Inflammatory bowel disease	Rectal exam, stool for occult blood Stool leukocytes and culture CBC Electrolytes CT—abdomen/pelvis
40 yo F presents with watery diarrhea and abdominal cramps. Last week she was on antibiotics for a UTI.	**Pseudomembranous (*Clostridium difficile*) colitis** Gastroenteritis Cryptosporidiosis Food poisoning Inflammatory bowel disease	Rectal exam Stool leukocytes, culture, occult blood *C. difficile* toxin in stool Electrolytes
25 yo M presents with watery diarrhea and abdominal cramps. He was recently in Mexico.	**Traveler's diarrhea** Giardiasis Amebiasis Food poisoning Hepatitis A	Rectal exam Stool leukocytes, culture, *Giardia* antigen, *Entamoeba histolytica* antigen Electrolytes AST/ALT/bilirubin/alkaline phosphatase Viral hepatitis serology
30 yo F presents with watery diarrhea and abdominal cramping and bloating. Her symptoms are aggravated by milk ingestion and are relieved by fasting.	**Lactose intolerance** Gastroenteritis Inflammatory bowel disease Irritable bowel syndrome Hyperthyroidism	Rectal exam Stool exam Hydrogen breath test TSH
33 yo M presents with watery diarrhea, diffuse abdominal pain, and weight loss over the past three weeks. He has not responded to antibiotics.	**Crohn's disease** Gastroenteritis Ulcerative colitis Celiac disease Pseudomembranous colitis Hyperthyroidism Small bowel lymphoma Carcinoid	Rectal exam Stool exam and culture CBC, electrolytes TSH CT—abdomen Colonoscopy Small bowel series Urinary 5-HIAA

Key History

Amount, duration, context (after severe vomiting, alcohol ingestion, nosebleed), associated symptoms (constitutional, nausea, abdominal pain, dyspepsia); medications (especially warfarin, NSAIDs); history of peptic ulcer disease, liver disease, abdominal aortic aneurysm repair, easy bleeding.

Key Physical Exam

Vital signs, including orthostatics; ENT, heart, lung, abdominal, and rectal exams.

Presentation	Differential	Workup
45 yo F presents with coffee-ground emesis for the last three days. Her stool is dark and tarry. She has a history of intermittent epigastric pain that is relieved by food and antacids.	**Bleeding peptic ulcer** Gastritis Gastric cancer Esophageal varices	Rectal exam CBC, electrolytes AST/ALT/bilirubin/alkaline phosphatase Endoscopy (including *H. pylori* testing if ulcer is confirmed)
40 yo F presents with epigastric pain and coffee-ground emesis. She has a history of rheumatoid arthritis that has been treated with aspirin. She is an alcoholic.	**Gastritis** Bleeding peptic ulcer Gastric cancer Esophageal varices Mallory-Weiss tear	Rectal exam CBC, electrolytes AST/ALT/bilirubin/alkaline phosphatase Barium swallow Endoscopy

Key History

Melena vs. bright blood; amount, duration, associated symptoms (constitutional, abdominal or rectal pain, tenesmus, constipation/diarrhea); trauma; prior history of similar symptoms; prior colonoscopy; medications (especially warfarin); history of easy bleeding or atherosclerotic vascular disease.

Key Physical Exam

Vital signs ± orthostatics; abdominal and rectal exams.

Presentation	Differential	Workup
67 yo M presents with blood in his stool, weight loss, and constipation. He has a family history of colon cancer.	**Colorectal cancer** Anal fissure Hemorrhoids Diverticulosis Ischemic bowel disease Angiodysplasia Upper GI bleeding Inflammatory bowel disease	Rectal exam CBC, PT/PTT AST/ALT/bilirubin/alkaline phosphatase CEA Colonoscopy CT—abdomen/pelvis Barium enema
33 yo F presents with rectal bleeding and diarrhea for the past week. She has had lower abdominal pain and tenesmus for several months.	**Ulcerative colitis** Crohn's disease Proctitis Anal fissure Hemorrhoids Diverticulosis Dysentery	Rectal exam CBC, PT/PTT AXR Colonoscopy CT—abdomen/pelvis Barium enema
58 yo M presents with bright red blood per rectum and chronic constipation. He consumes a low-fiber diet.	**Diverticulosis** Anal fissure Hemorrhoids Angiodysplasia Colorectal cancer	Rectal exam CBC, PT/PTT Electrolytes Colonoscopy CT—abdomen/pelvis

▶ HEMATURIA

Key History

Amount, duration, ± clots, associated symptoms (constitutional, renal colic, dysuria, irritative voiding symptoms); medications; history of vigorous exercise, trauma, smoking, stones, cancer, or easy bleeding.

Key Physical Exam

Vital signs; lymph nodes; abdominal exam; genitourinary and rectal exams; extremities.

Presentation	Differential	Workup
65 yo M presents with painless hematuria. He is a heavy smoker and works as a painter.	**Bladder cancer** Renal cell carcinoma Nephrolithiasis Acute glomerulonephritis Prostate cancer Coagulation disorder (i.e., factor VIII antibodies) Polycystic kidney disease	Genitourinary exam UA, urine cytology BUN/Cr, PSA, CBC, PT/PTT Cystoscopy U/S—renal/bladder CT—abdomen/pelvis IVP
35 yo M presents with painless hematuria. He has a family history of kidney problems.	**Polycystic kidney disease** Nephrolithiasis Acute glomerulonephritis (e.g., IgA nephropathy) UTI Coagulation disorder Bladder cancer	Genitourinary exam UA BUN/Cr, PSA, CBC, PT/PTT U/S—renal CT—abdomen/pelvis IVP
55 yo M presents with flank pain and blood in his urine without dysuria. He has experienced weight loss and fever over the past two months.	**Renal cell carcinoma** Bladder cancer Nephrolithiasis Acute glomerulonephritis Pyelonephritis Prostate cancer	Genitourinary, rectal exam UA, urine cytology, BUN/Cr, PSA, CBC, PT/PTT U/S—renal CT—abdomen/pelvis IVP

► OTHER URINARY SYMPTOMS

Key History

Duration, obstructive symptoms (hesitancy, diminished stream, sense of incomplete bladder emptying, straining, postvoid dribbling), irritative symptoms (urgency, frequency, nocturia), constitutional symptoms; bone pain; medications; history of UTIs, urethral stricture, or urinary tract instrumentation; stones, diabetes, alcoholism.

Key Physical Exam

Vital signs; abdominal exam (including suprapubic percussion to assess for a distended bladder); genital and rectal exams; focused neurologic exam.

Presentation	Differential	Workup
▪ 60 yo M presents with nocturia, urgency, weak stream, and terminal dribbling. He denies any weight loss, fatigue, or bone pain. He has had two episodes of urinary retention that required catheterization.	**Benign prostatic hyperplasia (BPH)** Prostate cancer UTI Bladder stones	Rectal exam UA CBC, BUN/Cr, PSA U/S—prostate (transrectal)
▪ 71 yo M presents with nocturia, urgency, weak stream, terminal dribbling, hematuria, and lower back pain over the past four months. He has also experienced weight loss and fatigue.	**Prostate cancer** BPH Renal cell carcinoma UTI Bladder stones	Rectal exam UA CBC, BUN/Cr, PSA U/S—prostate (transrectal) CT—pelvis IVP
▪ 18 yo M presents with a burning sensation during urination and urethral discharge. He recently had unprotected sex with a new partner.	**Urethritis** Cystitis Prostatitis	Genital ± rectal exam UA Urine culture Gram stain and culture of urethral discharge Chlamydia and gonorrhea PCR
▪ 45 yo diabetic F presents with dysuria, urinary frequency, fever, chills, and nausea over the past three days. There is left CVA tenderness on exam.	**Acute pyelonephritis** Nephrolithiasis Renal cell carcinoma Lower UTI (cystitis, urethritis)	UA Urine culture and sensitivity CBC, BUN/Cr U/S—renal CT—abdomen

▶ ERECTILE DYSFUNCTION (ED)

Key History

Duration, severity, ± nocturnal erections, libido, stress or depression, trauma, associated incontinence; medications (and recent changes); past medical history (hypertension, diabetes, high cholesterol, known atherosclerotic vascular disease, prior prostate surgery); smoking, alcohol and drug use.

Key Physical Exam

Vital signs; cardiovascular exam; genital and rectal exams.

Presentation	Differential	Workup
▪ 47 yo M presents with impotence that started three months ago. He has hypertension and was started on atenolol four months ago. He also has diabetes and is on insulin.	**Drug-related ED** ED caused by hypertension ED caused by diabetes mellitus Psychogenic ED Peyronie's disease	Genital exam Rectal exam Glucose CBC

Key History

Primary vs. secondary, duration, possible pregnancy, associated symptoms (headache, decreased peripheral vision, galactorrhea, hirsutism, virilization, hot flashes, vaginal dryness, symptoms of thyroid disease); history of anorexia nervosa, excessive dieting, vigorous exercise, pregnancies, D&Cs, uterine infections; drug use; medications.

Key Physical Exam

Vital signs; breast exam; complete pelvic exam.

Presentation	Differential	Workup
40 yo F presents with amenorrhea, morning nausea and vomiting, fatigue, and polyuria. Her last menstrual period was six weeks ago, and her breasts are full and tender. She uses the rhythm method for contraception.	**Pregnancy** Anovulatory cycle Hyperprolactinemia UTI Thyroid disease	Pelvic exam Urine hCG U/S—pelvis CBC, electrolytes UA, urine culture Prolactin, TSH Baseline Pap smear, cervical cultures, rubella antibody, HIV antibody, hepatitis B surface antigen, and VDRL/RPR
23 yo obese F presents with amenorrhea for six months, facial hair, and infertility for the past three years.	**Polycystic ovary syndrome** Thyroid disease Hyperprolactinemia Pregnancy Ovarian or adrenal malignancy Premature ovarian failure	Pelvic exam Urine hCG U/S—pelvis LH/FSH, TSH, prolactin Testosterone, DHEAS
35 yo F presents with amenorrhea, galactorrhea, visual field defects, and headaches for the past six months.	**Amenorrhea secondary to prolactinoma** Pregnancy Thyroid disease Premature ovarian failure Pituitary tumor	Pelvic and breast exam Urine hCG Prolactin LH/FSH, TSH MRI—brain
48 yo F presents with amenorrhea for the past six months accompanied by hot flashes, night sweats, emotional lability, and dyspareunia.	**Menopause** Pregnancy Pituitary tumor Thyroid disease	Pelvic exam Urine hCG LH/FSH, TSH, prolactin, testosterone, DHEAS CBC MRI—brain

Presentation	Differential	Workup
35 yo F presents with amenorrhea, cold intolerance, coarse hair, weight loss, and fatigue. She has a history of abruptio placentae followed by hypovolemic shock and failure of lactation two years ago.	**Sheehan's syndrome** Premature ovarian failure Pituitary tumor Thyroid disease Asherman's syndrome	Pelvic exam Urine hCG CBC LH/FSH, prolactin TSH, FT_4 ACTH MRI—brain Hysteroscopy
18 yo F presents with amenorrhea for the past four months. She has lost 95 pounds and has a history of vigorous exercise and cold intolerance.	**Anorexia nervosa**	CBC TSH FT_4 ACTH FSH LH
29 yo F presents with amenorrhea for the past six months. She has a history of occasional palpitations and dizziness. She lost her fiancé in a car accident.	**Anxiety-induced amenorrhea**	CBC TSH FT_4 ACTH Urine cortisol level Progesterone challenge test FSH/LH/estradiol levels

► VAGINAL BLEEDING

Key History

Pre- vs. postmenopausal, duration, amount; menstrual history and relation to last menstrual period; associated discharge, pelvic or abdominal pain, or urinary symptoms; trauma; medications (especially warfarin, contraceptives); history of easy bleeding or bruising; history of abnormal Pap smears.

Key Physical Exam

Vital signs; abdominal exam; complete pelvic exam.

Presentation	Differential	Workup
17 yo F presents with prolonged, excessive menstrual bleeding occurring irregularly over the past six months.	**Dysfunctional uterine bleeding** Coagulation disorders (e.g., von Willebrand's disease, hemophilia) Cervical cancer Molar pregnancy Hypothyroidism Diabetes mellitus	Pelvic exam Urine hCG Cervical cultures, Pap smear CBC, ESR, glucose PT/PTT Prolactin, LH/FSH TSH U/S—pelvis

Presentation	Differential	Workup
61 yo obese F presents with profuse vaginal bleeding over the past month. Her last menstrual period was 10 years ago. She has a history of hypertension and diabetes mellitus. She is nulliparous.	**Endometrial cancer** Cervical cancer Atrophic endometrium Endometrial hyperplasia Endometrial polyps Atrophic vaginitis	Pelvic exam Pap smear Endometrial biopsy U/S—pelvis Endometrial curettage Colposcopy Hysteroscopy
45 yo G5P5 F presents with postcoital bleeding. She is a cigarette smoker and takes OCPs.	**Cervical cancer** Cervical polyp Cervicitis Trauma (e.g., cervical laceration)	Pelvic exam Pap smear Colposcopy and biopsy
28 yo F who is eight weeks pregnant presents with lower abdominal pain and vaginal bleeding.	**Spontaneous abortion** Ectopic pregnancy Molar pregnancy	Pelvic exam Urine hCG U/S—pelvis CBC, PT/PTT Quantitative serum hCG
32 yo F presents with sudden onset of left lower abdominal pain that radiates to the scapula and back and is associated with vaginal bleeding. Her last menstrual period was five weeks ago. She has a history of PID and unprotected intercourse.	**Ectopic pregnancy** Ruptured ovarian cyst Ovarian torsion PID	Pelvic exam Urine hCG Cervical cultures U/S—pelvis Quantitative serum hCG

Key History

Amount, color, consistency, odor, duration; associated vaginal burning, pain, or pruritus; recent sexual activity; onset of last menstrual period; use of contraceptives, tampons, and douches; history of similar symptoms; history of STDs.

Key Physical Exam

Vital signs; abdominal exam; complete pelvic exam.

Presentation	Differential	Workup
28 yo F presents with a thin, grayish-white, foul-smelling vaginal discharge.	**Bacterial vaginosis** Vaginitis—candidal Vaginitis—trichomonal Cervicitis (chlamydia, gonorrhea)	Pelvic exam Wet mount Cervical cultures KOH prep ("whiff test") pH of vaginal fluid
30 yo F presents with a thick, white, cottage cheese–like, odorless vaginal discharge and vaginal itching.	**Vaginitis—candidal** Bacterial vaginosis Vaginitis—trichomonal	Pelvic exam KOH prep ("whiff test") Wet mount Cervical cultures pH of vaginal fluid
35 yo F presents with a malodorous, profuse, frothy, greenish vaginal discharge with intense vaginal itching and discomfort.	**Vaginitis—trichomonal** Vaginitis—candidal Bacterial vaginosis Cervicitis (chlamydia, gonorrhea)	Pelvic exam Wet mount Cervical cultures pH of the vaginal fluid KOH prep ("whiff test")

▶ DYSPAREUNIA

Key History

Duration, timing, associated symptoms (vaginal discharge, rash, painful menses, GI symptoms, hot flashes), adequacy of lubrication; libido; sexual history; history of sexual trauma or domestic violence; history of endometriosis, PID, or prior abdominal/pelvic surgeries.

Key Physical Exam

Vital signs; abdominal exam; complete pelvic exam.

Presentation	Differential	Workup
54 yo F c/o painful intercourse. Her last menstrual period was nine months ago. She has hot flashes.	**Atrophic vaginitis** Endometriosis Cervicitis Depression Domestic abuse	Pelvic exam Wet mount, KOH prep, cervical cultures U/S—pelvis

Presentation	Differential	Workup
37 yo F presents with dyspareunia, inability to conceive, and dysmenorrhea.	**Endometriosis** Cervicitis Vaginismus Vulvodynia PID Depression Domestic violence	Pelvic exam Wet mount, KOH prep, cervical cultures U/S—pelvis Laparoscopy

► ABUSE

Key History

Establish confidentiality; directly question about physical, sexual, or emotional abuse and about fear, safety, backup plan; history of frequent accidents/injuries, mental illness, drug use; firearms in the home.

Key Physical Exam

Vital signs; complete exam ± pelvic.

Presentation	Differential	Workup
28 yo F c/o multiple facial and bodily injuries. She claims that she fell on the stairs. She was hospitalized for some physical injuries seven months ago. She presents with her husband.	**Domestic violence** Osteogenesis imperfecta Substance abuse Consensual violent sexual behavior	XR—skeletal survey CT—maxillofacial Urine toxicology CBC
30 yo F presents with multiple facial and physical injuries. She was attacked and raped by two men.	**Rape**	Pelvic exam Urine hCG Wet mount, KOH prep, cervical cultures XR—skeletal survey CBC HIV antibody Viral hepatitis serologies

Key History

Location, quality, intensity, duration, pattern (small vs. large joints; number involved; swelling, redness, warmth), associated symptoms (constitutional, red eye, oral or genital ulceration, diarrhea, dysuria, rash, focal numbness/weakness), exacerbating and alleviating factors; trauma (including vigorous exercise); medications; DVT risk factors; alcohol and drug use; family history of rheumatic disease.

Key Physical Exam

Vital signs; HEENT and musculoskeletal exams; relevant neurovascular exam.

Presentation	Differential	Workup
▥ 30 yo F presents with wrist pain and a black eye after tripping, falling, and hitting her head on the edge of a table. She looks anxious and gives an inconsistent story.	**Domestic violence** Factitious disorder Substance abuse	XR—wrist CT—head Urine toxicology
▥ 30 yo F secretary presents with wrist pain and a sensation of numbness and burning in her palm and the first, second, and third fingers of her right hand. The pain worsens at night and is relieved by loose shaking of the hand. There is sensory loss in the same fingers. Exam reveals a positive Tinel's sign.	**Carpal tunnel syndrome** Median nerve compression in forearm or arm Radiculopathy of nerve roots C6 and C7 in cervical spine	Nerve conduction study EMG
▥ 28 yo F presents with pain in the interphalangeal joints of her hands together with hair loss and a butterfly rash on her face.	**Systemic lupus erythematosus (SLE)** Rheumatoid arthritis Psoriatic arthritis Parvovirus B19 infection	ANA, anti-dsDNA, ESR, C3, C4, rheumatoid factor (RF), CBC XR—hands UA
▥ 28 yo F presents with pain in the metacarpophalangeal joints of both hands. Her left knee is also painful and red. She has morning joint stiffness that lasts for an hour. Her mother had rheumatoid arthritis.	**Rheumatoid arthritis** SLE Disseminated gonorrhea Arthritis associated with inflammatory bowel disease Osteoarthritis	ANA, anti-dsDNA, ESR, RF, CBC XR—hands, left knee Cervical culture Arthrocentesis and synovial fluid analysis

Presentation	Differential	Workup
18 yo M presents with pain in the interphalangeal joints of both hands. He also has scaly, salmon-pink lesions on the extensor surface of his elbows and knees.	**Psoriatic arthritis** Rheumatoid arthritis SLE	RF, ANA, ESR CBC XR—hands XR—pelvis/sacroiliac joints Uric acid
65 yo F presents with inability to use her left leg and bear weight on it after tripping on a carpet. Onset of menopause was 20 years ago, and she did not receive HRT or calcium supplements. Her left leg is externally rotated, shortened, and adducted, and there is tenderness in her left groin.	**Hip fracture** Hip dislocation Pelvic fracture	XR—hip/pelvis CT or MRI—hip CBC Serum calcium and vitamin D Bone density scan (DEXA)
40 yo M presents with pain in the right groin after a motor vehicle accident. His right leg is flexed at the hip, adducted, and internally rotated.	**Hip dislocation—traumatic** Hip fracture	XR—hip CT or MRI—hip CBC PT/PTT Blood type and cross-match Urine toxicology and blood alcohol level
56 yo obese F presents with right knee stiffness and pain that increases with movement. Her symptoms have gradually worsened over the past 10 years. She noticed swelling and deformity of the joint and is having difficulty walking.	**Osteoarthritis** Pseudogout Gout Meniscal or ligament damage	XR—knee CBC ESR Knee arthrocentesis and synovial fluid analysis (cell count, Gram stain, culture, crystals) MRI—knee
45 yo M presents with right knee pain with swelling and redness.	**Septic arthritis** Gout Pseudogout Lyme arthritis Trauma Reiter's arthritis	CBC Knee arthrocentesis and synovial fluid analysis (see above) Blood, urethral cultures XR—knee Uric acid Lyme antibody
65 yo M presents with right foot pain. He has been training for a marathon.	**Stress fracture** Plantar fasciitis Foot sprain or strain	XR—foot Bone scan—foot MRI—foot

Presentation	Differential	Workup
65 yo M presents with pain in the heel of the right foot that is most notable with his first few steps and then improves as he continues walking. He has no known trauma.	**Plantar fasciitis** Heel fracture Splinter/foreign body	XR—heel Bone scan
55 yo M presents with pain in the elbow when he plays tennis. His grip is impaired as a result of the pain. There is tenderness over the lateral epicondyle as well as pain on resisted wrist dorsiflexion (Cozen's test) with the elbow in extension.	**Tennis elbow (lateral epicondylitis)** Stress fracture	XR—arm Bone scan MRI—elbow
27 yo F presents with painful wrists and elbows, a swollen and hot knee joint that is painful on flexion, a rash on her limbs, and vaginal discharge. She is sexually active with multiple partners and occasionally uses condoms.	**Disseminated gonorrhea** Rheumatoid arthritis SLE Psoriatic arthritis Reiter's arthritis	Knee arthrocentesis and synovial fluid analysis (cell count, Gram stain, culture) ANA, anti-dsDNA, ESR, RF, CBC Blood, cervical cultures XR—knee
60 yo F presents with pain in both legs that is induced by walking and is relieved by rest. She had cardiac bypass surgery six months ago and continues to smoke heavily.	**Peripheral vascular disease (intermittent claudication)** Leriche's syndrome (aortoiliac occlusive disease) Lumbar spinal stenosis (pseudoclaudication) Osteoarthritis	Ankle-brachial index Doppler U/S—lower extremity Angiography MRI—lumbar spine
45 yo F presents with right calf pain. Her calf is tender, warm, red, and swollen compared to the left side. She was started on OCPs two months ago for dysfunctional uterine bleeding.	**DVT** Baker's cyst rupture Myositis Cellulitis Superficial venous thrombosis	Doppler U/S—right leg CBC CPK D-dimer PT, aPTT, fibrinogen XR—right leg
60 yo F c/o left arm pain that started while she was swimming and was relieved by rest.	**Angina/MI** Tendonitis Osteoarthritis Shoulder dislocation	CPK-MB, troponin, ECG CBC ESR XR—shoulder CXR Echocardiography Stress test

Presentation	Differential	Workup
50 yo M presents with right shoulder pain after falling onto his outstretched hand while skiing. He noticed deformity of his shoulder and had to hold his right arm.	**Shoulder dislocation** Fracture of the humerus Rotator cuff injury	XR—shoulder XR—arm MRI—shoulder
55 yo M presents with crampy bilateral thigh and calf pain, fatigue, and dark urine. He is on simvastatin and clofibrate for hyperlipidemia.	**Rhabdomyolysis due to simvastatin or clofibrate** Polymyositis Inclusion body myositis Thyroid disease	CBC CPK Aldolase UA Urine myoglobin TSH

▶ LOW BACK PAIN

Key History

Location, quality, intensity, radiation, context (moving furniture, bending/twisting, trauma), timing (disturbs sleep), associated symptoms (especially constitutional, incontinence), exacerbating and alleviating factors; history of cancer, recurrent UTIs, diabetes, renal stones, IV drug use, smoking.

Key Physical Exam

Vital signs; neurologic exam (especially L4–S1 nerve roots); back palpation and range of motion (although rarely of diagnostic utility); hip exam (can refer pain to the back); consider rectal exam.

Presentation	Differential	Workup
45 yo F presents with low back pain that radiates to the lateral aspect of her left foot. Straight leg raising is positive. The patient is unable to tiptoe.	**Disk herniation** Lumbar muscle strain Tumor in the vertebral canal	XR—L-spine MRI—L-spine
45 yo F presents with low back pain that started after she cleaned her house. The pain does not radiate, and there is no sensory deficit or weakness in her legs. Paraspinal muscle tenderness and spasm are also noted.	**Lumbar muscle strain** Disk herniation Abdominal aortic aneurysm Vertebral compression fracture	XR—L-spine

Presentation	Differential	Workup
■ 45 yo M presents with pain in the lower back and legs during prolonged standing and walking. The pain is relieved by sitting and leaning forward (e.g., pushing a grocery cart).	**Lumbar spinal stenosis** Lumbar muscle strain Tumor in the vertebral canal Peripheral vascular disease	XR—L-spine MRI—L-spine (preferred) CT—L-spine Ankle-brachial index
■ 17 yo M presents with low back pain that radiates to the left leg and began after he fell on his knee during gym class. He also describes areas of loss of sensation in his left foot. The pain and sensory loss do not match any known distribution. He insists on requesting a week off from school because of his injury.	**Malingering** Lumbar muscle strain Disk herniation Knee or leg fracture Ankylosing spondylitis	XR—L-spine/knee MRI—L-spine

▶ CHILD WITH FEVER

(No child will be present; only the mother will be present to tell the story.)

Key History

Severity, duration, associated localizing symptoms, appetite, rash, sick contacts, day care, immunizations, past history.

Key Physical Exam

Vital signs; HEENT, neck, heart, lung, abdominal, and skin exams.

Presentation	Differential	Workup
■ 20-day-old M presents with fever, decreased breast-feeding, and lethargy. He was born at 36 weeks as a result of premature rupture of membranes.	**Neonatal sepsis** Meningitis Pneumonia UTI	Physical exam CBC, electrolytes UA Urine culture Blood culture CXR LP—CSF analysis

Presentation	Differential	Workup
3 yo M presents with a two-day history of fever and pulling on his right ear. He is otherwise healthy, and his immunizations are up to date. His older sister recently had a cold. The child attends a day care center.	**Acute otitis media** URI Meningitis UTI	Physical exam (including pneumatic otoscopy) CBC UA
12-month-old M presents with fever for the last two days accompanied by a maculopapular rash on his face and body. He has not yet received the MMR vaccine.	**Measles (or other viral exanthem)** Rubella Roseola Fifth disease Varicella Scarlet fever Meningitis	Physical exam CBC Viral antibodies/titers Throat swab for culture LP
4 yo M presents with diarrhea, vomiting, lethargy, weakness, and fever. The child attends a day care center where several children have had similar symptoms.	**Gastroenteritis** (viral, bacterial, parasitic) Food poisoning UTI URI Volvulus Intussusception	Physical exam Stool exam and culture CBC Electrolytes UA, urine culture AXR

► BEHAVIORAL PROBLEMS IN CHILDHOOD

(No child will be present; only the mother will be present to tell the story.)

Key History

Onset, severity, duration, triggers; physical violence or use of weapons; substance use, developmental history, changes in environment, school performance.

Key Physical Exam

Vital signs; neurologic exam.

Presentation	Differential	Workup
■ 9 yo M presents with a two-year history of angry outbursts both in school and at home. His mother complains that he runs around "as if driven by a motor." His teacher reports that he cannot sit still in class, regularly interrupts his classmates, and has trouble making friends.	**Attention-deficit hyperactivity disorder (ADHD)** Oppositional defiant disorder Manic episode Conduct disorder	Physical exam Mental status exam
■ 12 yo F presents with a two-month history of fighting in school, truancy, and breaking curfew. Her parents recently divorced, and she just started school in a new district. Before her parents divorced, she was an average student with no behavioral problems.	**Adjustment disorder** Substance intoxication/abuse/ dependence Manic episode Oppositional defiant disorder Conduct disorder	Physical exam Mental status exam Urine toxicology
■ 15 yo M presents with a one-year history of failing grades, school absenteeism, and legal problems, including shoplifting. His parents report that he spends most of his time alone in his room, adding that when he does go out, it is with a new set of friends.	**Substance abuse** Conduct disorder Oppositional defiant disorder Adjustment disorder	Urine toxicology Mental status exam
■ 5 yo M presents with a six-month history of temper tantrums that last 5–10 minutes and immediately follow a disappointment or a discipline. He has no trouble sleeping, has had no change in appetite, and does not display these behaviors when he is at day care.	**Age-appropriate behavior** ADHD Oppositional defiant disorder	Physical exam Mental status exam

SECTION IV

Practice Cases

This chapter consists of 41 commonly encountered cases that approximate those on the actual USMLE Step 2 CS exam. Each case consists of four parts:

1. **Doorway information sheet:** Designed to simulate the actual information that you will find on the doorway of each examination room, this sheet contains the opening scenario, vital signs, and the tasks you are required to perform during the exam. You should read this sheet just before starting the 15-minute encounter.

2. **Checklist/SP sheet:** This sheet outlines information that standardized patients (SPs) will use to guide them in their encounter and lists questions SPs might ask you, along with potential answers to these questions. Also included is a sample checklist that SPs will use to evaluate your performance.

3. **Blank patient note:** A blank form on which you can write your own note after the patient encounter.

4. **Sample patient note and discussion:** We have included a sample patient note that you can review after you have written your own, as well as a discussion of reasonable differential diagnoses and diagnostic tests to consider in each case.

Because the cases in this section are designed to simulate the actual exam, you can get the most out of them by practicing them with a friend who can act as an SP. To maximize the effectiveness of these practice cases, you should also time each encounter in accordance with the guidelines provided in Sections I and II and compare each of your patient notes with those provided in the text.

For a quicker self-review, you can try to formulate a patient note after reviewing the doorway sheet and the SP checklist and then compare your note with the sample note we have provided.

CASE 1
DOORWAY INFORMATION

Opening Scenario

Sharon Smith, a 48-year-old female, comes to the clinic complaining of abdominal pain.

Vital Signs

BP: 135/70 mmHg
Temp: 98.5°F (36.9°C)
RR: 16/minute
HR: 76/minute, regular

Examinee Tasks

1. Take a focused history.
2. Perform a focused physical exam (do not perform rectal, genitourinary, or female breast exam).
3. Explain your clinical impression and workup plan to the patient.
4. Write the patient note after leaving the room.

Checklist/SP Sheet

PATIENT DESCRIPTION

Patient is a 48 yo F, married with four children.

NOTES FOR THE SP

- Sit up on the bed.
- Show pain on palpation of the right upper abdomen that is exacerbated during inspiration.
- Exhibit epigastric tenderness on palpation.
- If ultrasound is mentioned by the examinee, ask, "What is the meaning of this word?"

CHALLENGING QUESTIONS TO ASK

"My father had pancreatic cancer. Could I have it too?"

SAMPLE EXAMINEE RESPONSE

"It's highly unlikely, as your symptoms are very unusual for pancreatic cancer. Regardless, some routine blood and x-ray tests should help us exclude that as a possibility."

Examinee Checklist

ENTRANCE:

☐ Examinee knocked on the door before entering.
☐ Examinee introduced self by name.
☐ Examinee identified his/her role or position.
☐ Examinee correctly used patient's name.
☐ Examinee made eye contact with the SP.

HISTORY:

☐ Examinee showed compassion for your pain.

☑ **Question**	**Patient Response**
☐ Chief complaint	Abdominal pain.
☐ Onset	Two weeks ago.
☐ Constant/intermittent	Well, I don't have the pain all the time. It comes and goes.
☐ Frequency	At least once every day.
☐ Progression	It is getting worse.
☐ Severity on a scale	When I have the pain, it is 7/10, and then it may go down to 0.
☐ Location	It is here (points to the epigastrium).
☐ Radiation	No.
☐ Quality	Burning.
☐ Alleviating factors	Food, antacids, and milk.
☐ Exacerbating factors	Heavy meals and hunger.
☐ Types of food that exacerbate pain	Heavy, fatty meals, like pizza.
☐ Relationship of food to pain	Well, usually the pain will decrease or stop completely when I eat, but it comes back after 2–3 hours.
☐ Previous episodes of similar pain	No.
☐ Nausea/vomiting	Sometimes I feel nauseated when I am in pain. Yesterday I vomited for the first time.
☐ Description of vomitus	It was a sour, yellowish fluid.
☐ Blood in vomitus	No.
☐ Diarrhea/constipation	No.
☐ Weight changes	No.
☐ Appetite changes	No.
☐ Change in stool color	No.
☐ Current medications	Maalox, ibuprofen (two pills 2–3 times a day if asked).
☐ Past medical history	I had a urinary tract infection one year ago, treated with amoxicillin, and arthritis in both knees. I take ibuprofen for pain.
☐ Past surgical history	I had two C-sections.
☐ Family history	My father died at 55 of pancreatic cancer. My mother is alive and healthy.
☐ Occupation	Housewife.
☐ Alcohol use	No.
☐ Illicit drug use	No.

☑ Question	Patient Response
☐ Tobacco	No.
☐ Sexual activity	With my husband (laughs).
☐ Drug allergies	No.

Physical Examination:

- ☐ Examinee washed his/her hands.
- ☐ Examinee asked permission to start the exam.
- ☐ Examinee used respectful draping.
- ☐ Examinee did not repeat painful maneuvers.

☑ Exam Component	Maneuver
☐ CV exam	Auscultation
☐ Pulmonary exam	Auscultation
☐ Abdominal exam	Inspection, auscultation, palpation (including Murphy's sign), percussion

Closure:

- ☐ Examinee discussed initial diagnostic impressions.
- ☐ Examinee discussed initial management plans:
  - ☐ Follow-up tests: Examinee mentioned the need for a rectal exam.
- ☐ Examinee asked if the patient has any other questions or concerns.

Sample Closure:

Mrs. Smith, there are a number of disorders that can cause pain similar to what you have described. Pain of this type is most commonly due to an ulcer, an abdominal infection, or a gallstone. We will have to run some tests to confirm the diagnosis and to rule out more serious illness. These tests will include a rectal exam, an ultrasound examination of your abdomen, blood tests, and possibly upper endoscopy, which involves examining your stomach by means of an optical instrument passed through your mouth. Once we have made the diagnosis, we will be able to treat your condition and help alleviate your pain. Do you have any questions for me?

History

Physical Examination

Differential Diagnosis

1.

2.

3.

4.

5.

Diagnostic Workup

1.

2.

3.

4.

5.

History

HPI: *48 yo F c/o intermittent, burning, nonradiating epigastric pain that started for the first time 2 weeks ago. The pain occurs at least once a day, usually 2–3 hours after meals. It is exacerbated by hunger and heavy, fatty food and is alleviated by milk, antacids, and other food. It reaches 7/10 in severity and then diminishes to 0/10. It is sometimes accompanied by nausea. The patient vomited once yesterday, an acidic, yellowish, nonbloody fluid. No diarrhea or constipation. No changes in weight or appetite. No changes in the color of the stool.*
ROS: *Negative except as above.*
Allergies: *NKDA.*
Medications: *Maalox, ibuprofen.*
PMH: *Arthritis in the knees, treated with ibuprofen. UTI last year, treated with amoxicillin.*
PSH: *Two C-sections.*
SH: *No smoking, no EtOH, no illicit drugs. Sexually active with husband only.*
FH: *Father died of pancreatic cancer at age 55.*

Physical Examination

Patient is in no acute distress.
VS: *WNL.*
Chest: *No tenderness, clear breath sounds bilaterally.*
Heart: *RRR; normal S1/S2; no murmurs, rubs, or gallops.*
Abdomen: *Soft, nondistended, C-section scar, epigastric tenderness without rebound, ⊕Murphy's sign, ⊕BS, no hepatosplenomegaly.*

Differential Diagnosis

1. Peptic ulcer disease
2. Cholecystitis
3. Gastritis
4. Functional or nonulcer dyspepsia
5. Perforated ulcer
6. Gastric cancer

Diagnostic Workup

1. Rectal exam, stool for occult blood
2. AST/ALT/bilirubin/alkaline phosphatase, lipase
3. U/S—abdomen
4. Upper endoscopy
5. HIDA scan
6. *H. pylori* antibody testing

CASE DISCUSSION

Differential Diagnosis

Although the causes of abdominal pain are many, this presentation should prompt you to ponder the common etiologies.

- **Peptic ulcer disease:** The history of NSAID use and burning epigastric pain alleviated by antacids and food are consistent with this diagnosis (although the clinical history cannot accurately distinguish duodenal from gastric ulcers).
- **Cholecystitis:** Several features suggest this diagnosis, but the pain in acute cholecystitis is usually unremitting and is not alleviated by milk or antacids. This patient's intermittent pain may be due to "biliary colic," representing transient obstruction of the cystic duct, usually due to gallstones.
- **Gastritis:** This can easily explain epigastric pain, nausea, and vomiting in patients taking NSAIDs.
- **Functional or nonulcer dyspepsia:** This is the most common cause of chronic dyspepsia. After thorough evaluation, no obvious organic etiology is discovered.
- **Perforated ulcer:** These patients appear toxic and have severe diffuse abdominal pain with rebound tenderness and involuntary guarding.
- **Gastric cancer:** Although this patient does not have early satiety, anorexia, weight loss, or a left supraclavicular mass (Virchow's node), it should be noted that signs and symptoms are minimal until late in the course of this rare disease.
- **Other etiologies:** Less likely possibilities include pancreatitis, atypical GERD, choledocholithiasis, mesenteric ischemia, and extra-abdominal causes.

Diagnostic Workup

- **Rectal exam, stool for occult blood:** May document occult blood loss due to peptic ulcer, gastritis, cancer, or other causes.
- **AST/ALT/bilirubin/alkaline phosphatase, lipase:** To look for evidence of hepatocellular injury, biliary obstruction, or pancreatitis.
- **U/S—abdomen:** A quick, inexpensive imaging technique with which to examine a patient with suspected acute cholecystitis (it may show stones, pericholecystic fluid, a thickened gallbladder wall, and a sonographic Murphy's sign).
- **Upper endoscopy:** Peptic ulcer, gastritis, and gastric cancer have lesions that can be visualized (biopsy is required for gastric cancer diagnosis and sometimes for *H. pylori* diagnosis).
- **HIDA (hepatobiliary) scan:** Can document obstruction of the cystic duct in acute cholecystitis; a positive scan shows absence of filling of the gallbladder. HIDA is usually ordered after ultrasound (i.e., when the easier but less sensitive Ultrasound does not establish the diagnosis of acute cholecystitis).
- **Noninvasive *H. pylori* testing:** Serologic tests for antibodies to *H. pylori* are adequate for diagnosis but not to document cure, as antibody levels often remain detectable after treatment (indicating exposure, not necessarily active infection). The urease breath test is a useful test with which to confirm *H. pylori* eradication in peptic ulcer disease.

Opening Scenario

Jessica Anderson, a 21-year-old female, comes to the ER complaining of abdominal pain.

Vital Signs

BP: 120/80 mmHg
Temp: 100.5°F (38.1°C)
RR: 20/minute
HR: 88/minute, regular

Examinee Tasks

1. Take a focused history.
2. Perform a focused physical exam (do not perform rectal, genitourinary, or female breast exam).
3. Explain your clinical impression and workup plan to the patient.
4. Write the patient note after leaving the room.

Checklist/SP Sheet

PATIENT DESCRIPTION

Patient is a 21 yo F, single with one child.

NOTES FOR THE SP

- Exhibit right lower abdominal tenderness on palpation.
- Show rebound tenderness (pain when the examinee removes his palpating hand).
- Demonstrate guarding (contraction of the abdominal muscles when palpating the RLQ).
- Experience pain in the RLQ when the examinee presses on the LLQ (Rovsing's sign).
- Manifest pain when the examinee extends your right hip (psoas sign).

CHALLENGING QUESTIONS TO ASK

- "My child is in the house alone. I must leave now."
- "I can't afford to stay in the hospital. Please give me a prescription for antibiotics so that I can leave."

SAMPLE EXAMINEE RESPONSE

"First we have to make sure that your illness isn't life threatening. Our social worker would be happy to work with you to ensure that your child is taken care of, as well as to address any financial concerns you may have."

Examinee Checklist

ENTRANCE:

- [ ] Examinee knocked on the door before entering.
- [ ] Examinee introduced self by name.
- [ ] Examinee identified his/her role or position.

☐ Examinee correctly used patient's name.

☐ Examinee made eye contact with the SP.

HISTORY:

☐ Examinee showed compassion for your pain.

☑ Question	Patient Response
☐ Chief complaint	Abdominal pain.
☐ Onset	This morning.
☐ Frequency	Strong, steady pain.
☐ Progression	It is getting worse.
☐ Severity on a scale	7/10.
☐ Location	It is here (points to the right lower abdomen).
☐ Radiation	No.
☐ Quality	Cramping.
☐ Alleviating factors	None.
☐ Exacerbating factors	Movement.
☐ Pain with ride to hospital	Yes.
☐ Precipitating events	None.
☐ Fever/chills	I've been a little hot since this morning, but no chills.
☐ Nausea/vomiting	I feel nauseated and vomited once two hours ago.
☐ Description of vomitus	It was a sour, yellowish fluid.
☐ Blood in vomitus	No.
☐ Diarrhea/constipation	Loose bowel movements this morning.
☐ Description of stool	Brown.
☐ Blood in stool	No.
☐ Urinary frequency/burning	No.
☐ Last menstrual period	Five weeks ago.
☐ Vaginal spotting	Yes, today is the first day of my menstrual period.
☐ Color of the spotting	Brownish.
☐ Vaginal discharge	No.
☐ Frequency of menstrual periods	Every four weeks; lasts for seven days.
☐ Starting menses	Age 13.
☐ Pads/tampons changed this day	Only one; usually 2–3 a day.
☐ Pregnancies	Three years ago.
☐ Problems during pregnancy/delivery	No, it was a normal delivery, and my child is healthy.

☑ Question	Patient Response
☐ Miscarriages/abortions	None.
☐ Current medications	Ibuprofen.
☐ Sexual activity	Yes.
☐ Contraceptives	Oral contraceptive pills. My boyfriend refuses to use condoms.
☐ Sexual partners	One partner; I met him two months ago.
☐ Over the last year	I had three sexual partners.
☐ History of STDs	Yes, I had some kind of infection a month ago, but I can't remember the name of it. The doctor gave me a shot and some pills for one week, and then it was over.
☐ Treatment of the partner	He refused the treatment.
☐ HIV test	No.
☐ Past medical history	None except for what I've mentioned.
☐ Past surgical history	None.
☐ Occupation	Waitress.
☐ Alcohol use	Two or three beers a week.
☐ Illicit drug use	No.
☐ Tobacco	One pack a day for the last six years.
☐ Drug allergies	No.

Physical Examination:

☐ Examinee washed his/her hands.
☐ Examinee asked permission to start the exam.
☐ Examinee used respectful draping.
☐ Examinee did not repeat painful maneuvers.

☑ Exam Component	Maneuver
☐ CV exam	Auscultation
☐ Pulmonary exam	Auscultation
☐ Abdominal exam	Inspection, auscultation, palpation, percussion, psoas sign, obturator sign, Rovsing's sign, CVA tenderness

Closure:

☐ Examinee discussed initial diagnostic impressions.
☐ Examinee discussed initial management plans:
    ☐ Follow-up tests: Examinee mentioned the need for rectal and pelvic exams.
    ☐ Discussed safe sex practices.

☐   Counseled regarding smoking cessation.
☐   Offered the assistance of social workers to help the patient identify available financial resources.
☐ Examinee asked if the patient has any other questions or concerns.

Sample Closure:

Ms. Anderson, your symptoms may be due to a problem with your reproductive organs, such as an infection in your fallopian tubes or a cyst on your ovaries. They might also result from a complicated pregnancy, as may be indicated if your pregnancy test comes back positive. Another possibility might be an infection in your appendix, which could require surgery. In order to ensure an accurate diagnosis, we will need to run some tests, including a blood test, a urinalysis, a pregnancy test, and possibly a CT scan of your abdomen and pelvis. I will also need to perform a rectal and pelvic exam. Since cigarette smoking is associated with a variety of diseases, I would advise you to quit smoking; we have many ways to help you if you are interested. I would also recommend that you use a condom every time you have intercourse in order to prevent STDs, including HIV, and to avoid pregnancy. We can have you meet with our social worker to discuss your social situation, and she can offer you a variety of resources. Do you have any questions for me?

PATIENT NOTE

History

Physical Examination

Differential Diagnosis

1.

2.

3.

4.

5.

Diagnostic Workup

1.

2.

3.

4.

5.

History

HPI: 21 yo G1P1 F c/o right lower abdominal pain that started this morning. The pain is 7/10, crampy, and constant. It is exacerbated by movement and does not radiate. It is accompanied by fever, nausea, vomiting, and loose stools. The patient noticed some brownish spotting this morning. No urinary symptoms; no abnormal vaginal discharge.

OB/GYN: LMP 5 weeks ago. Regular periods every 4 weeks lasting 7 days. Menarche at age 13. Uncomplicated NSVD at full term 3 years ago.

Allergies: NKDA.

Medications: Ibuprofen.

PMH: STD 1 month ago, possibly treated with ceftriaxone and doxycycline.

PSH: None.

SH: One PPD for 6 years, 2–3 beers/week, no illicit drugs. Unprotected sex with multiple partners.

Physical Examination

Patient is in pain.

VS: WNL except for temperature of 100.5°F.

Chest: No tenderness, clear breath sounds bilaterally.

Heart: RRR; normal S1/S2; no murmurs, rubs, or gallops.

Abdomen: Soft, nondistended, hypoactive BS, no hepatosplenomegaly. Direct and rebound RLQ tenderness, RLQ guarding, ⊕psoas sign, ⊕Rovsing's sign, ⊖obturator sign, no CVA tenderness.

Differential Diagnosis

1. PID
2. Appendicitis
3. Ruptured ectopic pregnancy
4. Ruptured ovarian cyst
5. Adnexal torsion
6. Gastroenteritis
7. Abortion
8. Endometriosis

Diagnostic Workup

1. Rectal exam
2. Pelvic exam
3. Urine hCG
4. Cervical cultures
5. UA
6. CBC
7. U/S—abdomen/pelvis
8. CT—abdomen/pelvis
9. Laparoscopy

Case Discussion

Differential Diagnosis

- **PID:** Suspicion is high for this diagnosis in a patient with multiple sexual partners and a history of STDs who presents with lower abdominal pain and fever. Other findings suggestive of PID include cervical motion tenderness, purulent cervical discharge, adnexal tenderness (usually bilateral), and fever > 101°F (38.3°C).
- **Appendicitis:** Acute right lower abdominal pain that is exacerbated by movement is compatible with this diagnosis. If peritoneal signs are present, patients will usually complain of pain with activity that jostles their abdomen (e.g., the ride to the hospital). Patients may also present with low-grade fever, nausea, vomiting, direct and rebound RLQ tenderness, RLQ guarding, a positive psoas sign, and a positive Rovsing's sign.
- **Ruptured ectopic pregnancy:** Even though this patient does not have previously documented PID (or previous tubal pregnancy), the crampy lower abdominal pain, nausea and vomiting, and vaginal spotting occurring after a five-week period of amenorrhea suggest this diagnosis. However, positive psoas and Rovsing's signs are not typical of ectopic pregnancy.
- **Ruptured ovarian cyst:** The sudden-onset unilateral lower abdominal pain, rebound tenderness, and guarding are consistent with this diagnosis. Rupture may occur at any time during the menstrual cycle, and symptoms may resemble a ruptured ectopic pregnancy as described above.
- **Adnexal torsion:** This presentation may be due to adnexal torsion, an uncommon complication that is most often associated with ovarian enlargement due to a benign mass.
- **Gastroenteritis:** Viral gastroenteritis presents with crampy abdominal pain, nausea and vomiting, low-grade fever, and diarrhea. It can be difficult to distinguish from appendicitis and gynecologic etiologies but is less likely in this case given the presence of rebound tenderness.
- **Abortion:** The fact that the patient's last menstrual period was only five weeks ago makes this less likely, but the crampy abdominal pain and vaginal spotting may signal an abortion. Furthermore, the presence of fever suggests possible septic abortion.
- **Endometriosis:** This is an unlikely diagnosis, in part because the patient has no history of chronic pelvic pain, dysmenorrhea, dyspareunia, or infertility, which are often associated. In a patient with established endometriosis, this presentation with acute severe pain, including rebound tenderness, could be due to rupture of an endometrioma ("chocolate cyst").

Diagnostic Workup

- **Rectal exam:** Elicits pain on the right side of the abdomen in acute appendicitis (not very specific).
- **Pelvic exam:** Look for cervical motion tenderness and discharge, uterine size, and adnexal masses or tenderness.
- **Urine hCG:** Positive in pregnancy. Urine and serum tests are equally sensitive, but obtaining quantitative hCG levels (available only via serum test) may help diagnose and treat ectopic pregnancy.
- **Cervical cultures:** *Neisseria gonorrhoeae* and *Chlamydia trachomatis*, the main causes of PID, are detected via DNA probes.
- **UA:** To rule out UTI.
- **CBC:** Findings are nonspecific, but leukocytosis may be seen in infection or appendicitis.
- **U/S—abdomen/pelvis:** Can help diagnose appendiceal or ovarian pathology. Transvaginal ultrasound can identify an intrauterine gestational sac when the time elapsed since the last menstrual period is 35 days (this corresponds to a β-hCG of about 1500); fluid in the cul-de-sac is nonspecific and may suggest ectopic pregnancy or a ruptured ovarian cyst.
- **CT—abdomen/pelvis:** Can detect the presence of appendiceal inflammation, abscess in appendicitis, or signs of other GI or gynecologic pathology.
- **Laparoscopy:** Can diagnose ectopic pregnancy (gold standard), ruptured ovarian cyst, ovarian torsion, PID ± tubo-ovarian abscess, appendicitis, etc.

Opening Scenario

Richard Green, a 74-year-old male, comes to the ER complaining of pain in his right arm.

Vital Signs

BP: 135/85 mmHg
Temp: 98.0°F (36.7°C)
RR: 12/minute
HR: 76/minute, regular

Examinee Tasks

1. Take a focused history.
2. Perform a focused physical exam (do not perform rectal, genitourinary, or female breast exam).
3. Explain your clinical impression and workup plan to the patient.
4. Write the patient note after leaving the room.

Checklist/SP Sheet

PATIENT DESCRIPTION
Patient is a 74 yo M.

NOTES FOR THE SP
- Sit up on the bed.
- Hold your right arm close to your body with your left hand and keep it internally rotated.
- Show pain when the examinee tries to move your right shoulder in any direction.
- Do not allow the examinee to bring your shoulder to its full range of motion in flexion, extension, abduction, or external rotation.

CHALLENGING QUESTIONS TO ASK
"Doctor, do you think I will be able to move my arm again like before?"

SAMPLE EXAMINEE RESPONSE
"I hope so, but first we need to find out exactly what is causing your problem."

Examinee Checklist

ENTRANCE:

- ☐ Examinee knocked on the door before entering.
- ☐ Examinee introduced self by name.
- ☐ Examinee identified his/her role or position.
- ☐ Examinee correctly used patient's name.
- ☐ Examinee made eye contact with the SP.

HISTORY:

☐ Examinee showed compassion for your pain.

☑ Question	Patient Response
☐ Chief complaint	Pain in the right arm.
☐ Onset	Three days ago.
☐ Precipitating events	I was playing with my grandchildren in the garden when I tripped and fell.
☐ Description of the fall	I tripped over a toy on the ground and fell on my hand. My arm was outstretched.
☐ Loss of consciousness	No.
☐ Location	The upper and middle parts of the arm.
☐ Weakness/paralysis	None.
☐ Numbness/loss of sensation	None.
☐ Progression of pain	I didn't feel any pain at the time, and then the pain started gradually. It is stable now, but it is still there.
☐ Pain anywhere else	No.
☐ Seen by a doctor since then	No.
☐ Any treatments	I used a sling and took some Tylenol, but the pain didn't get better.
☐ Alleviating factors	Not moving my arm and Tylenol.
☐ Exacerbating factors	Moving my arm.
☐ Reason for not seeking medical attention	Well, it wasn't that bad, and I thought it would get better on its own (looks anxious). Also, my son didn't have time to bring me to the hospital; he was busy.
☐ Living conditions	I live with my son. He is married and has three children. Life has been hard on him lately. He lost his job and is looking for a new one.
☐ Social history	I am a widower; my wife died three years ago, and since then I've lived with my son.
☐ Bad treatment in his son's house	No (looks anxious). They are all nice.
☐ Do you feel safe at home?	Yes (looks anxious).
☐ Current medications	Tylenol, albuterol inhaler.
☐ Allergies	Yes, I am allergic to aspirin.
☐ Past medical history	Asthma.
☐ Past surgical history	They removed my prostate two years ago. It was very difficult for me to urinate, but that has gotten much better. They said there was no evidence of cancer.
☐ Occupation	Retired schoolteacher.
☐ Alcohol use	No.

☑ Question	Patient Response
☐ Tobacco	No.
☐ Exercise	Every day I walk for 20 minutes to the grocery store and back.

Physical Examination:

- ☐ Examinee washed his/her hands.
- ☐ Examinee asked permission to start the exam.
- ☐ Examinee used respectful draping.
- ☐ Examinee did not repeat painful maneuvers.

☑ Exam Component	Maneuver
☐ Head and neck exam	Checked for bruises, neck movements
☐ CV exam	Auscultation
☐ Pulmonary exam	Auscultation
☐ Exam of the arms	Compared both arms in terms of strength, range of motion (shoulder, elbow, wrist), sensation, DTRs, pulses

Closure:

- ☐ Examinee discussed initial diagnostic impressions.
- ☐ Examinee discussed initial management plans:
  - ☐ Diagnostic tests.
  - ☐ Discussed alternative living options such as assisted living.
  - ☐ Offered social work assistance.
  - ☐ Offered a statement of support: "Your safety is my primary concern, and I am here for help and support when you need it."
- ☐ Examinee asked if the patient has any other questions or concerns.

Sample Closure:

Mr. Green, you may have a fractured bone, a simple sprain, or a dislocation of the shoulder joint. We will need to obtain an x-ray of your shoulder in order to help us make a diagnosis, and more precise imaging studies may be necessary as well. Your safety is my primary concern, and I am here to offer you help and support whenever you need it. Sometimes living with a family can be stressful for the whole household. Have you ever considered moving to an assisted-living community or to an apartment complex for seniors? If you are interested, I can arrange a meeting with our social worker, who can assess your social situation and help you find the resources you need. Do you have any questions for me?

PATIENT NOTE

History

Physical Examination

Differential Diagnosis

1.

2.

3.

4.

5.

Diagnostic Workup

1.

2.

3.

4.

5.

History

HPI: 74 yo M c/o pain in the right arm. The pain started 3 days ago, after he fell on his outstretched right hand. Treated at home with Tylenol and a sling, but pain persisted. No loss of consciousness before or after the fall. No paralysis or loss of sensation. The pain is in the upper and middle part of the arm, increases with any movement of the arm, and is alleviated by Tylenol and rest. When asked about the reason for the delay in seeking medical assistance, the patient looked anxious and stated that his son didn't have time to take him to the hospital.

ROS: Negative except as above.

Allergies: Aspirin.

Medications: Tylenol, albuterol inhaler.

PMH: Asthma, probable BPH s/p prostate surgery.

SH: No smoking, no EtOH. Widower for the last 3 years; lives with his son, who recently lost his job. Walks 20 minutes every morning.

Physical Examination

Patient is in no acute distress.

VS: WNL.

HEENT: Normocephalic, atraumatic, no bruises.

Neck: Supple, full range of motion in all directions, no bruises.

Chest: Clear breath sounds bilaterally.

Heart: RRR; normal S1/S2; no murmurs, rubs, or gallops.

Extremities: Nonlocalized tenderness over middle and upper right arm and right shoulder; pain and restricted range of motion on flexion, extension, abduction, and external rotation of right shoulder. Right elbow and wrist are normal. Pulses normal and symmetric in brachial and radial arteries. Unable to assess muscle strength due to pain. DTRs intact and symmetric. Sensation intact to pinprick and soft touch.

Differential Diagnosis

1. Humeral fracture
2. Osteoporosis
3. Shoulder dislocation
4. Elder abuse
5. Rotator cuff tear

Diagnostic Workup

1. XR—right shoulder and arm
2. MRI—shoulder
3. Bone density scan (DEXA)

CASE DISCUSSION

Differential Diagnosis

- **Humeral fracture:** Most commonly occurs in elderly persons, usually after a fall. The axillary nerve can be injured in a proximal humerus fracture, causing sensory loss along the lateral aspect of the deltoid region. The radial nerve can be injured in a fracture of the midshaft/distal third of the humerus, causing wrist drop.
- **Osteoporosis:** Suspect underlying osteoporosis in elderly patients (especially women) presenting with fractures following minimal trauma. The most common sites of osteoporotic fractures are the thoracic and lumbar vertebral bodies, the neck of the femur, and the distal radius.
- **Shoulder dislocation:** The glenohumeral joint is the most commonly dislocated joint in the human body. It most often dislocates anteriorly and usually results from a fall on an outstretched hand with forceful abduction, extension, and external rotation of the shoulder. On exam the arm is held in the neutral position, and movement is avoided owing to pain.
- **Elder abuse:** The history contains red flags (bruises, anxious behavior) that may indicate elder abuse. The American Medical Association has defined elder abuse as "an act or omission which results in harm or threatened harm to the health or welfare of an elderly person." The diagnosis of elder abuse is not readily made because more often than not, both the abuser and the victim may deny abuse. Thus, diagnosis is inferential in many cases, and supporting evidence must be sought.
- **Rotator cuff tear:** Patients usually present with nonspecific pain localized to the shoulder, but pain is often referred down the proximal lateral arm owing to shared innervation. There may be an inability to abduct or flex the shoulder. Patients may also demonstrate significant weakness in internal or external rotation strength.

Diagnostic Workup

- **XR—right shoulder and arm:** AP and lateral views that include the joints above and below the injury can show fracture or dislocation. An axillary view is useful to help diagnose proximal humeral fracture or dislocation.
- **MRI—shoulder:** Required to diagnose rotator cuff tears, labral disease, and other disorders.
- **Bone density scan (DEXA):** To diagnose and quantify osteoporosis.

Opening Scenario

Brian Davis, a 21-year-old male, comes to the office complaining of a sore throat.

Vital Signs

BP: 120/80 mmHg
Temp: 99.5°F (37.5°C)
RR: 15/minute
HR: 75/minute, regular

Examinee Tasks

1. Take a focused history.
2. Perform a focused physical exam (do not perform rectal, genitourinary, or female breast exam).
3. Explain your clinical impression and workup plan to the patient.
4. Write the patient note after leaving the room.

Checklist/SP Sheet

PATIENT DESCRIPTION
Patient is a 21 yo M.

NOTES FOR THE SP

- Be rude and defensive.
- Make most of your answers a curt "yes" or "no."
- Pretend that you have LUQ tenderness on abdominal palpation.

CHALLENGING QUESTIONS TO ASK
"Do you think I have AIDS?"

SAMPLE EXAMINEE RESPONSE
"That's a difficult question. Do you believe you have been exposed to HIV?"

Examinee Checklist

ENTRANCE:

☐ Examinee knocked on the door before entering.
☐ Examinee introduced self by name.
☐ Examinee identified his/her role or position.
☐ Examinee correctly used patient's name.
☐ Examinee made eye contact with the SP.

☐   Examinee showed compassion for your illness.

☑ Question	Patient Response
☐ Chief complaint	Sore throat.
☐ Onset	Two weeks ago.
☐ Runny nose	No.
☐ Fever/chills	Mild fever over the last two weeks, but I didn't take my temperature. No chills.
☐ Night sweats	No.
☐ Cough	No.
☐ Swollen glands and lymph nodes	Yes, in my neck (if asked); a little painful (if asked).
☐ Jaundice	No.
☐ Chest pain	No.
☐ Shortness of breat	No.
☐ Abdominal pain	I've had some discomfort here (points to LUQ) constantly since yesterday.
☐ Radiation	No.
☐ Severity on a scale	4/10.
☐ Relationship of food to pain	No.
☐ Alleviating/exacerbating factors	None.
☐ Nausea/vomiting	No.
☐ Change in bowel habits	No.
☐ Change in urinary habits	No.
☐ Headache	No.
☐ Fatigue	I have been feeling tired for the past two weeks.
☐ Ill contacts	My ex-girlfriend had the same thing two months ago. I don't know what happened to her, because we broke up around that time.
☐ Weight changes	Yes, I feel that I am losing weight, but I don't know how much.
☐ Appetite changes	I don't feel like eating anything at all.
☐ Current medications	Tylenol.
☐ Past medical history	I had gonorrhea four months ago. I took some antibiotics.
☐ Past surgical history	None.
☐ Family history	My father and mother are alive and in good health.
☐ Occupation	Last year in college.
☐ Alcohol use	Yes, on the weekends.

☑ Question	Patient Response
☐ Illicit drug use	No.
☐ Tobacco	Yes, I smoke one pack a day. I started when I was 15 years old.
☐ Sexual activity	I have a new girlfriend.
☐ Use of condoms	Yes.
☐ Active with men, women, or both	Men and women.
☐ Number of sexual partners during the last year	Two.
☐ History of STDs	I told you, I had gonorrhea four months ago, and I was cured after a course of antibiotics.
☐ Drug allergies	No.

Physical Examination:

☐ Examinee washed his/her hands.
☐ Examinee asked permission to start the exam.
☐ Examinee used respectful draping.
☐ Examinee did not repeat painful maneuvers.

☑ Exam Component	Maneuver
☐ Head and neck exam	Examined nose, mouth, throat, lymph nodes; checked for sinus tenderness
☐ CV exam	Auscultation
☐ Pulmonary exam	Auscultation
☐ Abdominal exam	Auscultation, palpation, percussion
☐ Skin/lymph node exam	Inspected for rashes, lesions, lymphadenopathy

Closure:

☐ Examinee discussed initial diagnostic impressions.
☐ Examinee discussed initial management plans:
    ☐ Follow-up tests (including consent for HIV testing).
    ☐ Discussed safe sex practices.
    ☐ Counseled regarding smoking cessation.
    ☐ Counseled to avoid contact sports in light of possible increased risk of traumatic splenic rupture.
☐ Examinee asked if the patient has any other questions or concerns.

Sample Closure:

Mr. Davis, it is likely that you have acquired the same infection your girlfriend had. This may be no more than a transient viral infection, or it may represent a more serious illness such as HIV. We will need to run a few tests in order to help us make the diagnosis. I would recommend that we obtain two HIV tests. An HIV viral load test can help diagnose a new HIV infection. An HIV antibody test can look for a preexisting infection. In any case, I would strongly recommend using condoms during intercourse to avoid unwanted pregnancy and to prevent STDs. Since infectious mononucleosis is one of the diseases that might account for your symptoms, I would also recommend that you avoid contact sports in light of the possible risk of traumatic rupture of your spleen, which could be fatal. Also, since cigarette smoking is associated with a variety of diseases, I would advise you to quit smoking; we have many ways to help you if you are interested. Do you have any questions for me?

PATIENT NOTE

History

Physical Examination

Differential Diagnosis

1.

2.

3.

4.

5.

Diagnostic Workup

1.

2.

3.

4.

5.

PATIENT NOTE

History

HPI: *21 yo M c/o sore throat for the last 2 weeks. Two weeks ago he had a mild fever and fatigue, but he denies any chills, runny nose, cough, night sweats, shortness of breath, or wheezing. The patient also notes LUQ abdominal pain since yesterday. The pain is 4/10 and constant with no radiation, no relation to food, and no alleviating or exacerbating factors. He has poor appetite and subjective weight loss. His ex-girlfriend had the same symptoms 2 months ago.*
ROS: *Negative except as above.*
Allergies: *NKDA.*
Medications: *Tylenol.*
PMH: *Gonorrhea 4 months ago, treated with antibiotics.*
SH: *One PPD since age 15; drinks heavily on weekends. Multiple female and male partners; uses condoms.*
FH: *Noncontributory.*

Physical Examination

Patient is in no acute distress.
VS: *WNL.*
HEENT: *Nose, mouth, and pharynx WNL.*
Neck: *Supple, no lymphadenopathy.*
Chest: *Clear breath sounds bilaterally.*
Heart: *RRR; normal S1/S2; no murmurs, rubs, or gallops.*
Abdomen: *Soft, nondistended, ⊕BS, no hepatosplenomegaly, mild LUQ tenderness on palpation.*
Skin: *No rash or lymphadenopathy.*

Differential Diagnosis

1. Infectious mononucleosis
2. Acute HIV infection
3. Viral pharyngitis
4. Bacterial pharyngitis

Diagnostic Workup

1. CBC
2. Peripheral smear
3. Monospot
4. Rapid streptococcal antigen
5. Throat culture
6. Anti-EBV antibodies
7. HIV antibody and viral load

CASE DISCUSSION

Differential Diagnosis

- **Infectious mononucleosis:** The differential diagnosis for "sore throat" includes many pathogens. This patient's LUQ pain suggests splenomegaly, which could limit the differential (for a unifying diagnosis) to an infectious mononucleosis caused by EBV or, less commonly, by CMV infection. Recall that the physical exam is notoriously insensitive for detecting splenomegaly and may be misleading, as in this case. However, this patient does not have other typical features of infectious mononucleosis, such as lymphadenopathy or exudative pharyngitis.
- **Group A streptococcal pharyngitis:** Clinical features in patients with sore throat that predict group A streptococcal pharyngitis include tonsillar exudates, tender anterior cervical lymphadenopathy, a history of fever (temperature > 100.4°F/38°C), and absence of cough. "Strep throat" must be recognized and treated in order to prevent acute rheumatic fever.
- **Other common etiologies:** Include viruses (including acute HIV infection, which is often associated with a generalized maculopapular rash), *Neisseria gonorrhoeae*, *Mycoplasma* (although lower respiratory symptoms usually predominate), rubella, and *Chlamydia trachomatis*.

Diagnostic Workup

- **CBC:** Findings are nonspecific, but leukocytosis may be seen in infection.
- **Peripheral smear:** Can reveal atypical lymphocytes in infectious mononucleosis.
- **Monospot (heterophil agglutination test):** Usually becomes positive in EBV-associated mononucleosis within four weeks of onset of illness.
- **Rapid streptococcal antigen:** Has high negative predictive value (i.e., it can accurately confirm the absence of group A streptococcal pharyngitis).
- **Throat culture:** The gold standard for diagnosing bacterial pharyngitis.
- **Anti-EBV antibodies:** Antibodies to various EBV antigens can be detected, such as IgM antibody to virus capsid antigen (VCA) and to nuclear antigen (EBNA). There is also a PCR to detect EBV in serum.
- **HIV antibody and viral load:** Check antibody to exclude preexisting HIV infection, and check viral load to help document acute infection.

Opening Scenario

Kenneth Klein, a 55-year-old male, comes to the clinic complaining of blood in his stool.

Vital Signs

BP: 130/80 mmHg
Temp: 98.5°F (36.9°C)
RR: 16/minute
HR: 76/minute, regular

Examinee Tasks

1. Take a focused history.
2. Perform a focused physical exam (do not perform rectal, genitourinary, or female breast exam).
3. Explain your clinical impression and workup plan to the patient.
4. Write the patient note after leaving the room.

Checklist/SP Sheet

PATIENT DESCRIPTION

Patient is a 55 yo M, married with two children.

NOTES FOR THE SP

If colonoscopy is mentioned by the examinee, ask, "What is the meaning of this word?"

CHALLENGING QUESTIONS TO ASK

"My father had colon cancer. Could I have it too?"

SAMPLE EXAMINEE RESPONSE

"It is a possibility. Tell me more about the symptoms you're having that concern you with regard to cancer."

Examinee Checklist

ENTRANCE:

☐ Examinee knocked on the door before entering.
☐ Examinee introduced self by name.
☐ Examinee identified his/her role or position.
☐ Examinee correctly used patient's name.
☐ Examinee made eye contact with the SP.

HISTORY:

☐ Examinee showed compassion for your illness.

☑ Question	Patient Response
☐ Chief complaint	Blood in stool.
☐ Onset	One month ago.
☐ Frequency	Every time I move my bowels, I see some blood mixed in with the stool.
☐ Description (blood before, during, or after defecation)	The blood is mixed in with the brown stool.
☐ Bright red or dark blood	Bright red.
☐ Pain during defecation	No.
☐ Constipation	Well, I have had constipation for a long time, and I keep taking laxatives. At first I used to get some relief, but now there is no benefit from them.
☐ Frequency of bowel movements	I have had two bowel movements a week for the last six months.
☐ Diarrhea	I have had diarrhea for the past two days.
☐ Urgency	No.
☐ Tenesmus (ineffectual spasms of the rectum, accompanied by the desire to empty the bowel)	A little.
☐ Frequency of diarrhea	Three times a day.
☐ Description of the diarrhea	Watery, brown, mixed with blood.
☐ Mucus in stool	No.
☐ Melena	No.
☐ Fever/chills	No.
☐ Abdominal pain	No.
☐ Nausea/vomiting	No.
☐ Diet	I eat a lot of junk food. I don't eat vegetables at all.
☐ Weight changes	I have lost about 10 pounds over the past six months.
☐ Appetite changes	My appetite has been the same.
☐ Recent travel	No, but I am thinking of going on a trip with my family next week. Do you think I should stay home?
☐ Contact with people with diarrhea	No.
☐ Exercise	I walk for half an hour every day.
☐ Urinary problems	No.
☐ Current medications	No. I used to take many laxatives, such as bisacodyl and phenolphthalein, but I stopped all of them when the diarrhea started.
☐ Past medical history (recent antibiotic use)	I had bronchitis three weeks ago; it was treated with amoxicillin.
☐ Past surgical history	Hemorrhoids resected four years ago.

☑ Question	Patient Response
☐ Family history	My father died at 55 of colon cancer. My mother is alive and healthy.
☐ Occupation	Lawyer.
☐ Alcohol use	No.
☐ Illicit drug use	No.
☐ Tobacco	No.
☐ Sexual activity	With my wife.
☐ Drug allergies	None.

Physical Examination:

☐ Examinee washed his/her hands.
☐ Examinee asked permission to start the exam.
☐ Examinee used respectful draping.
☐ Examinee did not repeat painful maneuvers.

☑ Exam Component	Maneuver
☐ CV exam	Auscultation
☐ Pulmonary exam	Auscultation
☐ Abdominal exam	Auscultation, palpation, percussion

Closure:

☐ Examinee discussed initial diagnostic impressions.
☐ Examinee discussed initial management plans:
    ☐ Follow-up tests: Examinee mentioned the need for a rectal exam.
☐ Examinee asked if the patient has any other questions or concerns.

Sample Closure:

Mr. Klein, the symptoms you describe may be due to readily treatable problems, such as hemorrhoids, an infection in your colon, or diverticulosis, or they may be a sign of more serious disease, such as colorectal cancer. It is crucial that we run some blood tests, a stool exam, and probably colonoscopy, which involves looking at your colon through a thin tube that contains a camera. I will also need to perform a rectal exam today. Once we make a diagnosis, we should be able to treat your problem. Do you have any questions for me?

History

Physical Examination

Differential Diagnosis	Diagnostic Workup
1.	1.
2.	2.
3.	3.
4.	4.
5.	5.

PATIENT NOTE

History

HPI: 55 yo M c/o bright red blood in stool. He has a history of constipation that started 6 months ago, consisting of 2 bowel movements a week. One month ago he noticed blood mixed with stool at every bowel movement. During the last 2 days he started to have tenesmus and watery brown diarrhea (3 times a day) mixed with blood. He has no urgency, no mucus in stool, and no pain during defecation. He denies any fever, chills, nausea, vomiting, abdominal pain, recent history of travel, or contact with ill persons. He recalls a 10-pound weight loss during the last 6 months despite a good appetite. His diet consists of a lot of junk food with no vegetables.

ROS: Negative except as above.

Allergies: NKDA.

Medications: Used to take many laxatives (bisacodyl, phenolphthalein) but stopped after the onset of diarrhea 2 days ago.

PMH: Bronchitis 3 weeks ago, treated with amoxicillin.

PSH: Hemorrhoids resected 4 years ago.

SH: No smoking, no EtOH, no illicit drugs. Sexually active with wife only.

FH: Father died of colon cancer at age 55.

Physical Examination

Patient is in no acute distress.

VS: WNL.

Chest: Clear breath sounds bilaterally.

Heart: RRR; normal S1/S2; no murmurs, rubs, or gallops.

Abdomen: Soft, nondistended, nontender, ⊕BS, no hepatosplenomegaly.

Differential Diagnosis

1. Colorectal cancer
2. Hemorrhoids
3. Diverticulosis
4. Angiodysplasia
5. Pseudomembranous (C. difficile) colitis
6. Other infectious colitis
7. Ulcerative colitis

Diagnostic Workup

1. Rectal exam, stool for occult blood
2. Stool for C. difficile toxin
3. Fecal leukocytes
4. CBC
5. Anoscopy
6. Flexible proctosigmoidoscopy
7. Colonoscopy
8. Double-contrast (air contrast) barium enema
9. CT—abdomen/pelvis

CASE DISCUSSION

Differential Diagnosis

Bright red blood that is mixed with brown stool suggests a distal colonic or anorectal source. Otherwise, this patient's presentation is complex, and the differential remains broad. His chronic constipation may simply be due to a low-fiber diet or to irritable bowel syndrome, but neither of these entities explains hematochezia and weight loss.

- **Colorectal cancer:** A positive family history coupled with the presence of blood in the stool, a change in bowel habits, and weight loss makes colorectal cancer a plausible diagnosis. Screening colonoscopy should have been offered to the patient at age 45 (10 years prior to the age when a first-degree family member was diagnosed).
- **Hemorrhoids:** Recurrent hemorrhoids may explain the patient's hematochezia, although more typical findings in hemorrhoids are fresh blood on the paper or dripped into the toilet bowl.
- **Diverticulosis:** This is the most common cause of major lower GI bleeding, but it usually presents with larger-volume bleeds occurring in discrete, self-limited episodes.
- **Angiodysplasia:** This is another common cause of lower GI tract bleeding, but as with diverticular disease, it cannot explain the other features of this patient's presentation.
- **Pseudomembranous (*C. difficile*) colitis:** It is important to ask all patients with acute diarrhea about recent antibiotic exposure, as symptoms of antibiotic-associated colitis may be delayed for up to 6–8 weeks. Stools rarely contain gross blood, however. The absence of fever and lower abdominal cramping also makes this diagnosis (and other forms of infectious colitis) less likely.
- **Ulcerative colitis:** The absence of abdominal pain and the very recent onset of diarrhea and tenesmus make inflammatory bowel disease a less likely etiology for this patient's month-long hematochezia.

Diagnostic Workup

- **Rectal exam, stool for occult blood:** Useful to detect masses and hemorrhoids. Always test for occult blood in stool.
- **Stool for *C. difficile* toxin:** Recall that one negative test does not exclude the diagnosis, as the assays are positive in only 80% of patients on the first stool sample and in 90% after two stool samples.
- **Fecal leukocytes:** Usually present in invasive bacterial infection and in inflammatory bowel disease. Variably present in *C. difficile* colitis.
- **CBC:** To investigate anemia. Also, leukocytosis could suggest infection or inflammatory bowel disease.
- **Anoscopy:** Can identify bleeding internal hemorrhoids, rectal ulcers, and traumatic lesions.
- **Flexible proctosigmoidoscopy:** If nondiagnostic, follow up with a barium enema or a colonoscopy.
- **Colonoscopy:** Should be the initial test performed in patients > 40 years of age presenting with hematochezia.
- **Double-contrast (air contrast) barium enema:** Not as accurate as colonoscopy for the diagnosis of polyps and cancer (and cannot diagnose angiodysplasia). Used mainly when colonoscopy is unavailable or contraindicated.
- **CT—abdomen/pelvis:** Contrast-enhanced exams can detect diverticulosis or masses but generally are not useful in the evaluation of GI bleeding.

Opening Scenario

Joseph Short, a 46-year-old male, comes to the ER complaining of chest pain.

Vital Signs

BP: 165/85 mmHg
Temp: 98.6°F (37°C)
RR: 22/minute
HR: 90/minute, regular

Examinee Tasks

1. Take a focused history.
2. Perform a focused physical exam (do not perform rectal, genitourinary, or female breast exam).
3. Explain your clinical impression and workup plan to the patient.
4. Write the patient note after leaving the room.

Checklist/SP Sheet

PATIENT DESCRIPTION

Patient is a 46 yo M.

NOTES FOR THE SP

- Lie on the bed and exhibit pain.
- Place your hands in the middle of your chest.
- Exhibit difficulty breathing.
- If ECG is mentioned by the examinee, ask, "What is an ECG?"

CHALLENGING QUESTIONS TO ASK

"Is this a heart attack? Am I going to die?"

SAMPLE EXAMINEE RESPONSE

"As you suspect, your symptoms are of considerable concern. We need to learn more about what's going on to know if your pain is life threatening."

Examinee Checklist

ENTRANCE:

- [ ] Examinee knocked on the door before entering.
- [ ] Examinee introduced self by name.
- [ ] Examinee identified his/her role or position.
- [ ] Examinee correctly used patient's name.
- [ ] Examinee made eye contact with the SP.

History:

☐ Examinee showed compassion for your pain.

☑ Question	Patient Response
☐ Chief complaint	Chest pain.
☐ Onset	Forty minutes ago.
☐ Precipitating events	Nothing; I was asleep and I woke up at 5:00 in the morning having this pain.
☐ Progression	Constant severity.
☐ Severity on a scale	7/10.
☐ Location	Middle of the chest.
☐ Radiation	To my neck and left arm.
☐ Quality	Pressure.
☐ Alleviating/exacerbating factors	Nothing.
☐ Shortness of breath	Yes.
☐ Nausea/vomiting	I feel nauseated, but I didn't vomit.
☐ Sweating	Yes.
☐ Associated symptoms (cough, wheezing, abdominal pain, diarrhea/constipation)	None.
☐ Previous episodes of similar pain	Yes, but not exactly the same.
☐ Onset	The past three months.
☐ Severity	Less severe.
☐ Frequency	Two to three episodes a week for 5–10 minutes.
☐ Precipitating events	Walking up the stairs, strenuous work, and heavy meals.
☐ Alleviating factors	Antacids.
☐ Associated symptoms	None.
☐ Current medications	Maalox, diuretic.
☐ Past medical history	Hypertension for five years, treated with a diuretic. High cholesterol, managed with diet; I have not been very compliant with the diet. GERD 10 years ago, treated with antacids.
☐ Past surgical history	None.
☐ Family history	My father died of lung cancer at age 72. My mother is alive and has a peptic ulcer. No early heart attacks.
☐ Occupation	Accountant.
☐ Alcohol use	Once in a while.
☐ Illicit drug use	Cocaine, once a week.
☐ Last time of cocaine use	Yesterday afternoon.

☑ Question	Patient Response
☐ Tobacco	Stopped three months ago.
☐ Duration	Twenty-five years.
☐ Amount	One pack a day.
☐ Sexual activity	Well, doctor, to be honest, I haven't had sex with my wife for the last three months, because I get this pain in my chest during sex.
☐ Exercise	No.
☐ Diet	My doctor gave me a strict diet last year to lower my cholesterol, but I always cheat.
☐ Drug allergies	No.

Physical Examination:

☐ Examinee washed his/her hands.
☐ Examinee asked permission to start the exam.
☐ Examinee used respectful draping.
☐ Examinee did not repeat painful maneuvers.

☑ Exam Component	Maneuver
☐ Neck exam	Looked for JVD, carotid auscultation
☐ CV exam	Inspection, auscultation, palpation
☐ Pulmonary exam	Auscultation, palpation, percussion
☐ Abdominal exam	Auscultation, palpation, percussion
☐ Extremities	Checked peripheral pulses, checked blood pressure in both arms, looked for edema and cyanosis

Closure:

☐ Examinee discussed initial diagnostic impressions.
☐ Examinee discussed initial management plans:
    ☐ Diagnostic tests.
    ☐ Lifestyle modification (diet, exercise).
☐ Examinee asked if the patient has any other questions or concerns.

Sample Closure:

Mr. Short, the source of your pain can be a cardiac problem such as a heart attack or angina, or it may be due to acid reflux, lung problems, or disorders related to the large blood vessels in your chest. It is crucial that we perform some tests in order to identify the source of your problem. We will start with an ECG and some blood work, but more complex tests may be needed as well. In the meantime, I would strongly recommend that you stop using cocaine, since use of this drug can lead to a variety of medical problems, including heart attacks. Do you have any questions for me?

PATIENT NOTE

History

Physical Examination

Differential Diagnosis

1.

2.

3.

4.

5.

Diagnostic Workup

1.

2.

3.

4.

5.

History

HPI: 46 yo M c/o chest pain. Chest pain started 40 minutes before the patient presented to the ER. The pain woke the patient from sleep at 5 A.M. with a steady 7/10 pressure sensation in the middle of his chest that radiated to the left arm and the neck. Nothing makes it worse or better. Nausea, sweating, and dyspnea are also present. Similar episodes have occurred during the past 3 months, 2–3 times/week. These episodes were precipitated by walking up the stairs, strenuous work, sexual intercourse, and heavy meals. Pain during these episodes was less severe, lasted for 5–10 minutes, and disappeared spontaneously or after taking antacids.
ROS: Negative except as above.
Allergies: NKDA.
Medications: Maalox, diuretic.
PMH: Hypertension for 5 years, treated with a diuretic. High cholesterol, managed with diet. GERD 10 years ago, treated with antacids.
SH: One PPD for 25 years; stopped 3 months ago. Occasional EtOH, occasional cocaine (last used yesterday afternoon). No regular exercise; poorly adherent to diet.
FH: Father died of lung cancer at age 72. Mother has peptic ulcers. No early coronary disease.

Physical Examination

Patient is in severe pain.
VS: BP 165/85 (both arms), RR 22.
Neck: No JVD, no bruits.
Chest: No tenderness, clear symmetric breath sounds bilaterally.
Heart: Apical impulse not displaced; RRR; normal S1/S2; no murmurs, rubs, or gallops.
Abdomen: Soft, nondistended, nontender, ⊕BS, no hepatosplenomegaly.
Extremities: No edema, peripheral pulses 2+ and symmetric.

Differential Diagnosis

1. Myocardial ischemia or infarction
2. Cocaine-induced myocardial ischemia
3. GERD
4. Aortic dissection
5. Pericarditis
6. Pneumothorax
7. Pulmonary embolism
8. Costochondritis

Diagnostic Workup

1. ECG
2. Cardiac enzymes (CPK, CPK-MB, troponin)
3. CXR
4. Transthoracic echocardiogram
5. Cardiac catheterization
6. Transesophageal echocardiogram
7. CT—chest with IV contrast
8. Upper endoscopy
9. Cholesterol panel

CASE DISCUSSION

Differential Diagnosis

- **Myocardial ischemia or infarction:** The patient has multiple cardiac risk factors (including smoking, hypertension, and hyperlipidemia), and his symptoms are classic for cardiac ischemia.
- **Cocaine-induced:** Cocaine can predispose to premature atherosclerosis or can induce myocardial ischemia and infarction by causing coronary artery vasoconstriction or by increasing myocardial energy requirements.
- **GERD:** Severe chest pain is atypical but not uncommon for GERD and may worsen with recumbency overnight. Other atypical symptoms may include chronic cough, wheezing, or dysphagia. The classic symptom of GERD is heartburn, which may be exacerbated by meals.
- **Aortic dissection:** With the sudden onset of severe chest pain, aortic dissection should be suspected given the high potential for death if missed (and the potential for harm if mistaken for acute MI and treated with thrombolytic therapy). However, the patient's pain is not the classic sudden tearing chest pain that radiates to the back. In addition, his peripheral pulses and blood pressures are not diminished or unequal, and there is no aortic regurgitant murmur (although physical exam findings have poor sensitivity and specificity to diagnose aortic dissection).
- **Pericarditis:** The absence of pain that changes with position or respiration and the absence of a pericardial friction rub make pericarditis less likely.
- **Pneumothorax:** This diagnosis should be entertained in a patient with acute chest pain and difficulty breathing, but it is less likely in this case given that breath sounds are symmetric.
- **Pulmonary embolism:** As above, this is on the differential for acute chest pain and difficulty breathing, but this patient has no apparent risk factors for pulmonary embolism.
- **Costochondritis (or other musculoskeletal chest pain):** This is more typically associated with pain on palpation or pleuritic pain.

Diagnostic Workup

- **ECG:** Acute myocardial ischemia, infarction, and pericarditis have characteristic changes on ECG.
- **Cardiac enzymes (CPK, CPK-MB, troponin):** Specific tests for myocardial tissue necrosis that can turn positive as early as 4–6 hours after onset of pain.
- **CXR:** A widened mediastinum suggests aortic dissection and may reveal other causes of chest pain, including pneumothorax and pneumonia.
- **Transthoracic echocardiogram (TTE):** Can demonstrate segmental wall motion abnormalities in suspected acute MIs (infarction is unlikely in the absence of wall motion abnormalities).
- **Cardiac catheterization:** Can diagnose and treat coronary artery disease.
- **Transesophageal echocardiogram (TEE):** Highly specific and sensitive for aortic dissection, and can be done rapidly at the bedside.
- **CT–chest with IV contrast:** Another rapidly available diagnostic study that can rule out aortic dissection or pulmonary embolism.
- **Upper endoscopy:** Can be used to document tissue damage characteristic of GERD. However, it can be normal in up to one-half of symptomatic patients; esophageal probe (pH and manometry measurements) together with endoscopic visualization constitutes an effective diagnostic technique.
- **Cholesterol panel:** Can identify a critical risk factor for cardiovascular disease.

CASE 7
DOORWAY INFORMATION

Opening Scenario

The mother of Josh White, a seven-month-old male child, comes to the office complaining that her child has a fever.

Examinee Tasks

1. Take a focused history.
2. Explain your clinical impression and workup plan to the mother.
3. Write the patient note after leaving the room.

Checklist/SP Sheet

PATIENT DESCRIPTION
The patient's mother offers the history; she is a fair historian.

NOTES FOR THE SP
Show concern regarding your child's situation.

CHALLENGING QUESTIONS TO ASK

- "Is my child going to be okay?"
- "Do you think I need to bring my child to the hospital?"

SAMPLE EXAMINEE RESPONSE
"Well, I will need to examine your child first. Although I suspect that he has a viral infection, I still need to make sure he does not have anything else."

Examinee Checklist

ENTRANCE:

- ☐ Examinee knocked on the door before entering.
- ☐ Examinee introduced self by name.
- ☐ Examinee identified his/her role or position.
- ☐ Examinee correctly used patient's name.
- ☐ Examinee made eye contact with the SP.

HISTORY:

- ☐ Examinee showed compassion for your child's illness.

☑ Question	Patient Response
☐ Chief complaint	My child has a fever.
☐ Onset	Yesterday.
☐ Temperature	I measured it, and it was 101.
☐ Runny nose	Yes.
☐ Ear pulling/ear discharge	No.
☐ Cough	No.
☐ Shortness of breath	I think so; he is breathing quickly and using stomach muscles to breathe.
☐ Difficulty swallowing	I don't know, but he hasn't eaten anything since yesterday and is refusing to drink from his bottle or my breast.
☐ Rash	No.
☐ Nausea/vomiting	No.
☐ Change in bowel habits or in stool color or consistency	No.
☐ Change in urinary habits or in urine smell or color, making normal number of wet diapers	No.
☐ Shaking (seizures)	No.
☐ How has the baby looked (lethargic, irritated, playful, etc.)?	He has looked tired and irritated since yesterday.
☐ Appetite changes	He is not eating anything at all.
☐ Ill contacts	His three-year-old brother had an upper respiratory tract infection one week ago, and he is fine now.
☐ Day care center	Yes.
☐ Ill contacts in day care center	I don't know.
☐ Vaccinations	Up to date.
☐ Last checkup	Two weeks ago, and everything was perfect with him.
☐ Birth history	It was a 40-week vaginal delivery with no complications.
☐ Child weight, height, and language development	Normal.
☐ Eating habits	I am breast-feeding him, and I give him all the vitamins that his pediatrician prescribes. He has refused my breast since yesterday. He also gets baby food three times a day.
☐ Sleeping habits	Last night he did not sleep well and cried when I laid him down.
☐ Current medications	Tylenol.
☐ Past medical history	Jaundice in the first week of life.
☐ Past surgical history	None.
☐ Drug allergies	No.

Physical Examination:

None.

Closure:

☐ Examinee discussed initial diagnostic impressions.
☐ Examinee discussed initial management plans:
    ☐ Follow-up tests.
☐ Examinee asked if the patient has any other questions or concerns.

Sample Closure:

Mrs. White, your child's fever may be due to a simple upper respiratory tract infection or to an ear infection caused by a virus or certain types of bacteria. I would like to see your baby so that I can determine the cause of his fever and make sure it is not due to anything more serious, such as meningitis. In addition to a detailed physical exam, your baby may need some blood tests, a urinalysis, and possibly a chest x-ray. Do you have any questions for me?

PATIENT NOTE

History

Physical Examination

Differential Diagnosis

1.

2.

3.

4.

5.

Diagnostic Workup

1.

2.

3.

4.

5.

History

HPI: *The source of information is the patient's mother. The mother of a 7-month-old M c/o her child having a fever of 101°F since yesterday. For the past day, the child has been tired, irritated, and breathing rapidly. The mother notes that yesterday the child also had a runny nose, did not sleep well, and refused her breast and baby food. There is a history of ill contact with his 3-year-old brother, who had a URI 1 week ago but is recovered now. The child goes to a day care center. The mother denies cough, ear pulling, ear discharge, or rash.*

ROS: *Negative except as above.*

Allergies: *NKDA.*

Medications: *Tylenol.*

PMH: *Jaundice in the first week of life.*

Birth history: *40-week vaginal delivery with no complications.*

Dietary history: *Breast-feeding and supplemental vitamins.*

Immunization history: *UTD.*

Developmental history: *Last checkup was 2 weeks ago and showed normal weight, height, hearing/vision, and developmental milestones.*

Physical Examination

None.

Differential Diagnosis

1. Viral URI
2. Pneumonia
3. Meningitis
4. UTI
5. Otitis media
6. Gastroenteritis
7. Occult bacteremia

Diagnostic Workup

1. Pneumatic otoscopy
2. Tympanometry
3. CBC with differential, blood culture, UA and urine culture
4. LP—CSF analysis
5. CT—head
6. CXR
7. Bronchoscopy
8. Serum antibody titers
9. U/S—renal
10. Voiding cystourethrogram

CASE DISCUSSION

Differential Diagnosis

- **Viral URI:** Possible clues suggesting this diagnosis as the source of fever include rhinorrhea and recent exposure to a sibling with URI. It is probably viral, self-limited, and benign, but lower respiratory tract infection must first be ruled out in light of the child's apparent dyspnea and tachypnea.
- **Pneumonia:** Fever, rhinorrhea, tachypnea, and dyspnea support this diagnosis, although cough is not present. The physical exam may find retractions, nasal flaring, grunting, dullness on chest percussion, and rales.
- **Meningitis:** Findings are often subtle and nonspecific and may be limited to fever, irritability, and poor feeding, as seen in this case. The physical exam may reveal a bulging fontanelle; meningeal signs may not be obvious in infants (nuchal rigidity and focal neurologic signs are more commonly seen in older children).
- **UTI:** Infants with UTI may not have symptoms referable to the urinary tract. Those who do may have dribbling or colic before and during voiding. Patients with high fever and CVA tenderness are presumed to have pyelonephritis until proven otherwise.
- **Otitis media:** Otalgia and ear drainage can suggest this diagnosis in an ill, febrile child but are often not present (as in this case). The physical exam is key and may reveal a hyperemic, bulging TM; loss of TM landmarks; and decreased TM mobility.
- **Gastroenteritis:** This patient has fever but no GI symptoms. Viral infection typically causes vomiting and/or watery diarrhea, whereas bacterial infection may cause fever, tenesmus, bloody diarrhea, and severe abdominal pain.
- **Occult bacteremia:** This is an important consideration for children with high fever (> 102°F/38.9°C) and no obvious source. There is a relatively high proportion of children with no identifiable fever source who will have a positive blood culture, which can progress to sepsis if untreated. An extensive workup (see below) is not necessarily indicated in this case, as fever is < 102°F (38.9°C).

Diagnostic Workup

- **Pneumatic otoscopy:** Key to look for the decreased TM mobility seen in otitis media.
- **Tympanometry:** Useful in infants > 6 months of age; confirms abnormal TM mobility in otitis media.
- **CBC with differential, blood culture, UA and urine culture:** Constitutes the "septic" or occult bacteremia workup in children with unexplained high fever. Notably, a WBC count > 15,000/μL is suggestive of occult bacteremia. UTI may be occult and must be investigated.
- **LP—CSF analysis:** Should be performed if there is any concern for meningitis. CSF analysis includes cell count and differential, glucose, protein, Gram stain, culture, latex agglutination for common bacterial antigens, and occasionally PCR for specific viruses.
- **CT—head:** Used mainly to rule out brain abscess or hemorrhage.
- **CXR:** To diagnose pneumonia.
- **Bronchoscopy:** A diagnostic aid in severe or refractory pneumonia cases.
- **Serum antibody titers:** To identify causative viruses in pediatric infections (not commonly used).
- **U/S—renal:** To look for anatomic anomalies that predispose to UTI.
- **Voiding cystourethrogram:** To look for vesicoureteral reflux in UTI.

CASE 8

DOORWAY INFORMATION

Opening Scenario

The mother of Maria Sterling, an 18-month-old female child, comes to the office complaining that her child has a fever.

Examinee Tasks

1. Take a focused history.
2. Explain your clinical impression and workup plan to the mother.
3. Write the patient note after leaving the room.

Checklist/SP Sheet

PATIENT DESCRIPTION

The patient's mother offers the history; the child is at home.

NOTES FOR THE SP

Show concern regarding your child's situation.

CHALLENGING QUESTIONS TO ASK

- "Do you think that I did the right thing by coming here and telling you about my child's fever?"
- "Is my child going to be okay?"

SAMPLE EXAMINEE RESPONSE

"You absolutely did the right thing. Maria may have an infection that needs antibiotics; we need to examine her here in the office and then decide whether she needs any more testing or treatment."

Examinee Checklist

ENTRANCE:

- ☐ Examinee knocked on the door before entering.
- ☐ Examinee introduced self by name.
- ☐ Examinee identified his/her role or position.
- ☐ Examinee correctly used patient's name.
- ☐ Examinee made eye contact with the SP.

HISTORY:

- ☐ Examinee showed compassion for your child's illness.

☑ Question	Patient Response
☐ Chief complaint	My child has a fever.
☐ Onset	Two days ago.
☐ Temperature	I measured it, and it was 101°F rectally.
☐ Runny nose	No.
☐ Ear pulling/ear discharge	Yes, she has been pulling at her right ear for two days.
☐ Cough	No.
☐ Shortness of breath	No.
☐ Difficulty swallowing	She feels pain while she is eating her food.
☐ Rash	Yes, she has some sort of rash on her face and chest.
☐ Description of the rash	Tiny red dots, some slightly elevated, over the chest, back, belly, and face. There is no rash on her arms or legs.
☐ Onset of rash and progression	It started two days ago on her face and then spread to her chest, back, and belly.
☐ Nausea/vomiting	No.
☐ Change in bowel habits or in stool color or consistency	No.
☐ Change in urinary habits or in urine smell or color	No.
☐ Shaking (seizures)	No.
☐ How has the child looked (lethargic, irritated, playful, etc.)?	She looks tired. She is not playing with her toys today and is not watching TV the way she usually does.
☐ Appetite changes	She is not eating as usual but is drinking milk.
☐ Ill contacts	No.
☐ Day care center	Yes.
☐ Ill contacts in day care center	I don't know.
☐ Vaccinations	Up to date.
☐ Last checkup	One month ago, and everything was normal.
☐ Birth history	It was a 40-week vaginal delivery with no complications.
☐ Child weight, height, and language development	Normal.
☐ Eating habits	Whole milk and solid food; I did not breast-feed my child.
☐ Sleeping habits	She has not slept well for two days.
☐ Hearing problems	No.
☐ Vision problems	No.
☐ Current medications	Tylenol.
☐ Past medical history	Three months ago she had an ear infection that was treated successfully with amoxicillin.
☐ Past surgical history	None.
☐ Drug allergies	No.

Physical Examination:

None.

Closure:

☐ Examinee discussed initial diagnostic impressions.
☐ Examinee discussed initial management plans:
   ☐ Follow-up tests.
☐ Examinee asked if the patient has any other questions or concerns.

Sample Closure:

Mrs. Sterling, it appears that your child is suffering from an infection that may be viral or bacterial. She may be suffering from an ear infection or meningitis. A physical exam and some blood tests will be needed to identify the source of infection and the type of virus or bacteria involved. Although most viral infections clear on their own, bacterial infections require antibiotics; however, such infections generally respond well to treatment. Do you have any questions for me?

PATIENT NOTE

History

Physical Examination

Differential Diagnosis

1.

2.

3.

4.

5.

Diagnostic Workup

1.

2.

3.

4.

5.

History

HPI: *The source of information is the patient's mother. The mother of an 18-month-old F c/o her child having a fever for 2 days. She notes that the child is tired and is not playing with her toys or watching TV as she usually does. The mother recalls that her child has been pulling at her right ear and having difficulty swallowing and sleeping for the past 2 days. The child also developed a maculopapular facial rash that then spread over the chest, back, and abdomen. There is no rash on her arms or legs. The child also has loss of appetite. She goes to a day care center, but there is no known history of ill contacts. The mother denies cough or ear discharge.*
ROS: *Negative except as above.*
Allergies: *NKDA.*
Medications: *Tylenol.*
PMH: *Otitis media 3 months ago, treated with amoxicillin.*
Birth history: *40-week vaginal delivery with no complications.*
Dietary history: *Formula milk and solid food. She was not breast-fed.*
Immunization history: *UTD.*
Developmental history: *Last checkup was 1 month ago and showed normal weight, height, hearing, vision, and developmental milestones.*

Physical Examination

None.

Differential Diagnosis

1. Otitis media
2. Meningococcal meningitis
3. Scarlet fever
4. Fifth disease or other viral exanthem
5. Varicella

Diagnostic Workup

1. Pneumatic otoscopy
2. Tympanometry
3. LP—CSF analysis
4. Platelets, PT/PTT, D-dimer, fibrin split products, fibrinogen
5. CBC with differential, blood culture, UA and urine culture
6. Throat culture
7. Parvovirus B19 IgM antibody
8. Skin lesion scrapings
9. Varicella antibody titer

CASE DISCUSSION

Differential Diagnosis

- **Otitis media:** Fever and otalgia suggest this diagnosis but are present in < 50% of patients. Physical exam is key and may reveal a hyperemic, bulging TM; loss of TM landmarks; and decreased TM mobility.
- **Meningococcal meningitis:** Fever, lethargy, and a possible petechial rash are suggestive of meningococcemia. Patients may also have headache, vomiting, photophobia, neck stiffness, and seizures. This is a severe, rapidly progressive, and sometimes fatal infection; the patient would appear very ill.
- **Scarlet fever:** This patient has fever, difficulty swallowing (i.e., possible pharyngitis), and a rash that started on her face and spread to the trunk. However, the description does not allow one to ascertain whether or not the rash consists of a diffuse erythema with punctate elevations resembling sandpaper that spares the area around the mouth. Also, scarlet fever is more common in school-age children.
- **Fifth disease or other viral exanthem:** In children, viruses commonly present with low-grade fever and rash. In general, viral exanthems are quite nonspecific in their appearance and are usually maculopapular and diffuse. Parvovirus B19 infection, or fifth disease, usually presents as intense, red facial flushing ("slapped cheek" appearance) that then spreads over the trunk and becomes more diffuse. Rubeola classically presents as 2–5 days of high fever followed by a diffuse rash. However, almost any virus can be accompanied by rash in the pediatric patient, and it is not always necessary to ascertain which virus is causing the illness. If the illness is prolonged or particularly troublesome, antibody titers can be ordered to determine the exact etiology of the illness.
- **Varicella:** Fever and rash, along with day care attendance, could be consistent with this infection. However, in varicella the lesions are present in various stages of development at any given time (i.e., red macules, vesicles, pustules, crusting), and the rash is intensely pruritic. The incidence of varicella has declined since vaccination began in the 1990s.

Diagnostic Workup

- **Pneumatic otoscopy:** Key to look for the decreased TM mobility seen in otitis media.
- **Tympanometry:** Useful in infants > 6 months of age; confirms abnormal TM mobility in otitis media.
- **LP–CSF analysis:** Should be performed if there is any concern for meningitis. CSF analysis includes cell count and differential, glucose, protein, Gram stain, culture, latex agglutination for common bacterial antigens, and occasionally PCR for specific viruses.
- **Platelets, PT/PTT, D-dimer, fibrin split products, fibrinogen:** Evidence of DIC is often seen in meningococcemia.
- **CBC with differential, blood culture, UA and urine culture:** To isolate *Neisseria meningitidis* and to screen for occult bacteremia or UTI.
- **Throat culture:** To isolate *Streptococcus pyogenes* (causes scarlet fever). The rash is pathognomonic for this diagnosis.
- **Parvovirus B19 IgM antibody:** The best marker of acute or recent infection in suspected fifth disease.
- **Skin lesion scrapings:** Varicella antigens are identified by PCR or direct immunofluorescence (DFA) of skin lesions. Also, a Tzanck smear may show multinucleated giant cells in varicella infection.
- **Varicella antibody titer:** May be useful in uncertain cases (look for a fourfold rise in antibody titer following acute infection).

Opening Scenario

Eric Glenn, a 26-year-old male, comes to the office complaining of cough.

Vital Signs

BP: 120/80 mmHg
Temp: 99.5°F (37.5°C)
RR: 15/minute
HR: 75/minute, regular

Examinee Tasks

1. Take a focused history.
2. Perform a focused physical exam (do not perform rectal, genitourinary, or female breast exam).
3. Explain your clinical impression and workup plan to the patient.
4. Write the patient note after leaving the room.

Checklist/SP Sheet

PATIENT DESCRIPTION

Patient is a 26 yo M.

NOTES FOR THE SP

- Cough as the examinee enters the room.
- Continue coughing every 3–4 minutes during the encounter.
- Chest auscultation: When asked to take a breath while the examinee is listening to your right chest, pretend to inhale by moving your shoulders up, but do not actually breathe in.
- Chest palpation: When the examinee palpates your right chest and asks you to say "99," turn your face to the right side, and say it in a coarse, deep voice.
- If asked about sputum, ask the examinee, "What does 'sputum' mean?"
- During the encounter, pretend to have a severe attack of coughing. Note whether the examinee offers you a glass of water or a tissue.

CHALLENGING QUESTIONS TO ASK

"Do I need antibiotics to get better?"

SAMPLE EXAMINEE RESPONSE

"Possibly. Antibiotics don't help with bronchitis because this condition is primarily caused by viruses that are not sensitive to antibiotics. However, if we find that you have pneumonia, antibiotics will be needed."

Examinee Checklist

- ☐ Examinee knocked on the door before entering.
- ☐ Examinee introduced self by name.
- ☐ Examinee identified his/her role or position.
- ☐ Examinee correctly used patient's name.
- ☐ Examinee made eye contact with the SP.

HISTORY:

- ☐ Examinee showed compassion for your illness.
- ☐ Examinee offered you a glass of water or a tissue during your severe bout of coughing.

☑ Question	Patient Response
☐ Chief complaint	Cough.
☐ Onset	One week ago.
☐ Preceding symptoms/events	Runny nose, fever, sore throat two weeks ago for one week, which then resolved.
☐ Fever/chills	Mild fever, but I didn't take my temperature; no chills.
☐ Sputum production	Small amounts of white mucus.
☐ Blood in sputum	No.
☐ Chest pain	Yes, I feel a sharp pain when I cough or take a deep breath.
☐ Location	Right chest.
☐ Quality	It is like a knife. I can't take a deep breath.
☐ Alleviating/exacerbating factors	It increases when I take a deep breath and when I cough. I feel better when I sleep on my right side.
☐ Radiation of pain	No.
☐ Severity on a scale	8/10.
☐ Night sweats	No.
☐ Exposure to TB	None.
☐ Pet, animal exposure	None.
☐ Recent travel	None.
☐ Last PPD	Never had it.
☐ Associated symptoms (shortness of breath, wheezing, abdominal pain, nausea/ vomiting, diarrhea/constipation)	None.
☐ Weight/appetite changes	No.
☐ Current medications	Tylenol.
☐ Past medical history	I had gonorrhea two years ago and was cured after a course of antibiotics.

☑ Question	Patient Response
☐ Past surgical history	None.
☐ Family history	My father and mother are alive and in good health.
☐ Occupation	Pizza delivery boy.
☐ Alcohol use	I drink a lot on the weekends. I never count.
☐ Illicit drug use	Never.
☐ Tobacco	Yes, I smoke one pack a day. I started when I was 15 years old.
☐ Sexual activity	Well, I've had many girlfriends. Every Saturday night, I pick up a new girl from the nightclub.
☐ Use of condoms	Nope, I don't enjoy it with a condom.
☐ Drug allergies	No.

Physical Examination:

☐ Examinee washed his/her hands.
☐ Examinee asked permission to start the exam.
☐ Examinee used respectful draping.
☐ Examinee did not repeat painful maneuvers.

☑ Exam Component	Maneuver
☐ Head and neck exam	Examined mouth, throat, lymph nodes
☐ CV exam	Auscultation, palpation
☐ Pulmonary exam	Auscultation, palpation, percussion
☐ Extremities	Inspection

Closure:

☐ Examinee discussed initial diagnostic impressions.
☐ Examinee discussed initial management plans:
    ☐ Follow-up tests.
    ☐ Discussed safe sex practices.
    ☐ Recommended HIV testing (and discussed consent).
☐ Examinee asked if the patient has any other questions or concerns.

Sample Closure:

Mr. Glenn, your cough is most likely due to an infection that can be either bacterial or viral in origin. Some of these infections can be manifestations of HIV, and given your sexual history, I would recommend that we test for it. Another reason for your cough may be acid reflux. The chest pain you are experiencing is probably due to irritation of your lung membranes by an infectious process. We are going to test your blood and sputum and will also obtain a chest x-ray in order to help us make a definitive diagnosis. In the meantime, I would strongly recommend that you use condoms during intercourse to prevent STDs such as HIV as well as to avoid unwanted pregnancies. Do you have any questions for me?

PATIENT NOTE

History

Physical Examination

Differential Diagnosis

1.

2.

3.

4.

5.

Diagnostic Workup

1.

2.

3.

4.

5.

History

HPI: 26 yo M c/o cough for 1 week. Two weeks ago the patient had a fever, runny nose, and sore throat. These symptoms resolved and were followed by a cough that has persisted. The cough is productive of small amounts of white mucus with no blood. The patient also notes a sharp, stabbing 8/10 pain in the right chest that occurs with and is exacerbated by coughing and deep inspiration. He has a mild fever but denies chills, night sweats, shortness of breath, or wheezing. The patient has not traveled recently and denies exposure to TB. There are no weight or appetite changes.

ROS: Negative except as above.

Allergies: NKDA.

Medications: Tylenol.

PMH: Gonorrhea 2 years ago, treated with antibiotics.

SH: One PPD since age 15; drinks heavily on weekends. Unprotected sex with multiple female partners.

FH: Noncontributory.

Physical Examination

Patient is in no acute distress.

VS: WNL.

HEENT: Nose, mouth, and pharynx WNL.

Neck: No JVD, no lymphadenopathy.

Chest: Increase in tactile fremitus and decrease in breath sounds on the right side. No rhonchi, rales, or wheezing.

Heart: Apical impulse not displaced; RRR; normal S1/S2; no murmurs, rubs, or gallops.

Extremities: No cyanosis or edema.

Differential Diagnosis

1. Upper respiratory infection (URI)
2. Acute bronchitis
3. Pneumonia
4. Pleurodynia
5. Aspiration

Diagnostic Workup

1. CXR
2. CBC
3. Sputum Gram stain and culture
4. Urine *Legionella* antigen, serum *Mycoplasma* PCR, cold agglutinin measurement
5. Bronchoscopy with bronchoalveolar lavage
6. Pulse oximetry or ABG
7. HIV antibody

CASE DISCUSSION

Differential Diagnosis

This young man's acute productive cough and pleuritic pain are likely caused by viral respiratory infection or pneumonia. Rarely, severe coughing can lead to a rib fracture, which in turn can cause severe pleuritis.

- **URI-associated cough:** Acute cough frequently follows URI ("postinfectious") and can commonly persist for 1–2 weeks (or up to 6–8 weeks in patients with underlying asthma). URIs range from rhinosinusitis to acute bronchitis.
- **Acute bronchitis:** Cough can also accompany acute URI.
- **Pneumonia:** Pleuritic pain may signal lower respiratory tract infection. This diagnosis is often confirmed by characteristic chest exam findings, which may be difficult to elicit in an otherwise healthy SP. Increased tactile fremitus suggests airspace consolidation, but there are no bronchial breath sounds or rales to help suggest a focal pneumonia. Also, the absence of dyspnea argues against this diagnosis.
- **Pleurodynia:** An uncommon acute illness usually caused by one of the coxsackieviruses. It occurs in summer and early fall and presents with acute severe paroxysmal pain of the thorax or abdomen that worsens with cough or breathing. Most patients recover within three days to one week.
- **Other etiologies:** Other causes of acute cough include aspiration (alcoholics, elderly, and neurologically impaired are at risk), pulmonary embolism (extremely rare in a young patient with no risk factors), and pulmonary edema (signs and symptoms of heart failure would be present). Given the patient's history of STD, he should be screened for HIV infection. Notably, there is no evidence of immunosuppression on exam (e.g., no thrush), and in *Pneumocystis jiroveci pneumonia*, cough is usually nonproductive and accompanied by dyspnea.

Diagnostic Workup

- **CXR:** To help diagnose pneumonia (i.e., to see infiltrates, effusion), although a normal film does not necessarily rule it out.
- **CBC:** In acute infection, can reveal leukopenia or leukocytosis.
- **Sputum Gram stain and culture:** Often low yield (due to contamination by oral flora and often discordant results between Gram stain and culture in pneumococcal pneumonia), but may help identify a microbiologic diagnosis in pneumonia.
- **Urine *Legionella* antigen, serum *Mycoplasma* PCR, cold agglutinin measurement:** To help diagnose specific causes of atypical pneumonia. Usually not useful in the initial evaluation of patients with community-acquired pneumonia.
- **Bronchoscopy with bronchoalveolar lavage:** An invasive test that is rarely necessary to diagnose community-acquired pneumonia, but a gold standard that is often used early when *P. jiroveci* infection is suspected.
- **Pulse oximetry or ABG:** May help determine the need for hospitalization.
- **HIV antibody:** Should be offered to all patients with risk factors for this infection.

Opening Scenario

Marilyn McLean, a 54-year-old female, comes to the office complaining of persistent cough.

Vital Signs

BP: 120/80 mmHg
Temp: 99.5°F (37.5°C)
RR: 15/minute
HR: 75/minute, regular.

Examinee Tasks

1. Take a focused history.
2. Perform a focused physical exam (do not perform rectal, genitourinary, or female breast exam).
3. Explain your clinical impression and workup plan to the patient.
4. Write the patient note after leaving the room.

Checklist/SP Sheet

PATIENT DESCRIPTION

Patient is a 54 yo F.

NOTES FOR THE SP

- Cough as the examinee enters the room.
- Continue coughing every 3–4 minutes during the encounter.
- Hold a tissue in your hand, with red staining to simulate blood. Don't show it to the examinee unless he/she asks you.
- If asked about sputum, ask the examinee, "What does 'sputum' mean?"
- During the encounter, pretend to have a severe attack of coughing. Note whether the examinee offers you a glass of water or a tissue.

CHALLENGING QUESTIONS TO ASK

"Will I get better if I stop smoking?"

SAMPLE EXAMINEE RESPONSE

"Well, we still have to sort out exactly what's making you sick. Stopping smoking should help your chronic cough, and over the long term it will significantly decrease your cancer risk."

Examinee Checklist

ENTRANCE:

☐ Examinee knocked on the door before entering.
☐ Examinee introduced self by name.

☐ Examinee identified his/her role or position.
☐ Examinee correctly used patient's name.
☐ Examinee made eye contact with the SP.

HISTORY:

☐ Examinee showed compassion for your illness.
☐ Examinee offered you a glass of water or a tissue during your severe bout of coughing.

☑ Question	Patient Response
☐ Chief complaint	Persistent cough.
☐ Onset	I've had a cough for years, especially in the morning. This past month, the cough has gotten worse, and it is really annoying me.
☐ Changes of the cough during the day	No.
☐ Progression of the cough during the last month	It is getting worse.
☐ Do you cough at night?	Yes, sometimes I can't sleep because of it.
☐ Alleviating/exacerbating factors	Nothing.
☐ Sputum production	Yes.
☐ Amount	Two teaspoonfuls, stable.
☐ Color	Yellowish mucus.
☐ Odor	None.
☐ Consistency	Thick and viscous.
☐ Blood	Yes, recently.
☐ Amount of blood	Streaks.
☐ Preceding symptoms/events	None.
☐ Fever/chills	Mild, especially at night. I didn't take my temperature. I have had no chills.
☐ Night sweats	Yes.
☐ Chest pain	No.
☐ Shortness of breath	Yes, when I walk up the stairs.
☐ Exposure to TB	Yes, I work in a nursing home, and several of our residents are under treatment for TB.
☐ Recent travel	None.
☐ Last PPD	Last year, before I started working in the nursing home. It was negative.
☐ Associated symptoms (wheezing, abdominal pain, nausea/vomiting, diarrhea/constipation)	None.
☐ Appetite changes	Yes, I don't have an appetite.

☑ Question	Patient Response
☐ Weight changes	Yes, I lost six pounds in the last two months.
☐ Fatigue	Yes, I don't have the energy that I had before.
☐ Since when	Two months ago.
☐ Current medications	Cough syrup "over the counter," multivitamins, albuterol inhaler.
☐ Past medical history	Chronic bronchitis.
☐ Past surgical history	Tonsillectomy and adenoidectomy, age 11.
☐ Family history	My father died of old age. My mother is alive and has Alzheimer's.
☐ Occupation	Nurse's aide.
☐ Alcohol use	None.
☐ Illicit drug use	Never.
☐ Tobacco	No, I stopped smoking two weeks ago.
☐ Duration	I smoked for the past 35 years.
☐ Amount	One to two packs a day.
☐ Sexual activity	With my husband.
☐ Drug allergies	No.

Physical Examination:

- ☐ Examinee washed his/her hands.
- ☐ Examinee asked permission to start the exam.
- ☐ Examinee used respectful draping.
- ☐ Examinee did not repeat painful maneuvers.

☑ Exam Component	Maneuver
☐ Head and neck exam	Inspected mouth, throat, lymph nodes
☐ CV exam	Auscultation
☐ Pulmonary exam	Auscultation, palpation, percussion
☐ Abdominal exam	Auscultation, palpation
☐ Extremities	Inspection

Closure:

- ☐ Examinee discussed initial diagnostic impressions.
- ☐ Examinee discussed initial management plans.
- ☐ Examinee asked if the patient has any other questions or concerns.

Sample Closure:

Mrs. McLean, your cough may be due to a lung infection that can be treated with antibiotics, or it may result from a more serious disorder such as cancer. We will need to obtain some blood and sputum tests as well as a chest x-ray in order to identify the source of your problem. In addition, we may find it necessary to conduct more sophisticated tests in the future. The fact that you work in a nursing home puts you at risk for acquiring tuberculosis, so we are going to test you for that as well. I would also recommend that you adhere to standard respiratory precautions while working with patients who are infected with TB. Do you have any questions for me?

PATIENT NOTE

History

Physical Examination

Differential Diagnosis

1.

2.

3.

4.

5.

Diagnostic Workup

1.

2.

3.

4.

5.

History

HPI: 54 yo F with a PMH of chronic bronchitis c/o worsening cough over the last month. The cough is productive of 2 teaspoonfuls of yellowish mucus, with occasional streaks of blood. Patient notes dyspnea on exertion. She also has fever and sweats at night. No chest pain or wheezing. No chills. The patient reports fatigue, decreased appetite, and a weight loss of 6 pounds during the last 2 months. No recent travel. Exposed to patients with TB in the nursing home, where she works as a nurse's aide. Her last PPD test was last year and was negative.
ROS: Negative except as above.
Allergies: NKDA.
Medications: OTC cough syrup, multivitamins, albuterol inhaler.
PMH: Per HPI.
PSH: Tonsillectomy and adenoidectomy, age 11.
SH: One to two PPD for 35 years; stopped 2 weeks ago. No EtOH. Sexually active with husband only.
FH: Noncontributory.

Physical Examination

Patient is in no acute distress.
VS: WNL.
HEENT: Mouth and pharynx WNL.
Neck: No JVD, no lymphadenopathy.
Chest: Clear breath sounds bilaterally; no rhonchi, rales, or wheezing; tactile fremitus normal.
Heart: Apical impulse not displaced; RRR; normal S1/S2; no murmurs, rubs, or gallops.
Abdomen: Soft, nontender, ⊕BS, no hepatosplenomegaly.
Extremities: No clubbing, cyanosis, or edema.

Differential Diagnosis

1. Pulmonary tuberculosis
2. Lung cancer
3. Lung abscess
4. Atypical pneumonia
5. Typical pneumonia
6. COPD exacerbation
7. Wegener's granulomatosis

Diagnostic Workup

1. CBC
2. c-ANCA
3. Blood cultures
4. PPD
5. Sputum Gram stain, AFB smear, routine and mycobacterial sputum cultures, and cytology
6. CXR—PA and lateral
7. CT—chest
8. Bronchoscopy
9. Lung biopsy

CASE DISCUSSION

Differential Diagnosis

- **Pulmonary tuberculosis:** Clinical suspicion is high for this given the constitutional symptoms, hemoptysis, and recent exposure to active TB. The patient should be placed in respiratory isolation immediately.
- **Lung cancer:** As noted above, constitutional symptoms and hemoptysis in a long-time smoker are worrisome for cancer.
- **Lung abscess:** A lung abscess due to anaerobic bacteria is usually associated with a gradual onset of fatigue, fever, night sweats, cough producing a foul-smelling expectoration, and weight loss. Symptoms evolve over a period of weeks or months (the time course in this case favors abscess over uncomplicated pneumonia). Other bacterial causes of lung abscess typically present more acutely.
- **Atypical pneumonia:** Refers to infection by *Mycoplasma pneumoniae*, *Chlamydia pneumoniae*, and *Legionella* species. These can all present similarly with an insidious onset of fever, malaise, headache, myalgia, sore throat, hoarseness, chest pain, and nonproductive cough. Sputum may be blood-streaked. GI symptoms may be prominent in *Legionella* infection, and severe ear pain due to bullous myringitis may complicate up to 5% of *Mycoplasma* infections. The presence of weight loss and night sweats makes atypical pneumonia less likely in this case.
- **Typical pneumonia:** Classic bacterial pneumonia begins with abrupt onset of fever, chills, pleuritic chest pain, and productive cough. Remember that signs of pulmonary consolidation on physical exam are absent in up to two-thirds of documented cases. The more subacute time course seen here makes this diagnosis less likely.
- **COPD exacerbation:** This patient's baseline productive cough is due to COPD/chronic bronchitis secondary to tobacco exposure. Exacerbations of chronic bronchitis are more acute and involve increased sputum production and/or increased wheezing and dyspnea. Night sweats and weight loss are not typical features of this diagnosis.
- **Wegener's granulomatosis:** This rare small-vessel vasculitis usually develops over 4–12 months and classically involves the triad of upper respiratory tract, lower respiratory tract, and renal disease (which usually does not cause symptoms before the diagnosis is established). Constitutional symptoms are common. The absence of chronic upper respiratory complaints (e.g., sinusitis or nasal crusting) makes this diagnosis less likely.
- **Other etiologies:** Other common, benign causes of chronic cough include postnasal drip, GERD, asthma, and ACE inhibitors.

Diagnostic Workup

- **CBC:** To identify leukocytosis in infection (nonspecific).
- **c-ANCA:** Highly specific (> 90%) and sensitive for active Wegener's granulomatosis.
- **Blood cultures:** May be useful in severe pneumonia to identify causative pathogenic bacteria.
- **PPD (tuberculin skin test):** Identifies individuals who have been infected with *Mycobacterium tuberculosis*, but does not distinguish between active and latent infection.
- **Sputum Gram stain, AFB smear, routine and mycobacterial sputum cultures, and cytology:** To identify a causative agent of infection or to help detect malignancy.
- **CXR—PA and lateral:** To look for apical cavitary disease in TB reactivation, noncalcified nodules in lung cancer, a cavity with an air-fluid level in lung abscess, a patchy infiltrative pattern in atypical pneumonia, lobar consolidation in typical pneumonia, and infiltrates, nodules, masses, or cavities in Wegener's granulomatosis.
- **CT—chest:** May demonstrate lesions unseen on CXR, and aids in characterizing the size, shape, and composition of lung and mediastinal pathology. Can also guide diagnostic procedures (e.g., percutaneous transthoracic biopsies) and assist in staging.
- **Bronchoscopy:** Useful in diagnosing and staging lung cancer and in diagnosing infections.
- **Lung biopsy:** Can lead to definitive diagnosis. A range of techniques can be used depending on the location of the tumor.

Opening Scenario

Gail Abbott, a 52-year-old female, comes to the office complaining of yellow eyes and skin.

Vital Signs

BP: 130/80 mmHg
Temp: 98.3°F (36.8°C)
RR: 15/minute
HR: 70/minute, regular

Examinee Tasks

1. Take a focused history.
2. Perform a focused physical exam (do not perform rectal, genitourinary, or female breast exam).
3. Explain your clinical impression and workup plan to the patient.
4. Write the patient note after leaving the room.

Checklist/SP Sheet

PATIENT DESCRIPTION

Patient is a 52 yo F.

NOTES FOR THE SP

- Sit up on the bed.
- Show signs of scratching.
- Exhibit RUQ tenderness on palpation.
- If ERCP, ultrasound, or MRI is mentioned, ask for an explanation.

CHALLENGING QUESTIONS TO ASK

"My father had pancreatic cancer. Could I have it too?"

SAMPLE EXAMINEE RESPONSE

"It's possible; that's why we always rule it out in patients with yellow eyes or skin. Your family history does put you at slightly increased risk, and we will keep that in mind."

Examinee Checklist

ENTRANCE:

☐ Examinee knocked on the door before entering.
☐ Examinee introduced self by name.
☐ Examinee identified his/her role or position.
☐ Examinee correctly used patient's name.
☐ Examinee made eye contact with the SP.

History:

☐ Examinee showed compassion for your pain.

☑ Question	Patient Response
☐ Chief complaint	Yellow eyes and skin.
☐ Onset	Three weeks ago.
☐ Color of stool	Light.
☐ Color of urine	Dark.
☐ Pruritus	I started itching two months ago; Benadryl used to help but not recently.
☐ Abdominal pain	Sometimes.
☐ Onset	It was around the same time that I noticed the change in the color of my eyes and skin.
☐ Constant/intermittent	Well, I don't have the pain all the time. It comes and goes.
☐ Frequency	At least once every day.
☐ Progression	It is the same.
☐ Severity on a scale	When I have the pain, it is 3/10, and then it may go down to 0.
☐ Location	It is here (points to the RUQ).
☐ Radiation	No.
☐ Quality	Dull.
☐ Alleviating factors	Tylenol. I take four pills every day just to make sure I do not feel the pain.
☐ Exacerbating factors	None.
☐ Relationship of food to pain	None.
☐ Previous episodes of similar pain	No.
☐ Nausea/vomiting	Sometimes I feel nauseated when I am in pain, but no vomiting.
☐ Diarrhea/constipation	No.
☐ Colonoscopy	Never.
☐ Blood transfusion	Yes, when I had a C-section 20 years ago.
☐ Fever, night sweats	No.
☐ Fatigue	Yes, recently.
☐ Weight changes	No.
☐ Appetite changes	I have no appetite.
☐ Joint pain	No.
☐ Travel history	I went to Mexico for a brief vacation about two months ago.
☐ Immunization before travel	No.

☑ Question	Patient Response
☐ Current medications	Tylenol, Synthroid.
☐ Similar episodes	No.
☐ Past medical history	Hypothyroidism.
☐ Past surgical history	I had two C-sections at ages 25 and 30 and a tubal ligation at age 35.
☐ Family history	My father died at 55 of pancreatic cancer. My mother is alive and healthy.
☐ Occupation	I work in a travel agency.
☐ Illicit drug use	No.
☐ Tobacco	No.
☐ Sexual activity	Yes, with my husband.
☐ Drug allergies	Penicillin, causes rash.
☐ How much alcohol do you drink?/ Tell me about your use of alcohol	One or two glasses of wine every day for 30 years.
☐ Have you ever felt a need to cut down on drinking?	No.
☐ Have you ever felt annoyed by criticism of your drinking?	No.
☐ Have you ever felt guilty about your drinking?	No, I heard that alcohol protects against heart disease.
☐ Have you ever had a drink early in the morning ("eye opener") to steady your nerves or get rid of a hangover?	No.
☐ Affecting job/relationships/legal problems	No.

Physical Examination:

- ☐ Examinee washed his/her hands.
- ☐ Examinee asked permission to start the exam.
- ☐ Examinee used respectful draping.
- ☐ Examinee did not repeat painful maneuvers.

☑ Exam Component	Maneuver
☐ HEENT	Inspected sclerae, under tongue
☐ CV exam	Auscultation
☐ Pulmonary exam	Auscultation
☐ Abdominal exam	Inspection, auscultation, palpation (including Murphy's sign), percussion, measurement of liver span

☑ Exam Component	Maneuver
☐ Extremities	Checked for asterixis, edema
☐ Skin	Looked for spider nevi, cutaneous telangiectasias, palmar erythema

Closure:

☐ Examinee discussed initial diagnostic impressions.
☐ Examinee discussed initial management plans.
☐ Examinee asked if the patient has any other questions or concerns.

Sample Closure:

Mrs. Abbott, the symptoms you describe are usually due to a disorder either in the liver itself or in the ducts that carry bile from the liver to your intestines. We will have to run some blood tests and conduct imaging studies such as ultrasound in order to determine the type of disease you have. Once we find the cause of your problem, we can devise an appropriate treatment plan. Until then, I would recommend that you stop drinking and limit your use of Tylenol, as both may negatively affect your liver. Do you have any questions for me?

History

Physical Examination

Differential Diagnosis

1.

2.

3.

4.

5.

Diagnostic Workup

1.

2.

3.

4.

5.

History

HPI: 52 yo F c/o yellow skin and eyes that started for the first time 3 weeks ago. Accompanied by light-colored stool and dark urine. Around the same time she also began having 3/10 RUQ pain that is dull and intermittent (at least daily), does not radiate, is unrelated to meals, and is relieved by Tylenol. There is associated anorexia, pruritus, and occasional nausea. She recently traveled to Mexico. No diarrhea, constipation, or weight loss. History of blood transfusion 20 years ago.

ROS: Negative except for fatigue.

Allergies: Penicillin, causes rash.

Medications: Tylenol, Synthroid.

PMH: Hypothyroidism.

PSH: Two C-sections, tubal ligation.

SH: No smoking, 1–2 glasses of wine/day for 30 years, CAGE 0/4, no illicit drugs. Sexually active with husband only.

FH: Father died of pancreatic cancer at age 55.

Physical Examination

Patient is in no acute distress.

VS: WNL.

HEENT: Sclerae icteric.

Chest: Clear breath sounds bilaterally.

Heart: RRR; normal S1/S2; no murmurs, rubs, or gallops.

Abdomen: Soft, nondistended, C-section scar. Mild RUQ tenderness without rebound or guarding, ⊖Murphy's, ⊕BS, no organomegaly or masses. No evidence of ascites.

Extremities: No asterixis, no edema.

Skin: Jaundice, excoriations due to scratching, no spiders/telangiectasias/palmar erythema.

Differential Diagnosis

1. Extrahepatic biliary obstruction:
   Pancreatic cancer
   Choledocholithiasis
   Cholangiocarcinoma
   Carcinoma of the ampulla
   Sphincter of Oddi dysfunction
2. Viral hepatitis
3. Acetaminophen liver toxicity
4. Alcoholic hepatitis
5. Primary biliary cirrhosis

Diagnostic Workup

1. AST/ALT/bilirubin/alkaline phosphatase
2. CBC
3. PT/PTT
4. Viral hepatitis serologies
5. Acetaminophen level
6. U/S—abdomen
7. CT—abdomen
8. MRCP/ERCP

CASE DISCUSSION

Differential Diagnosis

Jaundice results from hyperbilirubinemia, the cause of which may be hepatic or nonhepatic. The presence of a change in stool and urine color excludes unconjugated hyperbilirubinemia (e.g., that associated with hemolysis or Gilbert's syndrome). Thus, the predominantly conjugated hyperbilirubinemia suspected in this patient may be due to hepatocellular disease, drugs, sepsis, hereditary disorders such as Dubin-Johnson syndrome, or extrahepatic biliary obstruction. Cholangitis is ruled out by the absence of fever and chills associated with episodes of abdominal pain.

- **Extrahepatic biliary obstruction:** The patient's family history puts her at increased risk for pancreatic cancer, which classically presents with painless jaundice. However, her intermittent pain (suggesting intermittent biliary obstruction) narrows the differential to choledocholithiasis (stone in the common bile duct), cholangiocarcinoma, carcinoma of the ampulla, or sphincter of Oddi dysfunction.
- **Viral hepatitis:** The patient is at risk for hepatitis A (in light of her trip to Mexico) and chronic hepatitis C (remote blood transfusion). The intermittent nature of her RUQ pain makes acute hepatitis less likely.
- **Acetaminophen liver toxicity:** Suspect this in acute liver injury, and recognize that even moderate amounts of acetaminophen may overwhelm the metabolic capacity of a damaged liver (usually in alcoholics and in patients with chronic hepatitis or cirrhosis).
- **Alcoholic hepatitis:** The patient's symptoms are consistent with this diagnosis. Hepatomegaly is often present. Although she reports drinking only one or two glasses of wine daily, patients often underreport alcohol consumption.
- **Primary biliary cirrhosis:** This usually occurs in women aged 40–60, often with pruritus as a presenting symptom. However, jaundice is usually a late finding and is not associated with RUQ pain.

Diagnostic Workup

- **AST/ALT/bilirubin/alkaline phosphatase:** Can help differentiate a hepatocellular process (primarily associated with increased AST and ALT) from a cholestatic process (primarily associated with increased bilirubin and alkaline phosphatase).
- **CBC:** A low platelet count is often seen in chronic liver disease, due to portal hypertension and subsequent splenomegaly.
- **PT/PTT:** A coagulopathy is often seen in advanced liver disease, due to synthetic dysfunction and subsequent clotting factor deficiencies.
- **Viral hepatitis serologies:** Check hepatitis A IgM antibody to document recent infection. Other screening tests include hepatitis B surface antigen and hepatitis C antibody.
- **Acetaminophen level:** To diagnose acetaminophen overdose.
- **U/S—abdomen:** Used to diagnose biliary obstruction, stones, or intrahepatic tumors.
- **CT—abdomen:** A CT scan provides information similar to that above but is more expensive.
- **MRCP/ERCP:** Can identify the cause, location, and extent of biliary obstruction. ERCP is invasive but has the advantage of being both a diagnostic and a therapeutic tool in many cases. MRCP is a noninvasive MRI-based diagnostic substitute.

Opening Scenario

Virginia Black, a 65-year-old female, comes to the clinic complaining of forgetfulness and confusion.

Vital Signs

BP: 135/90 mmHg
Temp: 98.0°F (36.7°C)
RR: 16/minute
HR: 76/minute, regular

Examinee Tasks

1. Take a focused history.
2. Perform a focused physical exam (do not perform rectal, genitourinary, or female breast exam).
3. Explain your clinical impression and workup plan to the patient.
4. Write the patient note after leaving the room.

Checklist/SP Sheet

PATIENT DESCRIPTION

Patient is a 65 yo F, widowed with one daughter.

NOTES FOR THE SP

- The examinee will name three objects for you and ask you to recall them after a few minutes. Pretend that you are unable to do so.
- If asked, give the examinee a list of your current medications (a piece of paper with "nitroglycerin patch, hydrochlorothiazide, and aspirin" written on it).
- Pretend that you have some weakness in your left arm.
- Show an increase in DTRs of the left arm and leg.

CHALLENGING QUESTIONS TO ASK

"Do you think I have Alzheimer's disease?"

SAMPLE EXAMINEE RESPONSE

"I don't know; we still need to do more testing. Tell me what you know about Alzheimer's disease."

Examinee Checklist

ENTRANCE:

☐ Examinee knocked on the door before entering.
☐ Examinee introduced self by name.

- ☐ Examinee identified his/her role or position.
- ☐ Examinee correctly used patient's name.
- ☐ Examinee made eye contact with the SP.

HISTORY:

- ☐ Examinee showed compassion for your illness.

☑ Question	Patient Response
☐ Chief complaint	Difficulty remembering things.
☐ Onset	I can't remember exactly, but my daughter told me that I started forgetting last year.
☐ Progression	My daughter has told me that it is getting worse.
☐ Things that are difficult to remember	Turning off the stove, my phone number, my keys, the way to my home, the names of my friends.
☐ Daily activities (bathing, feeding, toileting, dressing, transferring into and out of chairs and bed)	I have some trouble with these, and I need help sometimes.
☐ Shopping	Well, I stopped shopping, since I've lost my way home so many times. My daughter shops for me.
☐ Cooking	I stopped cooking because I often left the stove on and accidentally started a fire once.
☐ Housework	I live with my daughter, but I keep forgetting where I put my stuff.
☐ Paying the bills	My daughter does this for me.
☐ Gait problems	No.
☐ Urinary incontinence	No.
☐ Feeling (sad, depressed)	I feel upset because of all of this.
☐ Difficulty sleeping	No.
☐ Headaches	No.
☐ Lightheadedness or feeling faint	Only if I stand up too quickly.
☐ Passing out	No.
☐ Falls	Yes, sometimes.
☐ Head trauma	I think so; I had a large bruise on the side of my head a while back.
☐ Did you see a doctor for that fall?	No, it was just a bruise.
☐ Any shaking or seizures	No.
☐ Visual changes	No.
☐ Weakness/numbness/paresthesias	Yes, I have weakness in my left arm from a stroke I had a long time ago.
☐ Speech difficulties	No.

☑ Question	Patient Response
☐ Heart problems	I had a heart attack a long time ago.
☐ Chest pain, shortness of breath, abdominal pain, nausea/vomiting, diarrhea/constipation	No.
☐ Weight changes	I've lost weight. I don't know how much.
☐ Appetite changes	I don't have an appetite.
☐ High blood pressure	Yes, for a long time.
☐ Current medications	I don't know their names. (Give the list to the examinee if he asks for it.)
☐ Past medical history	I think that's enough, isn't it?
☐ Past surgical history	I had a bowel obstruction a long time ago, and they removed part of my intestine.
☐ Family history	My father and mother died healthy a long time ago.
☐ Occupation	I retired after the death of my husband.
☐ Alcohol use	No.
☐ Illicit drug use	No.
☐ Tobacco	No.
☐ Social history	I live with my daughter.
☐ Sexual activity	Not since the death of my husband one year ago.
☐ Support systems (family, friends)	I have many friends who care about me, besides my daughter.
☐ Drug allergies	No.

Physical Examination:

☐ Examinee washed his/her hands.
☐ Examinee asked permission to start the exam.
☐ Examinee used respectful draping.
☐ Examinee did not repeat painful maneuvers.

☑ Exam Component	Maneuver
☐ Eye exam	Inspected pupils, fundus
☐ Neck exam	Carotid auscultation
☐ CV exam	Auscultation, orthostatic vital signs
☐ Pulmonary exam	Auscultation
☐ Abdominal exam	Palpation
☐ Neurologic exam	Mini-mental status exam, cranial nerves, motor exam, DTRs, gait, Romberg sign, sensory exam

Closure:

- ☐ Examinee discussed initial diagnostic impressions.
- ☐ Examinee discussed initial management plans:
    - ☐ Follow-up tests.
    - ☐ Need to obtain history directly from other family members.
    - ☐ Need to evaluate home safety and supervision.
    - ☐ Community resources that help the patient at home.
    - ☐ Offered support throughout her illness.
- ☐ Examinee asked if the patient has any other questions or concerns.

Sample Closure:

Mrs. Black, the symptoms you are having can be due to a number of disorders that can affect the brain, many of which are treatable. We need to run some tests in order to pinpoint the cause of your problem. I would also like to ask your permission to speak with your family. They can help me with your diagnosis, and I can answer any questions they might have about what is happening to you and how they can help. I would also like you and your family to meet with the social worker in order to assess your situation at home in terms of adequate supervision and home-safety measures. The social worker will inform you of all the resources that are available in the community to help people in your situation. If you would like, I can remain in close contact with you and your family to provide help and support. Do you have any questions for me?

PATIENT NOTE

History

Physical Examination

Differential Diagnosis

1.

2.

3.

4.

5.

Diagnostic Workup

1.

2.

3.

4.

5.

PATIENT NOTE

History

HPI: *65 yo F c/o difficulty remembering that started 1 year ago after the death of her husband and is getting progressively worse. This problem has affected her daily activities (bathing, feeding, toileting, dressing, transferring into and out of chairs and bed, shopping, cooking, managing money, using the telephone, cleaning the house). She has transient orthostatic lightheadedness and frequent falls, including at least 1 head injury for which she did not seek medical attention. The patient feels upset because of her difficulty. She has weight loss and no appetite. She denies headache, visual changes, gait problems, difficulty sleeping, or urinary incontinence.*
ROS: *Residual weakness in left arm after a stroke.*
Allergies: *NKDA.*
Medications: *HCTZ, aspirin, transdermal nitroglycerin.*
PMH: *Hypertension, stroke, MI. The patient cannot remember exactly when she had them.*
PSH: *Partial bowel resection due to obstruction many years ago.*
SH: *No smoking, no EtOH, no illicit drugs. She is a widow, is retired, lives with her daughter, and has a good support system (family, friends).*
FH: *Noncontributory.*

Physical Examination

Patient is in no acute distress.
VS: *WNL, no orthostatic changes.*
HEENT: *Normocephalic, atraumatic, PERRLA, no funduscopic abnormalities.*
Neck: *Supple, no carotid bruits.*
Chest: *Clear breath sounds bilaterally.*
Heart: *RRR; normal S1/S2; no murmurs, rubs, or gallops.*
Abdomen: *Soft, nondistended, nontender, no hepatosplenomegaly.*
Neuro: Mental status: *Alert and oriented × 3, spells backward but can't recall 3 objects.* Cranial nerves: *2–12 intact.* Motor: *Strength 5/5 in all muscle groups except 3/5 in left arm.* DTRs: *Asymmetric 3+ in left upper and lower extremities, 1+ in the right, ⊖Babinski bilaterally.* Cerebellar: *⊖Romberg.* Gait: *Normal.* Sensation: *Intact to pinprick and soft touch.*

Differential Diagnosis

1. Alzheimer's disease
2. Vascular ("multi-infarct") dementia
3. Depression with pseudodementia
4. Hypothyroidism
5. Vitamin B_{12} deficiency
6. Subdural hematoma

Diagnostic Workup

1. CBC
2. Electrolytes, calcium, glucose, BUN/Cr
4. Serum B_{12}, TSH, RPR
5. CT—head or MRI—brain
6. EEG or SPECT

CASE DISCUSSION

Differential Diagnosis

Dementia is an acquired, progressive impairment in cognitive function that includes amnesia plus some degree of aphasia, apraxia, agnosia, and/or impaired executive function. It is critical to obtain additional history from nondemented family members in order to establish an accurate time course of cognitive decline. The dementia syndromes are primarily clinical diagnoses reached after any partially reversible causes have been excluded.

- **Alzheimer's disease:** This is the most common cause of dementia. It usually has an insidious onset, with steady, progressive decline in cognitive function over years. The earliest findings are impairment in memory and visuospatial abilities. Alzheimer's disease is a clinical diagnosis.
- **Vascular ("multi-infarct") dementia:** This often coexists with Alzheimer's disease, and given the patient's history of atherosclerotic vascular disease (e.g., stroke, MI), it could certainly be contributing in this case. There is classically more of a stepwise deterioration in vascular dementia compared to the steady cognitive decline seen in Alzheimer's. Also, there may be an earlier loss of executive function and personality changes in vascular dementia.
- **Depression with pseudodementia:** The time course of cognitive decline following the death of the patient's husband may indicate depression, which can present atypically in the elderly and may mimic or, more commonly, coexist with dementia. However, it is more likely that her cognitive decline has been progressive for several years but became more noticeable to her children after her husband died.
- **Hypothyroidism:** This can cause neuropsychiatric symptoms (often a late finding) and must be ruled out in patients with dementia. However, there are no classic signs or symptoms to suggest hypothyroidism in this case.
- **Vitamin B_{12} deficiency:** A prior bowel resection (e.g., of the terminal ileum) may put the patient at risk for this deficiency. It can cause depression, irritability, paranoia, confusion, and dementia but is usually associated with other neurologic symptoms, such as paresthesias and leg weakness. On occasion, dementia may precede the characteristic megaloblastic anemia.
- **Subdural hematoma:** This should be ruled out given the patient's history of falls and head trauma. Even though her cognitive decline spans at least a year, it is possible that a comorbid chronic subdural hematoma could have exacerbated her mental status changes in recent weeks or months.

Diagnostic Workup

- **CBC:** To look for macrocytic anemia in vitamin B_{12} deficiency.
- **Electrolytes, calcium, glucose, BUN/Cr:** To screen for medical conditions that can present with cognitive dysfunction (e.g., hypernatremia, hypercalcemia, hyperglycemia, uremia).
- **Serum B_{12}, TSH, RPR:** To screen for partially reversible causes of dementia (the latter can be restricted to patients manifesting signs of neurosyphilis).
- **CT−head:** To look for a crescent-shaped, hyperdense extra-axial mass in subdural hematoma, intracerebral masses, strokes, or dilated ventricles (as in normal pressure hydrocephalus).
- **MRI−brain:** The most sensitive exam to look for focal CNS lesions or atrophy.
- **EEG or SPECT:** Used in rare cases to help differentiate delirium from depression or dementia.

Opening Scenario

Raymond Stern, a 56-year-old male, comes to the clinic for diabetes follow-up.

Vital Signs

BP: 139/85 mmHg
Temp: 98.0°F (36.7°C)
RR: 15/minute
HR: 75/minute, regular

Examinee Tasks

1. Take a focused history.
2. Perform a focused physical exam (do not perform rectal, genitourinary, or female breast exam).
3. Explain your clinical impression and workup plan to the patient.
4. Write the patient note after leaving the room.

Checklist/SP Sheet

PATIENT DESCRIPTION

Patient is a 56 yo M.

NOTES FOR THE SP

- Pretend that you have a loss of sharp and dull sensations, vibration sense, and position sense in both feet ("stocking" distribution).
- Pretend to have a normal knee jerk and absent ankle reflex.

CHALLENGING QUESTIONS TO ASK

"Will I lose my feet, doctor?"

SAMPLE EXAMINEE RESPONSE

"Not if we continue to keep your blood sugars and cholesterol well controlled. The nerve damage to your feet is uncomfortable but alone will not lead to amputation as long as you take the proper measures to protect your feet from injury. We'll discuss how to do that later in the visit."

Examinee Checklist

ENTRANCE:

☐ Examinee knocked on the door before entering.
☐ Examinee introduced self by name.
☐ Examinee identified his/her role or position.
☐ Examinee correctly used patient's name.
☐ Examinee made eye contact with the SP.

HISTORY:

☐ Examinee showed compassion for your illness.

☑ Question	Patient Response
☐ Chief complaint	I am here for a diabetes checkup. The last time I saw my doctor was six months ago.
☐ Onset	I have had diabetes mellitus for the last 25 years.
☐ Treatment	NPH insulin, 20 units in the morning and 15 units in the evening.
☐ Compliance with medications	I never miss any doses.
☐ Last blood sugar reading	Three days ago, and it was 135.
☐ Blood sugar monitoring	I have a blood sugar monitor at home, and I check my blood sugar twice a week. It usually ranges between 120 and 145.
☐ Last HbA$_{1c}$	The last was six months ago, and it was 7.
☐ Last time eyes were checked	One year ago, and there were no signs of diabetic eye disease.
☐ How he is feeling today	Good.
☐ Medication side effects	No.
☐ Heart symptoms (chest pain, palpitations)	Sometimes I feel my heart racing, and I start sweating.
☐ Description of these symptoms	It happens rarely if I miss a meal. I feel better after drinking orange juice.
☐ Pulmonary complaints (shortness of breath, cough)	No.
☐ Neurologic complaints (headaches, dizziness, weakness, numbness)	I have tingling and numbness in my feet all the time, especially at night; it's gotten worse over the past two months.
☐ Polyuria, dysuria, hematuria	No.
☐ Abdominal complaints (pain, dyspepsia, nausea)	No.
☐ Change in bowel habits	No.
☐ Visual problems (blurred vision)	No.
☐ Foot infection	No.
☐ Marital or work problems	No, my wife is great, and I am very happy in my job.
☐ Feelings of anxiety or stress	No.
☐ Weight changes	No.
☐ Appetite changes	No.
☐ Hypertension	No.
☐ History of hypercholesterolemia	Yes, it was diagnosed two years ago.
☐ Previous heart problems	I had a heart attack last year.
☐ History of TIA or stroke	No.

☑ Question	Patient Response
☐ Current medications	Insulin, lovastatin, aspirin, atenolol.
☐ Past medical history	Heart attack last year; high cholesterol for two years.
☐ Past surgical history	None.
☐ Family history	My father died at age 60 of a stroke. My mother is healthy.
☐ Occupation	Clerk.
☐ Diet	I eat everything that my wife cooks—meat, vegetables, etc. I don't follow any special diet.
☐ Exercise	No.
☐ Alcohol use	Yes, whiskey on the weekends.
☐ CAGE questions	No (to all four).
☐ Illicit drug use	No.
☐ Tobacco	No.
☐ Social history	I am married and live with my wife.
☐ Sexual activity	I am not doing my job the way I used to, but my wife understands and is supportive. They told me it is the diabetes. Is it?
☐ Type of sexual problem	I can't get it up, doc. I don't even wake up with erections anymore.
☐ Libido	Good.
☐ Duration	One or two years ago.
☐ Feelings of depression	No.
☐ Drug allergies	No.

Physical Examination:

- ☐ Examinee washed his/her hands.
- ☐ Examinee asked permission to start the exam.
- ☐ Examinee used respectful draping.
- ☐ Examinee did not repeat painful maneuvers.

☑ Exam Component	Maneuver
☐ Eye exam	Funduscopic exam
☐ Neck exam	Carotid auscultation
☐ CV exam	Palpation, auscultation
☐ Pulmonary exam	Auscultation
☐ Abdominal exam	Auscultation, palpation, percussion

☑ **Exam Component**	**Maneuver**
☐ Extremities	Inspected feet, peripheral pulses
☐ Neurologic exam	DTRs, Babinski's sign, sensation and strength in lower extremities

Closure:

☐ Examinee discussed initial diagnostic impressions.
☐ Examinee discussed initial management plans:
    ☐ Follow-up tests.
    ☐ Lifestyle modification (diet, exercise).
☐ Examinee asked if the patient has any other questions or concerns.

Sample Closure:

Mr. Stern, the palpitations and sweating you have experienced may be due to episodes of low blood sugar, which may have resulted from a higher-than-normal dose of insulin or from skipping or delaying meals. The numbness you describe in your feet is probably related to the effect of diabetes on your nervous system; better control of your blood sugar may help improve this problem. There are many factors, including diabetes, that can cause the erection difficulties you describe. I will need to perform an examination of your genital area and run some blood tests, and at some point we may also need to conduct some more complex tests to identify the cause of your problems. Do you have any questions for me?

PATIENT NOTE

History

Physical Examination

Differential Diagnosis

1.

2.

3.

4.

5.

Diagnostic Workup

1.

2.

3.

4.

5.

History

HPI: *56 yo M presents for diabetes follow-up. He has had diabetes mellitus for the last 25 years, treated with insulin. He is compliant with his medications and monitors his blood glucose level twice a week, with readings ranging between 120 and 145. His last HbA_{1c} 6 months ago was 7%. He occasionally has episodes of palpitations and diaphoresis that occur after missing meals and resolve after drinking orange juice. He also has tingling and numbness in his feet all the time, especially at night, worsening over the last 2 months. No weight or appetite changes. Does not follow any special diet. Also notes loss of erections for 2 years.*
ROS: *Negative except as above.*
Allergies: *NKDA.*
Medications: *Lovastatin, NPH insulin, aspirin, atenolol.*
PMH: *Hypercholesterolemia diagnosed 2 years ago; MI 1 year ago.*
PSH: *None.*
SH: *No smoking, drinks whiskey on weekends (CAGE 0/4), no illicit drugs. Works as a clerk. He is married and lives with his wife.*
FH: *Father died of a stroke at age 60.*

Physical Examination

Patient is in no distress.
VS: *WNL.*
HEENT: *PERRLA, no funduscopic abnormalities.*
Neck: *No carotid bruits, no JVD.*
Chest: *Clear breath sounds bilaterally.*
Heart: *Apical impulse not displaced; RRR; normal S1/S2; no murmurs, rubs, or gallops.*
Abdomen: *Soft, nondistended, nontender, ⊕BS, no bruits, no organomegaly.*
Extremities: *No edema, no skin breakdown, 2+ dorsalis pedis pulses.*
Neuro: *Motor: Strength 5/5 in bilateral lower extremities. DTRs: Symmetric 2+ knee jerks, absent ankle jerks and ⊖Babinski bilaterally. Sensation: Decreased pinprick; soft touch, vibratory, and position sense in bilateral lower extremities.*

Differential Diagnosis

1. Insulin-induced hypoglycemia
2. Peripheral neuropathy:
   Diabetic peripheral neuropathy
   Alcoholic peripheral neuropathy
3. Multiple myeloma
4. Diabetic autonomic neuropathy, vascular disease, or medication-induced erectile dysfunction

Diagnostic Workup

1. Genital exam
2. Serum glucose, HbA_{1c}
3. UA, urine microalbumin, BUN/Cr
4. CBC, SPEP
5. Doppler U/S—penis
6. Nerve conduction studies

CASE DISCUSSION

Differential Diagnosis

- **Insulin-induced hypoglycemia:** The patient's history suggests episodes of hypoglycemia. Typical signs and symptoms of hypoglycemia include sweating, tachycardia, palpitations, tremor, anxiety, weakness, confusion, and seizures. Maintaining tight glycemic control may occasionally result in hypoglycemia, and patients should be educated about how to recognize and treat this complication.
- **Peripheral neuropathy:** The differential for peripheral neuropathy includes hereditary, toxic, metabolic, infectious, inflammatory, and paraneoplastic disorders. No specific cause is determined in up to 50% of cases. The history and exam guide us to some of the common causes discussed below.
    - **Diabetic peripheral neuropathy:** Involvement of the peripheral nervous system in diabetes may lead to symmetric sensory or mixed polyneuropathy (among other patterns of neuropathy). Burning foot paresthesias that are worse at night and loss of ankle reflexes, as seen in this case, are classic.
    - **Alcoholic peripheral neuropathy:** This causes a distal sensorimotor polyneuropathy marked by painful leg paresthesias and is directly attributable to alcohol or to associated nutritional deficiencies (e.g., thiamine and vitamin B_{12}).
- **Multiple myeloma:** Myeloma or other paraproteinemias must be ruled out in a patient with peripheral neuropathy.
- **Erectile dysfunction:** In diabetics, this is usually related to vascular disease, autonomic neuropathy, or medications (e.g., antihypertensives) for associated conditions. In general, impotence unaccompanied by loss of libido suggests either a vascular or a neurologic cause. Alcohol also causes an autonomic neuropathy and may contribute to erectile dysfunction.

Diagnostic Workup

- **Genital exam:** To rule out Peyronie's disease (e.g., penile scarring or plaque formation).
- **Serum glucose, HbA$_{1c}$:** To assess glycemic control.
- **UA, urine microalbumin, BUN/Cr:** To screen for diabetic nephropathy.
- **CBC, SPEP:** To detect paraproteinemias (e.g., multiple myeloma); anemia is often associated.
- **Doppler U/S—penis:** A helpful noninvasive test to measure penile blood flow.
- **Nerve conduction studies:** To confirm that symptoms arise from a peripheral nerve origin and to indicate an axonal vs. demyelinating mechanism.
- **Other studies:** In select cases, other studies useful in evaluating peripheral neuropathy include ESR, BUN/Cr, TSH, liver enzymes, RF, ANA, hepatitis B and C serologies, RPR, HIV antibody, urine heavy metal screen, CSF exam, CXR, and cutaneous nerve biopsy (e.g., to diagnose amyloidosis).

Opening Scenario

Edward Albright, a 53-year-old male, comes to the ER complaining of dizziness.

Vital Signs

BP: 135/90 mmHg
Temp: 98.0°F (36.7°C)
RR: 16/minute
HR: 76/minute, regular

Examinee Tasks

1. Take a focused history.
2. Perform a focused physical exam (do not perform rectal, genitourinary, or female breast exam).
3. Explain your clinical impression and workup plan to the patient.
4. Write the patient note after leaving the room.

Checklist/SP Sheet

PATIENT DESCRIPTION

Patient is a 53 yo M, married with three children.

NOTES FOR THE SP

- Ask the examinee to speak loudly. Pretend that you have difficulty hearing in your left ear and that you hear him better when he talks close to your right ear.
- Refuse to walk if the examinee asks you to. Pretend that you are afraid of falling down. Walk only if the examinee explains why he would like to see your gait.

CHALLENGING QUESTIONS TO ASK

None.

Examinee Checklist

ENTRANCE:

☐ Examinee knocked on the door before entering.
☐ Examinee introduced self by name.
☐ Examinee identified his/her role or position.
☐ Examinee correctly used patient's name.
☐ Examinee made eye contact with the SP.

HISTORY:

☐ Examinee showed compassion for your illness.

☑ Question	Patient Response
☐ Chief complaint	I feel dizzy.
☐ Describe the meaning of dizziness	Well, I feel as if the room were spinning around me.
☐ Onset	Two days ago.
☐ Progression	It is getting worse.
☐ Constant/intermittent	It comes and goes.
☐ Duration	It lasts for 20–30 minutes.
☐ Timing	It can happen anytime.
☐ Positions that can elicit the dizziness (lying down, sitting, standing up)	When I get up from bed or lie down to sleep, but as I said, it can happen anytime.
☐ Positions that can relieve the dizziness	None.
☐ Tinnitus	No.
☐ Hearing loss (which ear, when)	Yes, I have difficulty hearing you in my left ear. This started yesterday.
☐ Fullness or pressure in the ears	No.
☐ Discharge from the ears	No.
☐ Falls	No, sometimes I feel unsteady as if I were going to fall down, but I don't fall.
☐ Nausea/vomiting	Yes, I feel nauseated, and I vomited several times.
☐ Recent infections	I have had really bad diarrhea. I've had it for the past three days, but it is much better today.
☐ Fever	No.
☐ Description of stool	It was a watery diarrhea with no blood.
☐ Abdominal pain	No.
☐ URI (runny nose, sore throat, cough)	No.
☐ Headaches	No.
☐ Head trauma	No.
☐ Current medications	Furosemide, captopril.
☐ Past medical history	High blood pressure, diagnosed seven years ago.
☐ Past surgical history	Appendectomy.
☐ Family history	No similar problem in the family.
☐ Occupation	Executive director of an insurance company.
☐ Alcohol use	Yes, I drink 2–3 beers a week.
☐ Illicit drug use	No.
☐ Tobacco	No.
☐ Sexual activity	Yes, with my wife.
☐ Drug allergies	No.

Physical Examination:

☐ Examinee washed his/her hands.
☐ Examinee asked permission to start the exam.
☐ Examinee used respectful draping.
☐ Examinee did not repeat painful maneuvers.

☑ Exam Component	Maneuver
☐ HEENT	Inspected for nystagmus, funduscopic exam, otoscopy, assessed hearing, Rinne and Weber tests, inspected mouth and throat
☐ CV exam	Auscultation, orthostatic vital signs
☐ Neurologic exam	Cranial nerves, motor exam, DTRs, gait, Romberg sign, tilt test (e.g., Dix-Hallpike maneuver)

Closure:

☐ Examinee discussed initial diagnostic impressions.
☐ Examinee discussed initial management plans:
   ☐ Follow-up tests.
☐ Examinee asked if the patient has any other questions or concerns.

Sample Closure:

Mr. Albright, the dizziness you are experiencing may be due to a problem in your ears or brain, or it may result from low blood pressure. We will have to run some tests in order to pinpoint the source of your symptoms. These may include some blood tests, a hearing evaluation, and an MRI that will yield detailed images of your brain. Until we find the cause of your problem, it is important that you be careful when you stand up quickly or walk unaccompanied, and you should be sure to make use of hand railings whenever possible. Do you have any questions for me?

PATIENT NOTE

History

Physical Examination

Differential Diagnosis

1.

2.

3.

4.

5.

Diagnostic Workup

1.

2.

3.

4.

5.

History

HPI: 53 yo M c/o intermittent dizziness that started 2 days ago. He feels the room spinning around him. The episodes occur at any time during the day, especially when he gets up from bed or lies down to sleep. They last for 20–30 minutes and are getting progressively worse. He has hearing loss in his left ear that started yesterday. He denies tinnitus, fullness in the ear, discharge, headache, or head trauma. No recent URI. He recalls having watery, nonbloody diarrhea over the past 3 days that resolved today.

ROS: Nausea and vomiting.
Allergies: NKDA.
Medications: Furosemide, captopril.
PMH: Hypertension, diagnosed 7 years ago.
PSH: Appendectomy.
SH: No smoking, 2–3 beers/week, no illicit drugs.
FH: Noncontributory.

Physical Examination

Patient is in no acute distress.
VS: WNL, no orthostatic changes.
HEENT: NC/AT, PERRLA, EOMI without nystagmus, no papilledema, no cerumen, TMs normal, mouth and oropharynx normal.
Heart: RRR; normal S1/S2; no murmurs, rubs, or gallops.
Neuro: Cranial nerves: 2–12 grossly intact except for decreased hearing acuity in the left ear. ⊕Rinne (air conduction > bone conduction on the left), Weber no lateralization, ⊖tilt test. Motor: Strength 5/5 throughout. DTRs: 2+ intact, symmetric, ⊖Babinski bilaterally. Cerebellar: ⊖Romberg, finger to nose normal. Gait: Normal.

Differential Diagnosis

1. Ménière's disease
2. Orthostatic hypotension due to dehydration
3. Benign paroxysmal positional vertigo
4. Labyrinthitis
5. Perilymphatic fistula
6. Acoustic neuroma

Diagnostic Workup

1. Dix-Hallpike maneuver
2. VDRL/RPR
3. Audiometry
4. MRI—brain
5. Brain stem auditory evoked potentials
6. Electronystagmography

CASE DISCUSSION

Differential Diagnosis

Vertigo signals vestibular disease, whereas lightheadedness and dysequilibrium are usually nonvestibular in origin. A central vestibular system lesion (e.g., vertebrobasilar insufficiency, brain stem and cerebellar tumors, MS) is unlikely in this patient given the presence of hearing loss and an otherwise normal neurologic exam. Vertigo syndromes due to peripheral lesions are discussed below. These cases are often accompanied by nausea and vomiting, and vertigo may be so severe that the patient is unable to walk or stand.

- **Ménière's disease:** This classically presents with episodic vertigo (usually lasting 1–8 hours) and low-frequency hearing loss as well as with features not seen in this case, such as tinnitus and a sensation of aural fullness. Symptoms result from distention of the endolymphatic compartment of the inner ear. Syphilis and head trauma are two known causes.
- **Orthostatic hypotension due to dehydration:** Risk factors for dehydration in this case include diarrhea and loop diuretic use. However, the patient does not complain of lightheadedness and is not objectively orthostatic.
- **Benign paroxysmal positional vertigo (BPPV):** This describes transient vertigo following changes in head position but is not associated with hearing loss.
- **Labyrinthitis:** This frequently follows a viral infection (usually URI) and is accompanied by hearing loss and tinnitus, but vertigo is usually continuous and lasts several days to a week.
- **Perilymphatic fistula:** This is a rare cause of vertigo and sensorineural hearing loss, usually resulting from head trauma or extensive barotrauma. Episodes of vertigo are fleeting, generally lasting seconds.
- **Acoustic neuroma:** Acoustic neuroma more commonly causes continuous dysequilibrium rather than episodic vertigo. As noted above, central lesions are unlikely in patients with vertigo, hearing loss, and an otherwise normal neurologic exam. However, an intracranial mass lesion must be ruled out in any patient with unilateral hearing loss.

Diagnostic Workup

- **Dix-Hallpike maneuver:** Used to diagnose BPPV (look for nystagmus, reproduction of vertigo).
- **VDRL/RPR:** To rule out syphilis, which can cause Ménière's disease.
- **Audiometry:** Useful to assess hearing function.
- **MRI—brain:** Required for the evaluation of central vestibular lesions.
- **Brain stem auditory evoked potentials:** Useful to help diagnose central vestibular disease.
- **Electronystagmography:** Useful to document characteristics of nystagmus that may differentiate central from peripheral vestibular system lesions.

Opening Scenario

Gary Mitchell, a 46-year-old male, comes to the office complaining of fatigue.

Vital Signs

BP: 120/85 mmHg
Temp: 98.2°F (36.8°C)
RR: 12/minute
HR: 65/minute, regular

Examinee Tasks

1. Take a focused history.
2. Perform a focused physical exam (do not perform rectal, genitourinary, or female breast exam).
3. Explain your clinical impression and workup plan to the patient.
4. Write the patient note after leaving the room.

Checklist/SP Sheet

PATIENT DESCRIPTION
Patient is a 46 yo M.

NOTES FOR THE SP

- Look sad, and don't smile.
- Speak and move slowly.
- Start yawning as the examinee enters the room.

CHALLENGING QUESTIONS TO ASK

- "I think that life is full of misery. Why do we have to live?"
- "I am afraid that I might have AIDS."

SAMPLE EXAMINEE RESPONSE

This patient clearly has more to say. Silence is appropriate here, or some small encouragement for the patient to continue talking. Alternatively, say, "It sounds as if you're losing hope. Have you thought about hurting yourself or tried to do so?" Or "Tell me more about your concern about AIDS."

Examinee Checklist

ENTRANCE:

☐ Examinee knocked on the door before entering.
☐ Examinee introduced self by name.
☐ Examinee identified his/her role or position.

☐ Examinee correctly used patient's name.
☐ Examinee made eye contact with the SP.

HISTORY:

☐ Examinee showed compassion for your illness.
☐ Examinee explored the patient's concern for AIDS (e.g., "Tell me more about that").

☑ Question	Patient Response
☐ Chief complaint	Feeling tired, no energy.
☐ Onset	Three months ago.
☐ Associated events	We had a car accident, and I failed to save my friend from the car before it blew up.
☐ Injuries related to the accident	No.
☐ Progression of the fatigue during the day	Same throughout the day.
☐ Affecting job/performance	Yes, I can't concentrate on my work anymore. I don't have the energy to work.
☐ Appetite changes	Loss of appetite.
☐ Weight changes	I have gained six pounds over the past three months.
☐ Feeling of depression	Yes, I feel sad and depressed all the time.
☐ Suicidal thoughts/plans/attempts	I think of death sometimes but have had no plans or attempts.
☐ Feelings of blame or guilt	No, it was an accident. I tried to help my friend but couldn't.
☐ Sleeping problems (falling asleep, staying asleep, early waking)	Well, I don't have problems falling asleep, but I wake up sometimes because of nightmares. I always see the accident, my friend calling for help, and the car blowing up. I feel so scared and helpless. I wake up very early in the morning and feel sleepy all day.
☐ Snoring	Yes.
☐ Loss of concentration	Yes, I can't concentrate on my work.
☐ Associated symptoms (fever, chills, chest pain, shortness of breath, abdominal pain, diarrhea/constipation)	No.
☐ Cold intolerance	Yes.
☐ Skin/hair changes	My hair is falling out more than usual.
☐ Current medications	None.
☐ Past medical history	Well, I had some burning during urination. I don't really remember the diagnosis that the doctor reached, but it started with the letter C. I took antibiotics for one week. This was five months ago.
☐ Past surgical history	None.
☐ Family history	My parents are alive and in good health.
☐ Occupation	Accountant.

☑ Question	Patient Response
☐ Alcohol use	Two to three beers a month.
☐ Illicit drug use	Never.
☐ Tobacco	One pack a day for 25 years.
☐ Exercise	No.
☐ Diet	The usual. I haven't changed anything in my diet in more than 10 years.
☐ Sexual activity	Not interested anymore. I have a girlfriend, and we have been together for the last six months. I don't use condoms because they make me feel uncomfortable. I have had several sexual partners in the past.
☐ Drug allergies	No.

Physical Examination:

☐ Examinee washed his/her hands.
☐ Examinee asked permission to start the exam.
☐ Examinee used respectful draping.
☐ Examinee did not repeat painful maneuvers.

☑ Exam Component	Maneuver
☐ Head and neck exam	Inspected conjunctivae, mouth and throat, lymph nodes; examined thyroid gland
☐ CV exam	Auscultation
☐ Pulmonary exam	Auscultation
☐ Abdominal exam	Auscultation, palpation, percussion
☐ Extremities	Inspection, checked DTRs

Closure:

☐ Examinee discussed initial diagnostic impressions.
☐ Examinee discussed initial management plans:
    ☐ Diagnostic tests.
    ☐ Lifestyle modification (diet, exercise, relaxation techniques, smoking cessation).
    ☐ Discussed safe sex practices.
    ☐ Discussed HIV testing and consent.
    ☐ Depression counseling:
        ☐ Helped the patient identify sources of support (e.g., trusted friends and loved ones) and provided information about community groups.
        ☐ Discussed the possible need for referral to a psychiatrist.
        ☐ Suicide contract (contact your physician or go to the ER for any suicidal thoughts or plans).
☐ Examinee asked if the patient has any other questions or concerns.

Sample Closure:

Mr. Mitchell, it would appear that your life has been very stressful lately, and my suspicion is that you may be clinically depressed. Before I make a definitive diagnosis, however, I would like to order some blood tests, including one for HIV, as you have risk factors for sexually transmitted diseases. Depending on the results of these tests, I may also ask you to participate in a study in which you fall asleep for a short time within a laboratory so that doctors can observe how you breathe while you are sleeping. Once we have completed these tests, we should have a better idea of what is causing your fatigue. In the meantime, I would strongly recommend that you quit smoking, exercise regularly, and participate in activities that you find relaxing. I would also like you to promise me that if you feel like hurting yourself, you will call someone who can help you or go immediately to an emergency department. Do you have any questions for me?

PATIENT NOTE

History

Physical Examination

Differential Diagnosis

1.

2.

3.

4.

5.

Diagnostic Workup

1.

2.

3.

4.

5.

History

HPI: 46 yo M c/o fatigue. The patient notes that this fatigue began 3 months ago, following an unsuccessful attempt to save his friend after a car accident. The fatigue is constant throughout the day. He has low energy and decreased ability to concentrate, which have adversely affected his job as an accountant. Over the past 3 months, the patient had a decrease in appetite but gained 6 pounds. He feels sleepy throughout the day, wakes up early in the morning, and has difficulty staying asleep because of recurrent nightmares about the accident. He also reports snoring. The patient can't tolerate cold weather and complains of hair loss. He denies constipation. He has lost his interest in sex and admits to being depressed and helpless, with suicidal thoughts but no plans or attempts. The patient denies feelings of blame or guilt.

ROS: Negative except as above.

Allergies: NKDA.

Medications: None.

PMH: Urethritis (possibly chlamydia), treated 5 months ago.

SH: One PPD for 25 years, 2 beers/month. History of unprotected sex with multiple female partners.

FH: Noncontributory.

Physical Examination

Patient is in no acute distress, looks tired with a flat affect, speaks and moves slowly.

VS: WNL.

HEENT: No conjunctival pallor, mouth and pharynx WNL.

Neck: No lymphadenopathy, thyroid normal.

Chest: Clear breath sounds bilaterally.

Heart: RRR; normal S1/S2; no murmurs, rubs, or gallops.

Abdomen: Soft, nondistended, nontender, ⊕BS, no hepatosplenomegaly.

Extremities: No edema, normal DTRs in lower extremities.

Differential Diagnosis

1. Depression
2. Adjustment disorder with depressed mood
3. Hypothyroidism
4. Obstructive sleep apnea
5. Post-traumatic stress disorder
6. HIV infection

Diagnostic Workup

1. CBC
2. TSH
3. Ambulatory nocturnal pulse oximetry
4. Polysomnography
5. HIV antibody
6. MRI—brain

CASE DISCUSSION

Differential Diagnosis

Fatigue is a common, nonspecific complaint with many etiologies, from simple overexertion to serious diseases such as cancer.

- **Depression:** Many classic symptoms are present in this patient. The mnemonic **SIG EM CAPS** helps recall them: Sleep disturbance, decreased Interest, feelings of Guilt, decreased Energy, depressed Mood, decreased Concentration, change in Appetite, Psychomotor agitation or slowing, and Suicidal ideation.
- **Adjustment disorder with depressed mood:** The stress of witnessing a friend's death may lead to maladaptive behavior, with depression as the predominant symptom.
- **Hypothyroidism:** This should be ruled out in a patient with fatigue for months. The cold intolerance, hair loss, and weight gain are additional nonspecific symptoms that suggest this diagnosis.
- **Obstructive sleep apnea:** Although the patient snores, this diagnosis is less likely given that his excessive daytime somnolence is occurring in the context of many other depressive symptoms. Nonetheless, obstructive sleep apnea is common and underdiagnosed, and it does occur in nonobese patients.
- **Post-traumatic stress disorder (PTSD):** This is characterized by (1) reexperiencing a traumatic event (e.g., flashbacks); (2) avoidance of stimuli associated with the trauma; and (3) increased arousal (e.g., anxiety, sleep disturbance, hypervigilance). Despite having nightmares about the accident, this patient does not sufficiently manifest the last two features of the disorder.
- **HIV infection:** Given his history of STDs, the patient should also be tested for this. However, it is highly unlikely that HIV infection accounts for his current depression (unless there are frontal lobe lesions due to infection or malignancy).

Diagnostic Workup

- **CBC:** To rule out anemia.
- **TSH:** A screening test for hypothyroidism.
- **Ambulatory nocturnal pulse oximetry:** An initial test to evaluate possible obstructive sleep apnea.
- **Polysomnography:** To diagnose obstructive sleep apnea.
- **HIV antibody:** To rule out HIV infection.
- **MRI—brain:** To rule out the exceedingly rare possibility that the patient's symptoms are due to an intracranial mass lesion.

Opening Scenario

Jessica Lee, a 32-year-old female, comes to the office complaining of fatigue.

Vital Signs

BP: 120/85 mmHg
Temp: 98.2°F (36.8°C)
RR: 13/minute
HR: 80/minute, regular

Examinee Tasks

1. Take a focused history.
2. Perform a focused physical exam (do not perform rectal, genitourinary, or female breast exam).
3. Explain your clinical impression and workup plan to the patient.
4. Write the patient note after leaving the room.

Checklist/SP Sheet

PATIENT DESCRIPTION

Patient is a 32 yo F, married with two children.

NOTES FOR THE SP

- Look anxious and pale.
- Exhibit bruises on the face and arms that elicit pain when touched.

CHALLENGING QUESTIONS TO ASK

"I am drinking a lot of water, doctor. What do you think the reason is?"

SAMPLE EXAMINEE RESPONSE

"I don't know for sure, but I want to run some tests. We need to make sure that you haven't developed diabetes."

Examinee Checklist

ENTRANCE:

- ☐ Examinee knocked on the door before entering.
- ☐ Examinee introduced self by name.
- ☐ Examinee identified his/her role or position.
- ☐ Examinee correctly used patient's name.
- ☐ Examinee made eye contact with the SP.

HISTORY:

- ☐ Examinee showed compassion for your illness.

✓ Question	Patient Response
☐ Chief complaint	Feeling tired, weak, no energy.
☐ Onset	Five months ago.
☐ Associated events	None.
☐ Progression of the fatigue during the day	I feel okay in the morning; then gradually I start feeling more and more tired and weak.
☐ Change in vision (double vision) during the day	No.
☐ Affecting job/performance	Yes, I don't have energy to work.
☐ Appetite changes	I have a very good appetite.
☐ Weight changes	No.
☐ Feeling of depression	Sometimes I feel sad.
☐ Cause of bruises	I fell down the stairs and hurt myself (looks anxious). It is my fault. I don't always pay attention.
☐ Being physically or emotionally hurt or abused by anybody	Well, sometimes when my husband gets angry with me, but he loves me very much, and he promises not to do it again.
☐ Feeling safe/afraid at home	Sometimes I feel afraid, especially when my husband gets drunk.
☐ Are the children being abused or threatened?	Well, he slapped my younger son the other day for breaking a glass. He should be more attentive.
☐ Suicidal thoughts/plans/attempts	No.
☐ Feelings of blame or guilt	Yes, I think I am being awkward. It is my fault.
☐ Presence of guns at home	No.
☐ Any family members who know about the abuse	No.
☐ Emergency plan	No.
☐ Sleeping problems (falling asleep, staying asleep, early waking, snoring)	No.
☐ Loss of concentration	Yes, I can't concentrate on my work.
☐ Menstrual period	Regular and heavy; lasts seven days.
☐ Last menstrual period	Two weeks ago.
☐ Urinary symptoms	I recently started to wake up at night to urinate.
☐ Polyuria	Yes, I have to go to the bathroom more often during the day.
☐ Pain during urination or change in the color of urine	No.
☐ Polydipsia	Yes, I feel thirsty all the time, and I drink a lot of water.
☐ Associated symptoms (fever, chills, chest pain, shortness of breath, abdominal pain, diarrhea/constipation, cold intolerance, skin/hair changes)	None.

☑ Question	Patient Response
☐ Current medications	None.
☐ Past medical history	None.
☐ Past surgical history	I fell and broke my arm a year ago.
☐ Family history	My father had diabetes and died of a heart attack. My mother is in a nursing home with Alzheimer's.
☐ Occupation	Nurse.
☐ Alcohol use	No.
☐ Illicit drug use	Never.
☐ Tobacco	No.
☐ Exercise	No.
☐ Diet	I am a vegetarian.
☐ Sexual activity	I don't feel any desire for sex, but we do it when my husband wants.
☐ Drug allergies	No.

Physical Examination:

☐ Examinee washed his/her hands.
☐ Examinee asked permission to start the exam.
☐ Examinee used respectful draping.
☐ Examinee did not repeat painful maneuvers.

☑ Exam Component	Maneuver
☐ Head and neck exam	Inspected conjunctivae, mouth and throat, lymph nodes; examined thyroid gland
☐ CV exam	Auscultation
☐ Pulmonary exam	Auscultation
☐ Abdominal exam	Auscultation, palpation, percussion
☐ Extremities	Inspection, motor exam, DTRs

Closure:

☐ Examinee discussed initial diagnostic impressions.
☐ Examinee discussed initial management plans:
    ☐ Diagnostic tests.
    ☐ Domestic violence counseling:
        ☐ "I care about your safety and I am always available for help and support."
        ☐ "Everything we discuss is confidential, but I must involve child protective services if your children are being abused."
        ☐ Support group information, including contact numbers or Web sites.
        ☐ Safety planning.
☐ Examinee asked if the patient has any other questions or concerns.

Sample Closure:

Ms. Lee, I am concerned about your safety and your relationship with your husband. I would like you to know that I am available to you for help and support whenever you need it. Although everything we discuss is confidential, I must involve child protective services if I have reason to believe that your children are being abused. I will bring back some telephone numbers and contact information for you regarding where you can go for help if you or your children are in a crisis or if you just want someone to talk to. I am also concerned about your frequent urination and thirst. I will run a simple blood test to see if you have any problems with your blood sugar or your hormones. Do you have any questions?

PATIENT NOTE

History

Physical Examination

Differential Diagnosis	Diagnostic Workup
1.	1.
2.	2.
3.	3.
4.	4.
5.	5.

History

HPI: 32 yo F c/o fatigue and weakness. The patient notes that the fatigue and weakness started 5 months ago. The fatigue increases gradually during the day. She complains of loss of energy and concentration that adversely affects her job as a nurse. After questioning about the bruises on her face and arms, she admits that her husband, who is an alcoholic, has beaten her. She also reports at least 1 episode of physical abuse directed at her youngest son. She tries to defend his actions, feels guilty, and blames herself. She has not reported this to anyone and has no emergency plan. She feels sad but denies suicidal ideation. The patient also complains of polyuria, polydipsia, and nocturia that also began 5 months ago. She denies burning on urination or change in the color of urine. Her last menstrual period was 2 weeks ago; the menstrual period is regular, q28 days, lasting for 7 days of heavy flow. No constipation, cold intolerance, or change in appetite or weight. No sleep problems.

ROS: Negative except as above.

Allergies: NKDA.

Medications: None.

SH: No smoking, no EtOH. Sexually active with her husband; decreased sexual desire.

FH: Diabetic father died from a heart attack; mother is in a nursing home with Alzheimer's disease.

Physical Examination

Patient is in no acute distress, looks anxious.

VS: WNL.

HEENT: Pale conjunctivae.

Neck: No lymphadenopathy, thyroid normal.

Chest: Clear breath sounds bilaterally.

Heart: RRR; normal S1/S2; no murmurs, rubs, or gallops.

Abdomen: Soft, nondistended, nontender, ⊕BS, no hepatosplenomegaly.

Extremities: Muscle strength 5/5 throughout; DTRs 2+; symmetric, painful bruises on both arms.

Differential Diagnosis

1. Domestic violence
2. Depression
3. Diabetes mellitus
4. Diabetes insipidus
5. Anemia
6. Myasthenia gravis
7. Hypothyroidism

Diagnostic Workup

1. CBC, iron level, TIBC, ferritin, serum B_{12}
2. Electrolytes
3. UA
4. Serum glucose, HbA_{1c}
5. TSH
6. MRI—brain (pituitary protocol)
7. DDAVP nasal spray test (vasopressin)

CASE DISCUSSION

Differential Diagnosis

- **Domestic violence:** The patient is clearly a victim of domestic violence and of her husband's alcoholism. This can explain many of her symptoms but not the polyuria and polydipsia.
- **Depression:** As above, depression likely coexists but does not account for the patient's recent polyuria and polydipsia (if objectively verified).
- **Diabetes mellitus (DM):** Aside from domestic violence issues, many of the patient's symptoms can be explained by new-onset diabetes. Her positive family history puts her at risk. She should also be asked about any recent vaginal yeast infections, which are a frequent complication of hyperglycemia (and may be its initial presenting symptom).
- **Diabetes insipidus (DI):** This is an uncommon disease characterized by polyuria (of low specific gravity) and polydipsia. It has many etiologies and is caused by a deficiency of or resistance to vasopressin.
- **Anemia:** This may also help explain her fatigue and weakness. Menstruating females often have an iron-deficiency anemia, and strict vegans may also have anemia related to vitamin B_{12} deficiency. Conjunctival pallor on exam has a high likelihood ratio for predicting a hematocrit < 30% (hemoglobin < 10 g/dL).
- **Myasthenia gravis:** Increasing fatigue as the day progresses is highly nonspecific. By contrast, this disease involves fluctuating muscle weakness and presents with ptosis, diplopia, difficulty in chewing or swallowing, respiratory difficulties, and/or limb weakness.
- **Hypothyroidism:** Nonspecific symptoms such as fatigue and weakness may suggest this common diagnosis. However, hypothyroidism does not explain polyuria, polydipsia, or the admitted physical abuse.

Diagnostic Workup

- **CBC, iron level, TIBC, ferritin, serum B_{12}:** Blood tests to investigate anemia.
- **Electrolytes:** Hypernatremia may be seen in DI.
- **UA:** Dilute urine is seen in DI, glycosuria in DM.
- **Serum glucose, HbA_{1c}:** To screen for DM.
- **TSH:** Thyroid disease must be ruled out in a patient with symptoms of depression.
- **MRI—brain (pituitary protocol):** To look for mass lesions in central DI.
- **DDAVP nasal spray test ("vasopressin challenge test"):** To confirm a clinical suspicion of central DI.

Opening Scenario

William Jordan, a 61-year-old male, comes to the office complaining of fatigue.

Vital Signs

BP: 135/85 mmHg
Temp: 98.6°F (37°C)
RR: 13/minute
HR: 70/minute, regular

Examinee Tasks

1. Take a focused history.
2. Perform a focused physical exam (do not perform rectal, genitourinary, or female breast exam).
3. Explain your clinical impression and workup plan to the patient.
4. Write the patient note after leaving the room.

Checklist/SP Sheet

PATIENT DESCRIPTION

Patient is a 61 yo M, married with three children.

NOTES FOR THE SP

- Look weak and sad, and sit leaning forward.
- Exhibit abdominal discomfort that increases when you lie on your back.
- Show pain on palpation of the epigastric area.

CHALLENGING QUESTIONS TO ASK

"I want to go on a trip with my wife. Can we do the tests after I come back?"

SAMPLE EXAMINEE RESPONSE

"It doesn't sound as if you're feeling well enough to be able to enjoy a trip. Let's do some initial blood tests, and then we can see how you're feeling and decide whether we're comfortable letting you go away."

Examinee Checklist

ENTRANCE:

- ☐ Examinee knocked on the door before entering.
- ☐ Examinee introduced self by name.
- ☐ Examinee identified his/her role or position.
- ☐ Examinee correctly used patient's name.
- ☐ Examinee made eye contact with the SP.

HISTORY:

☐   Examinee showed compassion for your illness.

☑ Question	Patient Response
☐ Chief complaint	Feeling tired, weak, low energy.
☐ Onset	Six months ago.
☐ Associated events	None.
☐ Progression of the fatigue during the day	The same throughout the day.
☐ Affecting job/performance	Yes, I don't have energy for my daily 30-minute walk with my dog, and even at work I am not as energetic as before.
☐ Appetite changes	I have a poor appetite.
☐ Weight changes	I lost eight pounds during the past six months.
☐ Change in bowel habits	No, I have a bowel movement twice or three times a week. It has been like this for the last 10 years.
☐ Blood in stool	No.
☐ Abdominal pain or discomfort	Yes, I do feel some discomfort here (points to the epigastric area).
☐ Onset of discomfort	Four months ago; it increased gradually.
☐ Quality	Vague, deep.
☐ Severity on a scale	4/10.
☐ Alleviating/exacerbating factors	Nothing makes it worse, but I feel better when I lean forward.
☐ Relationship to food	No.
☐ Radiation	I feel the discomfort reaching my back.
☐ Nausea/vomiting	Sometimes I feel nauseated.
☐ Feeling of depression	Yes, I feel sad.
☐ Reason for feeling sad	I don't know, really.
☐ Suicidal thoughts/plans/attempts	No.
☐ Feelings of blame, guilt, worthlessness	No.
☐ Sleeping problems (falling asleep, staying asleep, early waking, snoring)	I wake up unusually early in the morning. It has been like this for the past two months.
☐ Loss of concentration	Yes, I can't concentrate anymore while watching the news or playing cards with my friends.
☐ Loss of interest	I don't enjoy playing cards with my friends anymore. I feel that life is boring.

✓	Question	Patient Response
☐	Associated symptoms (fever/chills, chest pain, cough, shortness of breath, cold intolerance, skin/hair changes)	None.
☐	Current medications	Tylenol, but it is not helping.
☐	Past psychiatric history	No.
☐	Past medical history	No.
☐	Past surgical history	Appendectomy at age 16.
☐	Family history	My father died in a car accident and had diabetes, and my mother died of breast cancer.
☐	Occupation	Police officer, retired one year ago.
☐	Alcohol use	One or two beers 2–3 times a week.
☐	Illicit drug use	Never.
☐	Tobacco	I stopped it six months ago after 30 years of smoking one pack a day (because I felt disgusted, and smoking made me feel sick).
☐	Exercise	I walk 30 minutes every day.
☐	Diet	Regular; I like junk food.
☐	Sexual activity	Sexually active with my wife.
☐	Drug allergies	No.

Physical Examination:

- ☐ Examinee washed his/her hands.
- ☐ Examinee asked permission to start the exam.
- ☐ Examinee used respectful draping.
- ☐ Examinee did not repeat painful maneuvers.

✓	Exam Component	Maneuver
☐	Head and neck exam	Inspected conjunctivae, mouth and throat, lymph nodes; examined thyroid gland
☐	CV exam	Auscultation
☐	Pulmonary exam	Auscultation
☐	Abdominal exam	Auscultation, percussion, palpation (including rebound tenderness and Murphy's sign)
☐	Extremities	Inspection, palpation

Closure:

- ☐ Examinee discussed initial diagnostic impressions.
- ☐ Examinee discussed initial management plans:
    - ☐ Diagnostic tests.
    - ☐ Depression counseling:
        - ☐ Asked about patient's existing support system (friends, family).
        - ☐ Discussed available support systems in the hospital and community.
        - ☐ Coping skills: Exercise, relaxation techniques, spending more time with family and friends.
- ☐ Examinee asked if the patient has any other questions or concerns.

Sample Closure:

Mr. Jordan, your symptoms are consistent with a few different diagnoses. They may be caused by an ulcer that would resolve with a course of antibiotics and acid suppressors, or they may have a more serious cause, such as pancreatic cancer. I am going to schedule you for an abdominal ultrasound that may reveal the source of your pain, and I will also run some blood tests. I know you are concerned about your upcoming vacation, but the results of your tests should be back within a few days, and they should give us a good idea what is wrong with you. In the meantime, our social worker can meet with you to help you find ways to cope with the stress you have been experiencing in your life. Do you have any questions for me?

PATIENT NOTE

History

Physical Examination

Differential Diagnosis

1.

2.

3.

4.

5.

Diagnostic Workup

1.

2.

3.

4.

5.

History

HPI: *61 yo M c/o fatigue and weakness. The patient notes that the fatigue and weakness started 6 months ago. He feels tired all day. He has poor appetite and lost 8 pounds in the last 6 months. He also complains of occasional nausea and of a vague, deep epigastric discomfort that radiates to the back. This discomfort started 4 months ago and has gradually increased to a severity of 4/10. The discomfort decreases when he leans forward and increases when he lies on his back. There is no relationship of the pain to food. No change in bowel movements or blood in the stool. He feels sad sometimes, has lost interest in things that he used to enjoy, wakes up unusually early in the morning, and complains of low energy and concentration that have affected his daily activities and work. The patient denies suicidal ideation or plans. No feelings of guilt or worthlessness.*
ROS: *Negative except as above.*
Allergies: *NKDA.*
Medications: *Tylenol.*
PMH: *None.*
PSH: *Appendectomy at age 16.*
SH: *One PPD for 30 years; stopped 6 months ago. Drinks 1–2 beers 2–3 times/week. Sexually active with his wife.*
FH: *Father with diabetes, died accidentally. Mother died from breast cancer.*

Physical Examination

Patient is in no acute distress, looks sad.
VS: *WNL.*
HEENT: *No conjunctival pallor, mouth and pharynx normal.*
Neck: *Supple, no JVD, no lymphadenopathy, thyroid normal.*
Chest: *Clear breath sounds bilaterally.*
Heart: *RRR; normal S1/S2; no murmurs, rubs, or gallops.*
Abdomen: *Soft, nondistended, mild epigastric tenderness, no rebound tenderness, ⊖Murphy's, ⊕BS, no hepatosplenomegaly.*
Extremities: *No edema.*

Differential Diagnosis

1. Depression
2. Pancreatic cancer
3. Chronic pancreatitis
4. Peptic ulcer disease
5. Hypothyroidism

Diagnostic Workup

1. CBC, stool for occult blood
2. Glucose
3. Amylase, lipase
4. AST/ALT/bilirubin/alkaline phosphatase
5. TSH
6. AXR
7. CT or U/S—abdomen
8. Upper endoscopy

CASE DISCUSSION

Differential Diagnosis

- **Depression:** The patient has many classic symptoms of depression (**SIG EM CAPS**; see Case 15). Although it may be a somatic symptom of depression, his abdominal pain is of significant concern and warrants a thorough medical evaluation.
- **Pancreatic cancer:** The pattern and location of pain are worrisome for pancreatic disease, and weight loss raises a concern for malignancy. Depression may be its initial manifestation. Diarrhea, presumably due to malabsorption, is also an occasional early finding (not seen in this case).
- **Chronic pancreatitis:** The pattern and location of pain are consistent with this diagnosis, but usually there is a history of recurrent episodes of similar pain. The patient's alcohol use should be explored further, as alcoholism accounts for 70–80% of chronic pancreatitis.
- **Peptic ulcer disease:** Suspect this diagnosis in any patient with epigastric pain, although the complaint is neither sensitive nor specific enough to make a reliable diagnosis. It is important to note that many patients deny any relationship of the pain to meals. Weight loss, however, is unusual in uncomplicated ulcer disease and may suggest gastric malignancy.
- **Hypothyroidism:** Nonspecific symptoms such as fatigue and weakness may suggest this common diagnosis. Abdominal pain is unusual.

Diagnostic Workup

- **CBC, stool for occult blood:** To screen for blood loss in peptic ulcer.
- **Glucose:** To screen for pancreatic endocrine dysfunction (i.e., diabetes mellitus).
- **Amylase, lipase:** Nonspecific, but can be elevated in chronic pancreatitis or malignancy.
- **AST/ALT/bilirubin/alkaline phosphatase:** To look for evidence of obstructive jaundice (often seen in pancreatic cancer).
- **TSH:** Thyroid disease must be ruled out in a patient with symptoms of depression.
- **AXR:** To look for pancreatic calcification in chronic pancreatitis.
- **CT or U/S—abdomen:** To diagnose pancreatic cancer or other pathology.
- **Upper endoscopy:** To diagnose ulcer disease.

DOORWAY INFORMATION

Opening Scenario

Kelly Clark, a 35-year-old female, comes to the ER complaining of headache.

Vital Signs

BP: 135/90 mmHg
Temp: 98.6°F (37°C)
RR: 16/minute
HR: 76/minute, regular

Examinee Tasks

1. Take a focused history.
2. Perform a focused physical exam (do not perform rectal, genitourinary, or female breast exam).
3. Explain your clinical impression and workup plan to the patient.
4. Write the patient note after leaving the room.

Checklist/SP Sheet

PATIENT DESCRIPTION

Patient is a 35 yo F, married with three children.

NOTES FOR THE SP

Hold the right side of your head during the encounter and look as if you are in severe pain.

CHALLENGING QUESTIONS TO ASK

"Do you have anything that will make me feel better? Please, doctor, I am in pain."

SAMPLE EXAMINEE RESPONSE

"Yes, we have many options for medicines to relieve your pain, but first I need to learn as much as I can about your pain so that I can recommend the best medicine."

Examinee Checklist

ENTRANCE:

☐ Examinee knocked on the door before entering.
☐ Examinee introduced self by name.
☐ Examinee identified his/her role or position.
☐ Examinee correctly used patient's name.
☐ Examinee made eye contact with the SP.

HISTORY:

☐ Examinee showed compassion for your pain.

☑ Question	Patient Response
☐ Chief complaint	Headache.
☐ Onset	Two weeks ago.
☐ Constant/intermittent	Well, I don't have the pain all the time. It comes and goes.
☐ Frequency	At least once a day.
☐ Progression	It is getting worse (2–3 times a day).
☐ Severity on a scale	When I have the pain, it is 9/10 and prevents me from working.
☐ Location	It is here (points to the whole right side of the head).
☐ Duration	One or two hours.
☐ Radiation (changes its location)	No.
☐ Quality	Sharp and pounding.
☐ Aura (warning that the headache is about to come)	No.
☐ Timing (the same time every day/ morning/evening)	The headache may come at any time. I'm having one now.
☐ Relationship with menses	No.
☐ Alleviating factors	Resting in a quiet, dark room; sleep, aspirin.
☐ Exacerbating factors	Stress, light, and noise.
☐ Nausea/vomiting	Sometimes I feel nauseated when I am in pain. Yesterday I vomited for the first time.
☐ Headache wakes you up from sleep	No.
☐ Visual changes/tears/red eye	No.
☐ Weakness/numbness	No.
☐ Speech difficulties	No.
☐ Runny nose during the attack	No.
☐ Similar episodes before	Yes, in college I had a similar headache that was accompanied by nausea.
☐ Weight/appetite changes	No.
☐ Joint pain/fatigue	Occasional aches and pains treated with ibuprofen.
☐ Stress	Yes, I am working on a new project that I have to finish this month. Last month was a disaster. I worked hard on my designs, but they were rejected, and I have to start all over again.
☐ Head trauma	No.
☐ Last menstrual period	Two weeks ago.
☐ Current medications	Ibuprofen.

☑ Question	Patient Response
☐ Past medical history	An episode of sinusitis four months ago, treated with amoxicillin (but the pain was different from the one I have now).
☐ Past surgical history	Tubal ligation eight years ago.
☐ Family history	My father died at age 65 of a brain tumor. My mother is alive and has migraines.
☐ Occupation	Engineer.
☐ Alcohol use	No.
☐ Illicit drug use	No.
☐ Tobacco use	No.
☐ Social history	I live with my husband and three children.
☐ Sexual activity	With my husband.
☐ Use of OCPs	No, I had a tubal ligation after my third child eight years ago.
☐ Drug allergies	No.

Physical Examination:

- ☐ Examinee washed his/her hands.
- ☐ Examinee asked permission to start the exam.
- ☐ Examinee used respectful draping.
- ☐ Examinee did not repeat painful maneuvers.

☑ Exam Component	Maneuver
☐ HEENT	Palpation (head, facial sinuses, temporomandibular joints), funduscopic exam; inspected nose, mouth, teeth, and throat
☐ Neck exam	Inspection, palpation
☐ CV exam	Auscultation
☐ Pulmonary exam	Auscultation
☐ Neurologic exam	Cranial nerves, muscle strength, DTRs

Closure:

- ☐ Examinee discussed initial diagnostic impressions.
- ☐ Examinee discussed initial management plans.
- ☐ Examinee asked if the patient has any other questions or concerns.

Sample Closure:

Ms. Clark, it sounds as if your symptoms are due to a migraine headache, so the first thing I will do is prescribe some medications that will help you with your pain. To ensure that there isn't something else going on, however, I would like to get a CT scan of your head to determine if there is a mass or a vascular problem that is causing your headache. A blood test may also show if you have problems other than migraine. Do you have any questions for me?

PATIENT NOTE

History

Physical Examination

Differential Diagnosis

1.

2.

3.

4.

5.

Diagnostic Workup

1.

2.

3.

4.

5.

History

HPI: *35 yo F c/o daily headaches for 2 weeks. These headaches occur 2–3 times a day and last for 1–2 hours. The pain is sharp and pounding. It is located on the right hemisphere of the head, with no radiation or preceding aura. The pain reaches 9/10 in severity and prevents the patient from continuing her activities. Headaches are exacerbated by stress, light, and noise and are alleviated by resting in a dark room, sleep, and aspirin. The pain is sometimes accompanied by nausea and vomiting. No changes in weight or appetite.*
ROS: *Occasional aches and pains.*
Allergies: *NKDA.*
Medications: *Ibuprofen.*
PMH: *Headaches at age 20, accompanied by nausea. One episode of sinusitis 4 months ago, treated with amoxicillin.*
PSH: *Tubal ligation 8 years ago.*
SH: *No smoking, no EtOH, no illicit drugs. Patient is an engineer, lives with husband and three children, and is sexually active with husband only.*
FH: *Father died of a brain tumor at age 65. Mother has migraines.*

Physical Examination

Patient is in severe pain.
VS: *WNL.*
HEENT: *NC/AT, nontender to palpation, PERRLA, EOMI, no papilledema, no nasal congestion, no pharyngeal erythema or exudates, dentition good.*
Neck: *Supple, no lymphadenopathy.*
Chest: *Clear breath sounds bilaterally.*
Heart: *RRR; normal S1/S2; no murmurs, rubs, or gallops.*
Neuro: Mental status: *Alert and oriented* × 3, *good concentration.* Cranial nerves: *2–12 grossly intact.* Motor: *Strength 5/5 throughout.* DTRs: *2+ intact, symmetric.*

Differential Diagnosis

1. Migraine
2. Tension headache
3. Depression
4. Pseudotumor cerebri
5. Intracranial mass lesion
6. Cluster headache
7. Sinusitis

Diagnostic Workup

1. CBC
2. CT—head or MRI—brain
3. LP
4. CT—sinus

CASE DISCUSSION

Differential Diagnosis

- **Migraine:** Despite lacking an aura, the patient's presentation is classic for this diagnosis.
- **Tension headache:** This is often associated with stress but is usually bilateral and squeezing. It lasts from hours to days and gets worse as the day progresses.
- **Depression:** Headaches may be worse on arising in the morning and are associated with other symptoms of depression.
- **Pseudotumor cerebri:** Headaches can be focal but are usually accompanied by diplopia and other visual symptoms. Exam should reveal papilledema but can be normal during the first few days after onset of illness.
- **Intracranial mass lesion**: One-third of patients with brain tumors present with a primary complaint of headache. Headache is nonspecific and may mimic features of migraine. Certain brain tumors may have a familial basis.
- **Cluster headache:** This involves unilateral periorbital pain, often accompanied by ipsilateral nasal congestion, rhinorrhea, lacrimation, redness of the eye, and/or Horner's syndrome. Episodes of daily pain occur in clusters and often awaken patients at night. However, this rarely occurs in women (a similar entity seen in women is termed *chronic paroxysmal hemicrania*).
- **Sinusitis:** This is a rare cause of headache. There are no signs or symptoms of sinus or respiratory infection in this case.

Diagnostic Workup

- **CBC:** To look for leukocytosis, a nonspecific sign of infection or inflammation. Mild normocytic anemia and thrombocytosis may also be seen in temporal arteritis.
- **CT—head or MRI—brain:** Headache syndromes are largely clinical diagnoses. Neuroimaging is generally reserved for patients with acute severe headache, chronic unexplained headache, or abnormalities on neurologic exam. MRI provides greater anatomic detail, but CT is preferred to rule out acute bleeds.
- **LP:** To look for elevated opening pressure in pseudotumor. CSF is otherwise normal. RBCs and xanthochromia can be seen in subarachnoid hemorrhage (perform if suspicion is high despite a negative CT scan).
- **CT—sinus:** To look for sinusitis.

Opening Scenario

Carl Fisher, a 57-year-old male, comes to the ER complaining of bloody urine.

Vital Signs

BP: 130/80 mmHg
Temp: 98.5°F (36.9°C)
RR: 13/minute
HR: 72/minute, regular

Examinee Tasks

1. Take a focused history.
2. Perform a focused physical exam (do not perform rectal, genitourinary, or female breast exam).
3. Explain your clinical impression and workup plan to the patient.
4. Write the patient note after leaving the room.

Checklist/SP Sheet

PATIENT DESCRIPTION

Patient is a 57 yo M.

NOTES FOR THE SP

- Show pain when the examinee checks for CVA tenderness on the right.
- If the examinee mentions prostate disease, ask, "What's prostate disease?"

CHALLENGING QUESTIONS TO ASK

"They told me this is because of my old age. Is that true?"

SAMPLE EXAMINEE RESPONSE

"No. Bloody urine is rarely normal."

Examinee Checklist

ENTRANCE:

☐ Examinee knocked on the door before entering.
☐ Examinee introduced self by name.
☐ Examinee identified his/her role or position.
☐ Examinee correctly used patient's name.
☐ Examinee made eye contact with the SP.

HISTORY:

☐ Examinee showed compassion for your illness.

☑ **Question**	**Patient Response**
☐ Chief complaint	I have blood in my urine, doctor.
☐ How did he know it was blood?	It was bright red and later had some clots.
☐ Onset	Yesterday morning.
☐ Progression	That was the only time it has ever happened; my urine is back to normal.
☐ Pain/burning on urination	None.
☐ Fever	None.
☐ Abdominal/flank pain	None.
☐ Polyuria, frequency	Yes.
☐ Straining during urination	Yes.
☐ Nocturia	Yes.
☐ Weak stream	Yes.
☐ Dribbling	Yes.
☐ Onset of the previous symptoms	Two years ago. They told me I am getting old; am I?
☐ History of renal stones	No.
☐ Associated symptoms (nausea/vomiting, diarrhea/constipation)	None.
☐ Constitutional symptoms (weight loss, appetite changes, night sweats)	None.
☐ Previous similar episodes	No.
☐ Current medications	Allopurinol.
☐ Past medical history	Gout.
☐ Past surgical history	Appendectomy at age 23.
☐ Family history	My father died at age 80 because of a kidney problem. My mother is alive and healthy.
☐ Occupation	Painter.
☐ Alcohol use	A couple of beers after work, 2–3 times a week.
☐ Illicit drug use	No.
☐ Tobacco	Yes, I have smoked one pack a day for thirty years.
☐ Sexual activity	I have a new girlfriend; I met her last month in the bar.
☐ Sexual orientation	Women only.
☐ Use of condoms	Sometimes, if they're available.

☑ Question	Patient Response
☐ History of STDs	I have herpes. The last attack was several months ago. The lesions stay for several days and resolve without treatment.
☐ HIV test	Never.
☐ Drug allergies	No.

Physical Examination:

☐ Examinee washed his/her hands.
☐ Examinee asked permission to start the exam.
☐ Examinee used respectful draping.
☐ Examinee did not repeat painful maneuvers.

☑ Exam Component	Maneuver
☐ CV exam	Auscultation
☐ Pulmonary exam	Auscultation
☐ Abdominal exam	Auscultation, palpation, percussion, checked for CVA tenderness
☐ Extremities	Inspection

Closure:

☐ Examinee discussed initial diagnostic impressions.
☐ Examinee discussed initial management plans:
    ☐ Suggested a genital exam.
    ☐ Suggested a rectal exam for the prostate.
    ☐ Diagnostic tests.
☐ Examinee asked if the patient has any other questions or concerns.

Sample Closure:

Mr. Fisher, the blood in your urine could be caused by a variety of factors, so I would like to do a few tests in order to tease out an answer. First I will draw some blood, and then I will perform a genital exam as well as a rectal exam in order to assess your prostate. I will then order a urine test to look for signs of infection. Depending on the results we obtain, I may also order some imaging studies to determine if there is a stone in your urinary tract, an anatomic abnormality, or a tumor. Do you have any questions for me?

PATIENT NOTE

History

Physical Examination

Differential Diagnosis

1.

2.

3.

4.

5.

Diagnostic Workup

1.

2.

3.

4.

5.

History

HPI: *57 yo male c/o 1 episode of painless hematuria yesterday morning. He has no fever, no abdominal or flank pain, and no dysuria. No history of renal stones. He has a 2-year history of straining on urination, polyuria, nocturia, weak urinary stream, and dribbling. No nausea, vomiting, diarrhea, or constipation. No change in appetite or weight loss. No previous similar episodes.*
ROS: *Negative except as above.*
Allergies: *NKDA.*
Medications: *Allopurinol.*
PMH: *Gout; genital herpes that recurred several months ago.*
PSH: *Appendectomy, age 23.*
SH: *One PPD for 30 years, 2 beers 2–3 times/week, no illicit drugs. Works as a painter. Heterosexual, has a new partner, and uses condoms occasionally.*
FH: *Father died from kidney disease at age 80.*

Physical Examination

Patient is in no acute distress.
VS: *WNL.*
Chest: *Clear breath sounds bilaterally.*
Heart: *RRR; normal S1/S2; no murmurs, rubs, or gallops.*
Abdomen: *Soft, nondistended, nontender, ⊕BS, no hepatosplenomegaly. Mild right CVA tenderness.*
Extremities: *No edema.*

Differential Diagnosis

1. Bladder cancer
2. Urolithiasis
3. BPH
4. Prostate cancer
5. Renal cell carcinoma
6. Glomerulonephritis
7. UTI

Diagnostic Workup

1. Genital exam
2. Rectal exam
3. UA
4. Urine culture
5. Urine cytology
6. BUN/Cr
7. PSA
8. U/S—renal
9. Cystoscopy
10. CT—abdomen/pelvis
11. IVP

CASE DISCUSSION

Differential Diagnosis

A useful mnemonic for the differential diagnosis of hematuria is **HITTERS**—etiologies include **H**ematologic or coagulation disorders, **I**nfection, **T**rauma, **T**umor, **E**xercise, **R**enal disorder, and **S**tones. Gynecologic sources may need to be excluded in women. The passage of clots often localizes the source of bleeding to the lower urinary tract. Gross hematuria in adults represents malignancy until proven otherwise.

- **Bladder cancer:** Hematuria and irritative voiding symptoms are consistent with this diagnosis, and the patient's cigarette smoking and possible occupational exposure to industrial solvents are risk factors. However, the finding of right CVA tenderness is unusual and could be a sign of upper urinary tract disease.
- **Urolithiasis:** Despite the presence of hematuria and CVA tenderness, this very common diagnosis is unlikely in the absence of sudden, severe colicky flank pain. Pain may migrate to the groin and is not alleviated by changes in position.
- **BPH:** The patient's urinary symptoms are classic for this diagnosis except that hematuria (if present) is usually microscopic. Again, CVA tenderness may signal upper urinary tract pathology.
- **Prostate cancer:** As above, this diagnosis is plausible but is hard to reconcile with the presence of CVA tenderness (could postulate metastasis to a right posterior rib).
- **Renal cell carcinoma:** The classic triad is hematuria, flank pain, and a palpable mass. Constitutional symptoms may be prominent. The patient's other urinary symptoms may be due to coexisting BPH.
- **Glomerulonephritis:** The absence of hypertension or signs of volume overload (e.g., edema) argues against intrinsic renal disease. However, remember that IgA nephropathy is the most common acute glomerulonephritis and most commonly presents with an episode of gross hematuria. Presentation is usually concurrent with URI, GI symptoms, or a flulike illness.
- **UTI:** This can cause hematuria but is uncommon in males. The patient has no other symptoms to suggest acute infection.

Diagnostic Workup

- **Genital exam:** To exclude a urologic source of bleeding in men.
- **Rectal exam:** To detect masses as well as prostatic enlargement or nodules.
- **UA:** To assess hematuria, pyuria, bacteriuria, etc. Dysmorphic RBCs or casts are signs of glomerular disease. The absence of hematuria does not rule out urolithiasis.
- **Urine culture:** To exclude UTI.
- **Urine cytology:** Has variable sensitivity in detecting bladder cancers, depending on the tumor's grade and stage. Examine three voided samples to maximize sensitivity.
- **BUN/Cr:** To evaluate kidney function.
- **PSA:** The serum level correlates with the volume of both benign and malignant prostatic tissue. Can be normal in about 20% of patients who have nonmetastatic prostate cancer.
- **U/S—renal:** Can detect bladder and renal masses and stones, but is operator dependent and is less sensitive in detecting ureteral disease.
- **Cystoscopy:** The gold standard for the diagnosis of bladder cancer.
- **CT—abdomen/pelvis:** To evaluate the urinary tract. Can identify neoplasms and a variety of benign conditions such as stones.
- **IVP:** Provides an assessment of the kidneys, ureters, and bladder but is generally being replaced by CT—urogram to avoid contrast administration.

Opening Scenario

James Miller, a 54-year-old male, comes to the clinic for hypertension follow-up.

Vital Signs

BP: 135/90 mmHg
Temp: 98.0°F (36.7°C)
RR: 16/minute
HR: 70/minute, regular

Examinee Tasks

1. Take a focused history.
2. Perform a focused physical exam (do not perform rectal, genitourinary, or female breast exam).
3. Explain your clinical impression and workup plan to the patient.
4. Write the patient note after leaving the room.

Checklist/SP Sheet

PATIENT DESCRIPTION
Patient is a 54 yo M.

NOTES FOR THE SP
Don't mention impotence unless the examinee asks whether you are having any side effects from your medications or whether you have any other concerns.

CHALLENGING QUESTIONS TO ASK
"I think it is my age. Isn't that right, doctor?"

SAMPLE EXAMINEE RESPONSE
"No, I don't think it's because of your age. I worry more about your medications. However, testosterone levels can decrease with age, and we will check for that."

Examinee Checklist

ENTRANCE:

☐ Examinee knocked on the door before entering.
☐ Examinee introduced self by name.
☐ Examinee identified his/her role or position.
☐ Examinee correctly used patient's name.
☐ Examinee made eye contact with the SP.

HISTORY:

☐ Examinee showed compassion for your illness.

☑ Question	Patient Response
☐ Chief complaint	I am here to check on my blood pressure.
☐ Onset	Last year I found out that I have hypertension.
☐ Treatment	The doctor started me on hydrochlorothiazide, but my blood pressure stayed high. He added propranolol six months ago.
☐ Compliance with medications	Well, sometimes I forget to take the pills, but in general I take them regularly.
☐ Last blood pressure checkup	Six months ago.
☐ How he is feeling today	Good.
☐ Home monitoring of blood pressure	No.
☐ Any other symptoms (fatigue, headaches, dizziness, blurred vision, nausea, palpitations, chest pain, shortness of breath, urinary changes, weakness, bowel movement changes, sleep problems)	No.
☐ Medication side effects	Over the past four months I started having problems in my sexual performance. A friend told me it is the propranolol, but I think it is my age. Isn't that right, doctor?
☐ Description of the problem	I have a weak erection.
☐ Severity on 1–10 scale, where 1 is flaccid and 6 is adequate for penetration	About a 4.
☐ Early-morning or nocturnal erections	No.
☐ Libido	That's weak too, doc. I'm just not as interested in sex as I used to be.
☐ Marital or work problems	No, my wife is great and I am very happy in my job.
☐ Feelings of depression	No.
☐ Feelings of anxiety or stress	No.
☐ Any leg or buttock pain while walking or resting	No.
☐ Weight changes	No.
☐ Appetite changes	No.
☐ Diabetes	No.
☐ History of hypercholesterolemia	Yes, it was diagnosed last year.
☐ Previous heart problems	No.
☐ History of TIA or stroke	No.
☐ Current medications	Propranolol, hydrochlorothiazide, lovastatin.
☐ Past medical history	None.
☐ Past surgical history	None.

✓	Question	Patient Response
☐	Family history	My father died at age 50 of a heart attack. My mother is healthy, but she has Alzheimer's disease. She is in a nursing home now.
☐	Occupation	Schoolteacher.
☐	Diet	I eat a lot of junk food.
☐	Exercise	No.
☐	Alcohol use	Yes, 3–4 beers a week.
☐	Illicit drug use	No.
☐	Tobacco	No.
☐	Social history	I am married and live with my wife.
☐	Sexual activity	I had a wonderful sex life with my wife until four months ago, when I started having this problem that I told you about. I think I am getting old.
☐	Drug allergies	No.

Physical Examination:

- ☐ Examinee washed his/her hands.
- ☐ Examinee asked permission to start the exam.
- ☐ Examinee used respectful draping.
- ☐ Examinee did not repeat painful maneuvers.

✓	Exam Component	Maneuver
☐	Head and neck exam	Funduscopic exam, carotid auscultation
☐	CV exam	Palpation, auscultation
☐	Pulmonary exam	Auscultation
☐	Abdominal exam	Auscultation, palpation
☐	Extremities	Inspection, palpation of peripheral pulses
☐	Neurologic exam	DTRs, Babinski's sign, sensation and strength in bilateral lower extremities

Closure:

- ☐ Examinee discussed initial diagnostic impressions.
- ☐ Examinee discussed initial management plans:
    - ☐ Follow-up tests: Examinee mentioned the need for genital and rectal exams.
    - ☐ Lifestyle modification (diet, exercise, alcohol cessation).
    - ☐ Changing propranolol to another antihypertensive medication that does not cause erectile dysfunction.
- ☐ Examinee asked if the patient has any other questions or concerns.

Sample Closure:

Mr. Miller, your blood pressure level was 135/90 when we measured it earlier today, which is close to our target of 130/80. However, it would be even better if we could get it down to around 120/80. Fortunately, that should be feasible with lifestyle changes such as decreasing your salt and fat intake and increasing the amount of exercise you are doing. As for your problems with your erection, this is a very common side effect of one of the blood pressure medications you are taking. For this reason, I would like to give you a medication other than propranolol to control your blood pressure. I am also going to order some blood tests to make sure that your problem is not due to any other medical condition. In addition, I would like to perform a genital exam as well as a rectal exam to assess your prostate. Do you have any questions for me?

PATIENT NOTE

History

Physical Examination

Differential Diagnosis

1.

2.

3.

4.

5.

Diagnostic Workup

1.

2.

3.

4.

5.

PATIENT NOTE

History

HPI: 54 yo M here for follow-up of his hypertension that was diagnosed last year. He was initially started on HCTZ; propranolol was added 6 months ago. He is fairly compliant with his medications. He does not monitor his blood pressure at home. His last blood pressure checkup was 6 months ago. He is feeling well except for erectile dysfunction and decreased libido noted 4 months ago. No leg claudication or any previous history of heart problems, stroke, TIA, or diabetes. No marital or work problems. No depression, anxiety, appetite or weight changes, or history of trauma.
ROS: Negative except as above.
Allergies: NKDA.
Medications: HCTZ, propranolol, lovastatin.
PMH: Hypertension, hypercholesterolemia diagnosed 1 year ago.
PSH: None.
SH: No smoking, 3–4 beers/week, no illicit drugs. Works as a schoolteacher; married and lives with his wife.
FH: Father died of a heart attack at age 50. Mother is in a nursing home due to Alzheimer's disease.

Physical Examination

Patient is in no acute distress.
VS: WNL.
HEENT: No funduscopic abnormalities.
Neck: No carotid bruits, no JVD.
Chest: Clear breath sounds bilaterally.
Heart: Apical impulse not displaced; RRR; normal S1/S2; no murmurs, rubs, or gallops.
Abdomen: Soft, nondistended, nontender, ⊕BS, no bruits, no organomegaly.
Extremities: No edema, no hair loss or skin changes. Radial, brachial, femoral, dorsalis pedis, and posterior tibialis 2+ and symmetric.
Neuro: Motor: Strength 5/5 in bilateral lower extremities. Sensation: Intact to pinprick and soft touch in lower extremities. DTRs: Symmetric 2+ in lower extremities, ⊖Babinski bilaterally.

Differential Diagnosis

1. Drug-induced erectile dysfunction (ED)
2. Hypogonadism
3. ED caused by vascular disease
4. Depression
5. Alcohol-related ED
6. Peyronie's disease

Diagnostic Workup

1. Genital exam
2. Rectal exam
3. Serum glucose
4. Testosterone
5. LH/FSH
6. Prolactin, TSH
7. Ferritin
8. MRI—brain
9. Doppler U/S—penis
10. Dynamic cavernosography
11. BUN/Cr, electrolytes, cholesterol, UA, ECG

CASE DISCUSSION

Differential Diagnosis

- **Drug-induced erectile dysfunction (ED):** Antihypertensives (but rarely diuretics) and alcohol are commonly associated with ED. β-blockers may also result in loss of libido.
- **Hypogonadism:** Testosterone deficiency has many underlying etiologies but, as with other endocrine problems, is attributable to either central (due to insufficient gonadotropin secretion by the pituitary) or end-organ disease (pathology in the testes themselves). In addition to diminished libido and possible ED, there are often associated symptoms such as hot flushes, fatigue, and depression.
- **ED caused by vascular disease:** Hypertension and hyperlipidemia are risk factors for atherosclerotic vascular disease, but there are no historical or physical findings (e.g., angina, leg claudication, diminished pulses, hair loss, or thin, shiny skin) to suggest its presence in this case. For example, arterial insufficiency involving the terminal aorta is a common cause of ED but is usually accompanied by vascular claudication of the legs (Leriche's syndrome).
- **Depression:** Psychogenic causes can lead to loss of libido and loss of erections and are suggested when nocturnal or early-morning erections are preserved (not seen in this case). This patient denies other depressive symptoms, but further exploration of his feelings about his demented, nursing-home-bound mother may be more revealing.
- **Alcohol-related ED:** The use of alcohol (as well as tobacco and illicit drugs) is associated with an increased risk of ED.
- **Peyronie's disease:** Fibrous plaque of the tunica albuginea can lead to penile scarring and ED.

Diagnostic Workup

- **Genital exam:** To rule out Peyronie's disease (e.g., see penile scarring or plaque formation).
- **Rectal exam:** To detect masses or prostatic abnormalities.
- **Serum glucose:** To screen for diabetes, a possible contributor to ED.
- **Testosterone level:** To screen for hypogonadism.
- **LH/FSH:** Gonadotropin levels should be checked in patients with low or borderline testosterone levels. Levels are elevated ("hypergonadotropic") in the setting of testicular pathology and are low ("hypogonadotropic") in the setting of pituitary or hypothalamic disease.
- **Prolactin, TSH:** To screen for other abnormalities of pituitary function in patients with hypogonadotropic hypogonadism.
- **Ferritin:** To screen for hemochromatosis, a common condition; ED can be an early manifestation due to iron deposition in the pituitary gland causing hypogonadotropic hypogonadism.
- **MRI—brain:** To rule out a pituitary or hypothalamic lesion in patients presenting with hypogonadotropic hypogonadism.
- **Doppler U/S—penis:** To assess blood flow in the cavernous arteries.
- **Dynamic cavernosography:** To determine the site and extent of venous leak (suspected in patients with normal arterial inflow).
- **BUN/Cr, electrolytes, cholesterol, UA, ECG:** Useful in the longitudinal care of hypertension and hyperlipidemia. To screen for kidney disease, for LVH or prior silent MIs, for response to cholesterol-lowering medication, and for complications of medical therapy (e.g., diuretic-induced hypokalemia).

CASE 21
DOORWAY INFORMATION

Opening Scenario

Kathleen Moore, a 33-year-old female, comes to the clinic complaining of knee pain.

Vital Signs

BP: 130/80 mmHg
Temp: 99.5°F (37.5°C)
RR: 16/minute
HR: 76/minute, regular

Examinee Tasks

1. Take a focused history.
2. Perform a focused physical exam (do not perform rectal, genitourinary, or female breast exam).
3. Explain your clinical impression and workup plan to the patient.
4. Write the patient note after leaving the room.

Checklist/SP Sheet

PATIENT DESCRIPTION
Patient is a 33 yo F, divorced with two daughters.

NOTES FOR THE SP

- Pretend to have pain when the examinee moves your left knee in all directions.
- Do not allow the examinee to fully flex or extend your left knee.
- Paint your left knee red to make it look inflamed.

CHALLENGING QUESTIONS TO ASK
"Do you think I will be able to walk on my knee like before?"

SAMPLE EXAMINEE RESPONSE
"Most likely, but that depends on the underlying problem and your response to treatment."

Examinee Checklist

ENTRANCE:

- [ ] Examinee knocked on the door before entering.
- [ ] Examinee introduced self by name.
- [ ] Examinee identified his/her role or position.
- [ ] Examinee correctly used patient's name.
- [ ] Examinee made eye contact with the SP.

HISTORY:

- [ ] Examinee showed compassion for your pain.

☑ Question	Patient Response
☐ Chief complaint	Left knee pain.
☐ Onset	Two days ago.
☐ Function	I can't move it. I use a cane to walk.
☐ Redness	Yes.
☐ Swelling of the joint	Yes.
☐ Alleviating factors	Rest and Tylenol help a little bit.
☐ Exacerbating factors	Moving my knee and walking.
☐ History of trauma to the knee	No.
☐ Other joint pain	Yes, my wrists and fingers are always painful and stiff. Five years ago I had a painful, swollen big toe on my left foot.
☐ Duration of the pain in the fingers	Six months.
☐ Stiffness in the morning/duration	Yes, for an hour.
☐ Photosensitivity	No.
☐ Rashes	No.
☐ Oral ulcers	I had many in my mouth last month, but they've resolved now.
☐ Fatigue	Yes, I've had no energy to work and have felt tired all the time for the past six months.
☐ Fever/chills	I feel hot now, but I have no chills.
☐ Hair loss	No.
☐ Cold temperature causing problems with the fingers	Sometimes my fingers become pale and then blue when they are exposed to cold weather or cold water.
☐ Heart symptoms (chest pain, palpitations)	No.
☐ Pulmonary complaints (shortness of breath, cough)	No.
☐ Neurologic complaints (seizures, weakness, numbness)	No.
☐ Urinary problems (hematuria)	No.
☐ Abdominal pain	No.
☐ History of recent tick bite	No.
☐ Pregnancies	I have two daughters. Both were delivered by C-section.
☐ Miscarriages/abortions	I had two spontaneous abortions a long time ago.
☐ Last menstrual period	Two weeks ago.
☐ Weight changes	I've lost about 10 pounds over the past six months.
☐ Appetite changes	I don't have a good appetite.

☑ Question	Patient Response
☐ Current medications	I used Tylenol to relieve my pain, but it is not working as well anymore.
☐ Past medical history	None.
☐ Past surgical history	Two C-sections at ages 23 and 25.
☐ Family history	My mother has rheumatoid arthritis and is living in a nursing home. I don't know my father.
☐ Occupation	Waitress.
☐ Alcohol use	I don't drink a lot, usually 2–4 beers a week except for weekends, when I don't count.
☐ CAGE questions	No (to all four).
☐ Last alcohol ingestion	Four days ago.
☐ Illicit drug use	No.
☐ Tobacco	Yes, one pack a day for the past 20 years.
☐ Sexual activity	I am sexually active with a new boyfriend whom I met two months ago.
☐ Use of condoms	Occasionally.
☐ Number of sexual partners during the last year	Four.
☐ Active with men, women, or both	Men only.
☐ Vaginal discharge	No.
☐ History of STDs	Yes, I had gonorrhea one year ago. I took antibiotics and was fine.
☐ Drug allergies	No.

Physical Examination:

☐ Examinee washed his/her hands.
☐ Examinee asked permission to start the exam.
☐ Examinee used respectful draping.
☐ Examinee did not repeat painful maneuvers.

☑ Exam Component	Maneuver
☐ Mouth exam	Inspection
☐ Musculoskeletal exam	Inspection and palpation (compared both knees, including range of motion); examined other joints (shoulders, elbows, wrists, hands, fingers, hips, ankles)
☐ Hair and skin exam	Inspection
☐ CV exam	Auscultation

☑ Exam Component	Maneuver
☐ Pulmonary exam	Auscultation
☐ Abdominal exam	Auscultation, palpation, percussion

Closure:

☐ Examinee discussed initial diagnostic impressions.
☐ Examinee discussed initial management plans:
    ☐ Follow-up tests: Examinee mentioned the need for a pelvic exam.
    ☐ Discussed safe sex practices.
☐ Examinee asked if the patient has any other questions or concerns.

Sample Closure:

Ms. Moore, there are a few things that could be causing your knee pain, such as gout, an infection, or rheumatoid arthritis. In order to find out, I would like to draw fluid from your knee and then draw some blood. Sometimes infections from the pelvis can spread to other parts of your body, such as your knee, and for that reason I would also like to do a pelvic exam. These tests will likely reveal the source of your pain. You mentioned earlier that you don't always use condoms. I know condoms may be difficult to use regularly, but they are important in helping to control the spread of STDs. Do you have any questions for me?

History

Physical Examination

Differential Diagnosis

1.

2.

3.

4.

5.

Diagnostic Workup

1.

2.

3.

4.

5.

History

HPI: 33 yo F c/o left knee pain that started 2 days ago and is causing difficulty walking. She has swelling and redness in her left knee and mild fever but no chills. She denies trauma. She has a history of fatigue and painful wrists and fingers and has experienced 1-hour morning stiffness over the past 6 months. She also recalls multiple oral ulcers that resolved last month. She describes Raynaud's phenomenon but denies rash, photosensitivity, hair loss, or recent tick bites. She recalls a 10-pound weight loss over the past 6 months and has no appetite.
ROS: Negative except as above.
Allergies: NKDA.
Medications: Tylenol.
PMH: Episode of acute left big toe arthritis 5 years ago; gonorrhea 1 year ago.
PSH: Two C-sections.
SH: One PPD for 20 years. Usually drinks 2–4 beers/week; on weekends drinks more; last ingestion 4 days ago; CAGE 0/4. No illicit drugs. Sexually active with multiple partners; inconsistent condom use.
FH: Mother has rheumatoid arthritis and lives in a nursing home.

Physical Examination

Patient is in no acute distress but favors the left knee.
VS: WNL.
HEENT: No oral lesions.
Chest: Clear breath sounds bilaterally.
Heart: RRR; normal S1/S2; no murmurs, rubs, or gallops.
Abdomen: Soft, nondistended, ⊕BS, no hepatosplenomegaly.
Extremities: Erythema, tenderness, pain, and restricted range of motion on flexion and extension of left knee compared to right knee. Shoulder, elbow, wrist, hand, finger, hip, and ankle joints WNL bilaterally.

Differential Diagnosis

1. Gout
2. Pseudogout
3. SLE
4. Rheumatoid arthritis
5. Gonococcal septic arthritis
6. Nongonococcal septic arthritis
7. Osteoarthritis

Diagnostic Workup

1. Pelvic exam and cervical cultures
2. Knee aspiration and synovial fluid analysis
3. XR—left knee and both hands
4. CBC
5. ANA, anti-dsDNA, RF
6. Blood culture

CASE DISCUSSION

Differential Diagnosis

- **Gout:** This acute, usually monoarticular, crystal-induced arthritis rarely occurs in premenopausal women, but the patient's history of first MTP arthritis ("podagra") is classic for gout. Alcohol ingestion causes hyperuricemia and may precipitate an acute attack. Foot, ankle, and knee joints are also commonly affected. Gout does not explain her hand arthralgias, but osteoarthritis is common and may coexist.

- **Pseudogout:** Another crystal-induced arthritis, pseudogout frequently involves the knees and wrists but is usually seen in patients > 60 years of age.

- **SLE:** Joint symptoms (usually symmetric peripheral arthralgias), constitutional symptoms, and Raynaud's phenomenon may be early manifestations of this disease. Unilateral knee involvement is not typical. The diagnosis requires at least four of the following 11 criteria: malar ("butterfly") rash, discoid rash, symmetric arthritis, photosensitivity, oral ulcers, serositis, renal disease, CNS involvement, hematologic disorders (her fatigue may be due to anemia), immunologic abnormalities (her history of spontaneous abortions may signal the presence of antiphospholipid antibodies), or ANA positivity. More testing needs to be done before SLE can be diagnosed in this case.

- **Rheumatoid arthritis:** This is suggested in a patient with a positive family history, symmetric small joint arthritis (e.g., fingers, wrists), prolonged morning stiffness, and systemic symptoms (low-grade fever, anorexia, weight loss, fatigue, and weakness). However, this patient's hand joints were not red, warm, swollen, or tender on exam. Monoarthritis is also uncommon but is occasionally seen early in the course of the disease.

- **Gonococcal septic arthritis:** This occurs in healthy hosts, most commonly young women (women are much more likely than men to have asymptomatic genitourinary gonococcal infection, which allows the bug to mutate and disseminate). The knee is the most frequently involved joint, but the monoarthritis (or tenosynovitis) is usually preceded by a few days of migratory polyarthralgias. Also, this patient does not have the characteristic rash, which consists of small necrotic pustules on the extremities (including the palms and soles).

- **Nongonococcal septic arthritis:** This occurs suddenly, usually affects the knee or wrist, and is most commonly caused by *S. aureus*. However, it is a disease of an abnormal host; previous joint damage and IV drug use are key risk factors not present in this case.

- **Osteoarthritis:** Onset is insidious, joint stiffness brief, and joint inflammation minimal, all of which are incongruent with this patient's presentation. Also, osteoarthritis spares the wrist and MCP joints and is not associated with constitutional symptoms.

Diagnostic Workup

- **Pelvic exam and cervical cultures:** Necessary to investigate gonococcal infection and are often positive in the absence of symptoms (urine, anorectal, and throat cultures may also be necessary).

- **Knee aspiration, Gram stain, culture, and inspection for crystals:** In most cases of acute monoarthritis, joint aspiration must be performed to rule out septic arthritis. Inflammatory joint synovial fluid contains > 3000 WBCs/μL, and septic joint fluid often contains > 50,000 cells/μL. The demonstration of needle-shaped, negatively birefringent crystals or rhomboid-shaped, weakly positively birefringent crystals confirms gout or pseudogout, respectively.

- **XR—left knee and both hands:** Specific changes in rheumatoid arthritis include symmetric joint space narrowing, marginal bony erosions, and periarticular demineralization. However, x-rays are usually normal during the first six months of illness. In gout, look for punched-out cortical erosions and a sclerotic joint margin. In pseudogout, look for calcified articular cartilage ("chondrocalcinosis"). In osteoarthritis, look for joint space narrowing, marginal osteophytes, subchondral osteosclerosis, and occasionally subchondral cysts.

- **CBC:** Look for anemia, leukopenia, and/or thrombocytopenia in SLE, or leukocytosis in acute gout and septic arthritis.

- **Immunologic tests:** ANA is a highly sensitive (but nonspecific) screening test for SLE. A negative test essentially excludes the disease. If ANA is positive, investigate antibody against double-stranded DNA (**anti-dsDNA**), antibody against the Smith antigen, anticardiolipin antibodies, and lupus anticoagulant to help confirm SLE. **RF** is present in > 75% of patients with rheumatoid arthritis.

- **Blood culture:** An important test in septic arthritis.

Opening Scenario

Charles Andrews, a 66-year-old male, comes to the clinic complaining of a tremor.

Vital Signs

BP: 135/90 mmHg
Temp: 98.6°F (37°C)
RR: 16/minute
HR: 70/minute, regular

Examinee Tasks

1. Take a focused history.
2. Perform a focused physical exam (do not perform rectal, genitourinary, or female breast exam).
3. Explain your clinical impression and workup plan to the patient.
4. Write the patient note after leaving the room.

Checklist/SP Sheet

PATIENT DESCRIPTION

Patient is a 66 yo M.

NOTES FOR THE SP

- Exhibit mild muscle rigidity in your wrists and arms—that is, when the examinee tries to move your wrists and arms, stiffen them and move them slowly.
- Lean your back forward slightly and walk in small, shuffling steps.
- Exhibit a resting hand tremor (pill rolling) that disappears with movement.

CHALLENGING QUESTIONS TO ASK

"Do you think I will get better?"

SAMPLE EXAMINEE RESPONSE

"I think your tremor will improve with medication, but I don't know how long the improvement will last. The tremor may be a sign of a larger movement disorder called Parkinson's disease, and we need to do more evaluation to explore that possibility."

Examinee Checklist

ENTRANCE:

☐ Examinee knocked on the door before entering.
☐ Examinee introduced self by name.
☐ Examinee identified his/her role or position.

☐ Examinee correctly used patient's name.
☐ Examinee made eye contact with the SP.

HISTORY:

☐ Examinee showed compassion for your illness.

☑ Question	Patient Response
☐ Chief complaint	I have a tremor in this hand (points to right hand).
☐ Location	Only in the right hand.
☐ Duration	I noticed it about six months ago, but it seems to be getting worse recently.
☐ Context	It shakes when I'm just sitting around doing nothing. It usually stops when I hold out the remote control to change the channel.
☐ Alleviating factors	None.
☐ Exacerbating factors	It seems more severe when I am really tired.
☐ Associated symptoms (falls, headaches, TIA symptoms, drooling, changes in voice or handwriting, difficulty with ADLs/IADLs, depression, constipation, rash, etc.)	No, I don't think so. My wife says I've slowed down, but I think that's just because I retired last year. (If asked what your wife means, say that she is frustrated because it is your job to push the grocery cart, but you can't keep up with her in the store anymore.)
☐ Prior history of similar symptoms	Well, back in college I occasionally had a hand tremor after pulling an all-nighter and drinking lots of coffee. The tremor was in both hands, but it was worse in the right. It seemed faster than the one I have now.
☐ Caffeine intake	One cup of coffee every morning. I used to drink three cups a day, but I've cut back over the past few months.
☐ Alcohol use	None. Both of my parents were alcoholics, so I never touch it.
☐ Past medical history	High cholesterol, treated with diet. Asthma, treated with an albuterol inhaler as needed.
☐ History of head trauma	No.
☐ Family history	My parents died in a car accident in their 40s, and my sister is healthy.
☐ Social history	I am married and live with my wife.
☐ Occupation	Retired chemistry professor.
☐ Exercise	No, I'm really not very active anymore.
☐ Tobacco	No.
☐ Illicit drug use	No.
☐ Current medications	Albuterol inhaler as needed. (If asked, say that you have not used it in more than a year.)
☐ Drug allergies	No.

Physical Examination:

- ☐ Examinee washed his/her hands.
- ☐ Examinee asked permission to start the exam.
- ☐ Examinee used respectful draping.
- ☐ Examinee did not repeat painful maneuvers.

☑ Exam Component	Maneuver
☐ CV exam	Auscultation
☐ Pulmonary exam	Auscultation
☐ Neurologic exam	Mental status, cranial nerves, motor exam (including muscle tone), DTRs, cerebellar, gait, sensory exam

Closure:

- ☐ Examinee discussed initial diagnostic impressions.
- ☐ Examinee discussed initial management plans:
  - ☐ Follow-up tests.
  - ☐ Discussed possible need to compare an old handwriting sample with a present sample.
  - ☐ Physician support throughout the patient's illness.
- ☐ Examinee asked if the patient has any other questions or concerns.

Sample Closure:

Mr. Andrews, I am sorry to have to tell you this, but on the basis of your history and physical exam, it would appear that you have Parkinson's disease. With medications your symptoms may improve, but eventually they will return. One indicator of disease progression involves looking closely at your handwriting. Do you think you could bring an old sample of your handwriting along with you on your next visit? You should also know that about 25% of the time, patients will present with your symptoms and not have Parkinson's. For this reason, I would like to run a few tests, including some imaging studies of your head and some blood tests. Although we won't have those results before you leave today, I will print out a comprehensive patient pamphlet that will give you resources to help answer your questions as they come up. I want you to know that I will be here to treat you and to help you every step of the way. Do you have any questions for me?

PATIENT NOTE

History

Physical Examination

Differential Diagnosis	Diagnostic Workup
1.	1.
2.	2.
3.	3.
4.	4.
5.	5.

History

HPI: *66 yo M c/o right hand tremor for 6 months. It occurs at rest and seems to be getting worse recently. The tremor is exacerbated by fatigue, and there are no alleviating factors (he does not drink alcohol). Reducing his caffeine intake to 1 cup of coffee daily did not seem to help. He denies associated symptoms but does say that his wife complains that he has "slowed down" since retiring last year. Specifically, he seems to be walking more slowly recently (time course unspecified, but within the past year). He had a hand tremor when very fatigued back in college, but it was bilateral and faster than his present tremor.*
ROS: *Negative except as above.*
Allergies: *NKDA.*
Medications: *Albuterol MDI prn (no use in past year).*
PMH: *High cholesterol, treated with diet. Mild asthma.*
SH: *No smoking, no EtOH, no illicit drugs. He is a retired chemistry professor, married and lives with his wife.*
FH: *Noncontributory.*

Physical Examination

Patient is in no acute distress.
VS: *WNL.*
Chest: *Clear breath sounds bilaterally.*
Heart: *RRR; normal S1/S2; no murmurs, rubs, or gallops.*
Neuro: Mental status: *Alert and oriented × 3.* Cranial nerves: *2–12 grossly intact.* Motor: *Right hand resting tremor, about 6 Hz, "pill rolling," improves or disappears during purposeful action or posture. Mild muscle rigidity in both wrists and arms, but no frank cogwheeling. Strength 5/5 throughout.* DTRs: *Symmetric 2+ in all extremities.* Cerebellar: *⊝Romberg, rapid alternating movements and heel-to-shin test normal and symmetric.* Gait: *Bradykinetic, takes small steps. Walks with back slightly bent forward.* Sensation: *Intact to soft touch and pinprick.*

Differential Diagnosis

1. Parkinson's disease
2. Essential tremor
3. Physiologic tremor
4. Midbrain lesion
5. Drug-induced tremor
6. Psychogenic tremor
7. Wilson's disease
8. Hyperthyroidism

Diagnostic Workup

1. TSH
2. Heavy metal screen
3. MRI—brain
4. Ceruloplasmin, slit lamp examination for Kayser-Fleischer rings, AST/ALT, CBC, 24-hour urinary copper, liver biopsy

CASE DISCUSSION

Differential Diagnosis

- **Parkinson's disease (PD):** This is the most common cause of resting tremor (i.e., it is evident with the affected body part supported and completely at rest but improves or subsides with voluntary activity), although some patients with PD also have a postural-action tremor that is indistinguishable from essential tremor (ET, see below). Tremor is usually low frequency (4–6 Hz), begins in one upper extremity, and may later involve the other extremities as well. Leg tremor is more commonly due to PD than to ET. The face, lips, and jaw may be involved, but in contrast to ET, PD does not produce head tremor. Along with the tremor, the patient's bradykinesia and rigidity suggest PD.

- **Essential tremor (ET):** This is the most common neurologic cause of postural tremor (i.e., tremor that is apparent when the arms are held outstretched) or action tremor (i.e., tremor that increases at the end of goal-directed activity such as finger-to-nose testing). Approximately 50% of cases are familial. Tremor is usually high frequency and often asymmetrically involves the distal upper extremity. The head, voice, chin, trunk, and legs can also be involved. ET is not associated with other neurologic signs and is improved following the ingestion of small amounts of alcohol. Differentiation from the classic resting tremor of PD is usually straightforward, as in this case.

- **Physiologic tremor:** This refers to a very low amplitude, high-frequency (10–12 Hz) tremor present in normal individuals. The tremor is often not visible, but when enhanced by medications or other medical conditions, it is the most common cause of postural and action tremors. Conditions that can enhance physiologic tremor include anxiety, excitement, sleep deprivation/fatigue, hypoglycemia, caffeine intake, alcohol withdrawal, thyrotoxicosis, fever, and pheochromocytoma.

- **Midbrain lesion:** Midbrain injury due to stroke, trauma, or demyelinating disease is a rare cause of a solitary asymmetric resting tremor.

- **Drug-induced tremor:** Many medications can enhance physiologic tremor, notably β-agonists (such as albuterol), nicotine, theophylline, TCAs, lithium, valproic acid, and corticosteroids. Mercury and arsenic exposure may also contribute to tremor. Neuroleptics and metoclopramide can cause drug-induced parkinsonism, but tremor is often absent in these cases.

- **Psychogenic tremor:** This often manifests with varying frequency and either becomes more irregular or subsides entirely when the patient is asked to perform a complex, repetitive motor task with the contralateral limb.

- **Wilson's disease:** This can cause resting tremor (among other manifestations) but is not considered in patients > 40 years of age.

- **Hyperthyroidism:** This is associated with fine tremor along with a variety of other classic signs and symptoms.

Diagnostic Workup

- **TSH:** To screen for hyperthyroidism.
- **Heavy metal screen:** To screen for mercury and arsenic toxicity via urine or blood tests.
- **MRI—brain:** To rule out a structural lesion, particularly in the midbrain or basal ganglia.
- **Ceruloplasmin, slit lamp examination for Kayser-Fleischer rings, AST/ALT, CBC, 24-hour urinary copper, liver biopsy:** These tests comprise the screening tests (and diagnostic tests, in the case of liver biopsy) used to evaluate for suspected Wilson's disease. As noted above, the patient's advanced age precludes consideration of Wilson's disease in this case.

Opening Scenario

Jay Keller, a 49-year-old male, comes to the ER complaining of passing out a few hours earlier.

Vital Signs

BP: 135/90 mmHg
Temp: 98.0°F (36.7°C)
RR: 16/minute
HR: 76/minute, regular

Examinee Tasks

1. Take a focused history.
2. Perform a focused physical exam (do not perform rectal, genitourinary, or female breast exam).
3. Explain your clinical impression and workup plan to the patient.
4. Write the patient note after leaving the room.

Checklist/SP Sheet

PATIENT DESCRIPTION

Patient is a 49 yo M, married with three children.

NOTES FOR THE SP

None.

CHALLENGING QUESTIONS TO ASK

"Do you think I have a brain tumor?"

SAMPLE EXAMINEE RESPONSE

"I think it's unlikely. To make absolutely sure, however, we will do a CT scan, which is a special x-ray test of the brain. That will help us see the structure of the brain and rule out any bleeding or tumor."

Examinee Checklist

ENTRANCE:

☐ Examinee knocked on the door before entering.
☐ Examinee introduced self by name.
☐ Examinee identified his/her role or position.
☐ Examinee correctly used patient's name.
☐ Examinee made eye contact with the SP.

HISTORY:

☐ Examinee showed compassion for your illness.

☑ Question	Patient Response
☐ Chief complaint	I passed out.
☐ Describe what happened	This morning I was taking the groceries to the car with my wife when I suddenly fell down and blacked out.
☐ Loss of consciousness before, during, or after the fall	I think I lost consciousness and then fell down on the ground.
☐ Duration of loss of consciousness	My wife told me that I did not respond to her for several minutes.
☐ Palpitations before the fall	Yes, just before I fell down, my heart started racing.
☐ Sensing something unusual before losing consciousness (sounds, lights, smells, etc.)	No.
☐ Spinning/lightheadedness	I felt lightheaded right before the fall.
☐ Shaking (seizure)	Yes, my wife told me that my arms and legs started shaking after I fell down.
☐ Duration of shaking	Maybe 30 seconds.
☐ Bit tongue	No.
☐ Lost control of the bladder	No.
☐ Weakness/numbness	No.
☐ Speech difficulties	No.
☐ Confusion after regaining consciousness	No.
☐ Headaches	No.
☐ Chest pain, shortness of breath	No.
☐ Abdominal pain, nausea/vomiting, diarrhea/constipation	No.
☐ Head trauma	No.
☐ Similar falls, lightheadedness, or passing out before	No.
☐ Gait abnormality	No.
☐ Weight changes	No.
☐ Appetite changes	No.
☐ Current medications	Hydrochlorothiazide, captopril, aspirin, atenolol.
☐ Past medical history	High blood pressure for the last 15 years; heart attack one year ago.
☐ Past surgical history	Appendectomy.
☐ Family history	My father died from a heart attack at age 55, and my mother died in good health.

☑ Question	Patient Response
☐ Occupation	Clerk in a video store.
☐ Alcohol use	Yes, I drink 3–4 beers a week.
☐ CAGE questions	No (to all four).
☐ Illicit drug use	No.
☐ Tobacco	No, I stopped a year ago. I had smoked one pack a day for the previous 25 years.
☐ Sexual activity	Yes, with my wife.
☐ Drug allergies	No.

Physical Examination:

- ☐ Examinee washed his/her hands.
- ☐ Examinee asked permission to start the exam.
- ☐ Examinee used respectful draping.
- ☐ Examinee did not repeat painful maneuvers.

☑ Exam Component	Maneuver
☐ Head and neck exam	Inspection (head, mouth), carotid auscultation and palpation, thyroid exam
☐ CV exam	Palpation, auscultation, orthostatic vital signs
☐ Pulmonary exam	Auscultation
☐ Extremities	Palpated peripheral pulses
☐ Neurologic exam	Mental status, cranial nerves (including funduscopic exam), motor exam, DTRs, cerebellar, Romberg test, gait, sensory exam

Closure:

- ☐ Examinee discussed initial diagnostic impressions.
- ☐ Examinee discussed initial management plans:
    - ☐ Follow-up tests.
- ☐ Examinee asked if the patient has any other questions or concerns.

Sample Closure:

Mr. Keller, I need to run some tests on you in order to determine the reason you passed out this morning, so I am going to get a CT scan of your head to look for bleeding or masses, and I will then order some blood tests to look for infections or electrolyte abnormalities. You mentioned that your heart was racing just before you passed out, so I will also ask you to wear a heart monitor for 24 hours. Doing so is just like having a constant ECG, and it will allow us to detect any abnormal heartbeats you might have. We will start with these tests and then go from there. Do you have any questions for me?

PATIENT NOTE

History

Physical Examination

Differential Diagnosis

1.

2.

3.

4.

5.

Diagnostic Workup

1.

2.

3.

4.

5.

History

HPI: 49 yo M c/o 1 episode of syncope that occurred a few hours ago. He was taking the groceries to the car with his wife when he suddenly felt lightheaded, had palpitations, lost consciousness, and fell down. He was unconscious for several minutes. His wife recalls that his arms and legs started shaking for 30 seconds after he fell down. He denies subsequent confusion, weakness or numbness, speech difficulties, tongue biting, or incontinence.
ROS: Negative except as above.
Allergies: NKDA.
Medications: HCTZ, captopril, aspirin, atenolol.
PMH: Hypertension for the last 15 years; MI 1 year ago.
PSH: Appendectomy.
SH: One PPD for 25 years; quit 1 year ago. Drinks 2–3 beers/week, CAGE 0/4, no illicit drugs.
FH: Father died from an MI at age 55.

Physical Examination

Patient is in no acute distress.
VS: WNL, no orthostatic changes.
HEENT: NC/AT, PERRLA, no funduscopic abnormalities, no tongue trauma.
Neck: Supple, no carotid bruits, 2+ carotid pulses with good upstroke bilaterally, thyroid normal.
Chest: Clear breath sounds bilaterally.
Heart: Apical impulse not displaced; RRR; normal S1/S2; no murmurs, rubs, or gallops.
Extremities: Symmetric 2+ brachial, radial, and dorsalis pedis pulses bilaterally.
Neuro: Cranial nerves: 2–12 grossly intact. Motor: Strength 5/5 throughout. Sensation: Intact to pinprick and soft touch bilaterally. DTRs: Symmetric 2+ in upper and lower extremities, ⊖Babinski bilaterally. Cerebellar: Romberg, finger to nose normal. Gait: Normal.

Differential Diagnosis

1. Convulsive syncope
2. Vasovagal syncope
3. Cardiac arrhythmia
4. Drug-induced orthostatic hypotension
5. Seizure
6. Aortic stenosis

Diagnostic Workup

1. CBC, electrolytes
2. CXR
3. CT—head or MRI—brain
4. ECG and Holter monitor
5. Echocardiography
6. Prolactin
7. EEG

CASE DISCUSSION

Differential Diagnosis

- **Convulsive syncope:** Seizure-like activity often occurs after syncope and is due to global cerebral hypoperfusion. There is no EEG correlate, and a seizure workup is not required.
- **Vasovagal syncope:** This often occurs in the setting of emotional stress or pain and may be due to excessive vagal tone with resulting hypotension. Syncope is often heralded by nausea, sweating, tachycardia, pallor, and feeling "faint." This is also the mechanism of syncope in postmicturition syncope.
- **Cardiac arrhythmia:** Cardiac syncope typically occurs without warning, although a history of palpitations may indicate the presence of an underlying arrhythmia. This patient's history of MI increases his risk of developing ventricular tachycardia, and β-blocker therapy may contribute to bradyarrhythmia.
- **Drug-induced orthostatic hypotension:** The patient's antihypertensive medications increase his risk for orthostatic hypotension and syncope. However, lightheadedness and syncope in this condition is usually postural (i.e., occurs when getting up from a lying or seated position), and this patient's orthostatic vital signs were normal.
- **Seizure:** Seizures usually occur unpredictably in a manner unrelated to posture or exertion. They may stem from a variety of causes, including metabolic factors, trauma, vascular factors, and brain tumors. Tonic-clonic seizures are often accompanied by tongue biting, incontinence, and prolonged confusion or drowsiness postictally.
- **Aortic stenosis:** This and other mechanical causes (e.g., hypertrophic obstructive cardiomyopathy, atrial myxoma) are commonly exertional or postexertional and occur without warning. The lack of a murmur and other physical findings makes this unlikely in this case.

Diagnostic Workup

- **CBC, electrolytes:** To rule out anemia, evidence of hyperviscosity, or electrolyte imbalance that could lead to arrhythmia or other causes of syncope.
- **CXR:** To rule out lung mass, cardiomyopathy, or other pathology.
- **CT–head:** The test of choice to exclude intracranial hemorrhage. Also rules out tumor, trauma, prior stroke, or abscess.
- **MRI–brain:** Provides better anatomic detail than CT. Indicated when focal neurologic signs and symptoms are present. MRA is helpful when vertebrobasilar insufficiency is suspected (i.e., when syncope is accompanied by other brain stem signs).
- **ECG and Holter or event monitor:** To evaluate possible arrhythmia.
- **Echocardiography:** To rule out mechanical causes of syncope (e.g., severe aortic stenosis, atrial myxoma, severe LVH with small residual cavity size, and hypertrophic obstructive cardiomyopathy).
- **Prolactin:** Often elevated within 30–60 minutes following a generalized seizure (it is useless after that time interval). Must be compared to baseline prolactin levels.
- **EEG:** To evaluate suspected seizure activity.

Opening Scenario

Kristin Grant, a 30-year-old female, comes to the office complaining of weight gain.

Vital Signs

BP: 120/85 mmHg
Temp: 98.0°F (36.7°C)
RR: 13/minute
HR: 65/minute, regular
BMI: 30

Examinee Tasks

1. Take a focused history.
2. Perform a focused physical exam (do not perform rectal, genitourinary, or female breast exam).
3. Explain your clinical impression and workup plan to the patient.
4. Write the patient note after leaving the room.

Checklist/SP Sheet

PATIENT DESCRIPTION

Patient is a 30 yo F.

NOTES FOR THE SP

None.

CHALLENGING QUESTIONS TO ASK

"I want to go back to smoking because I believe that I have started gaining weight since I quit."

SAMPLE EXAMINEE RESPONSE

"I understand that your weight is very important to you, but it's clear that the health consequences of smoking far outweigh those associated with weight gain. We also need to determine what else might be contributing to your weight gain and then discuss strategies to deal with it."

Examinee Checklist

ENTRANCE:

☐ Examinee knocked on the door before entering.
☐ Examinee introduced self by name.
☐ Examinee identified his/her role or position.
☐ Examinee correctly used patient's name.
☐ Examinee made eye contact with the SP.

HISTORY:

☐ Examinee showed compassion for your illness.

☑	Question	Patient Response
☐	Chief complaint	I am gaining weight.
☐	Onset	Three months ago.
☐	Pounds gained	Twenty pounds.
☐	Cold intolerance	Yes.
☐	Skin/hair changes	My hair is falling out more than usual, and I feel that my skin has become dry.
☐	Voice change	No.
☐	Constipation	No.
☐	Appetite changes	I have a good appetite.
☐	Fatigue	No.
☐	Depression	No.
☐	Sleeping problems (falling asleep, staying asleep, early waking, snoring)	No.
☐	Associated symptoms (fever/chills, chest pain, shortness of breath, abdominal pain, diarrhea)	No.
☐	Last menstrual period	One week ago.
☐	Frequency of menstrual periods	I used to get my period every four weeks, but recently I've been getting it every six weeks or more. The period lasts seven days.
☐	Start of change in cycle	Six months ago.
☐	Pads/tampons changed a day	It was 2–3 a day, but the blood flow is becoming less, and I use only one a day now.
☐	Age at menarche	Age 13.
☐	Pregnancies	I have one child; he is 10 years old.
☐	Problems during pregnancy/delivery	No, it was a normal delivery, and my child is healthy.
☐	Miscarriages/abortions	None.
☐	Hirsutism	No.
☐	Current medications	Lithium.
☐	Past medical history	I have bipolar disorder. I was started on lithium six months ago; I haven't had any problems since then.
☐	Past surgical history	None.
☐	Family history of obesity	My mother and sister are obese.
☐	Occupation	Housekeeper.
☐	Alcohol use	None.
☐	Illicit drug use	Never.
☐	Tobacco	I quit smoking three months ago. I had smoked two packs a day for 10 years.

☑ Question	Patient Response
☐ Exercise	No.
☐ Diet	The usual. I haven't changed anything in my diet in more than 10 years. Donuts, lots of coffee during the day, chicken, steak, Chinese food, and salad.
☐ Sexual activity	With my husband.
☐ Contraceptives	My husband had a vasectomy two years ago.
☐ Drug allergies	No.

Physical Examination:

☐ Examinee washed his/her hands.
☐ Examinee asked permission to start the exam.
☐ Examinee used respectful draping.
☐ Examinee did not repeat painful maneuvers.

☑ Exam Component	Maneuver
☐ Head exam	Inspected conjunctivae, mouth, and throat
☐ Neck exam	Palpated lymph nodes, thyroid gland
☐ CV exam	Auscultation
☐ Pulmonary exam	Auscultation
☐ Abdominal exam	Auscultation, palpation, percussion
☐ Extremities	Inspection, checked DTRs

Closure:

☐ Examinee discussed initial diagnostic impressions.
☐ Examinee discussed initial management plans:
    ☐ Diagnostic tests.
    ☐ Lifestyle modification (diet, exercise, relaxation techniques, smoking cessation support).
☐ Examinee asked if the patient has any other questions or concerns.

Sample Closure:

Ms. Grant, most smokers gain an average of five pounds once they have quit. You have gained 20 pounds. This may well have resulted from your smoking cessation, but bear in mind that the health risk posed by smoking is far worse than the risk you might incur from excessive weight gain. In addition, there may be other reasons for your weight gain; for example, it may be related to your thyroid gland or may represent a side effect of the lithium you have been taking. I would like to draw some blood to measure your thyroid function and lithium levels. In the meantime, in addition to stopping smoking, you should continue to promote a healthier lifestyle. Try eating fewer fatty foods and consuming healthier foods such as fruits and vegetables. An exercise program of only 30 minutes three times a week can also improve your health. I would also recommend that you cut down on your weekend drinking, as alcohol is full of calories but lacks any nutritional value. Do you have any questions for me?

PATIENT NOTE

History

Physical Examination

Differential Diagnosis

1.

2.

3.

4.

5.

Diagnostic Workup

1.

2.

3.

4.

5.

History

HPI: 30 yo F c/o weight gain of 20 pounds over the past 3 months after she stopped smoking. She has a good appetite and reports no change in her diet. For 6 months she has experienced oligomenorrhea and hypomenorrhea, dry skin, and cold intolerance. No voice change, no constipation, no hirsutism, no depression, no fatigue, and no sleep problems.

OB/GYN: Last menstrual period last week. See HPI for other.

ROS: Negative except as above.

Allergies: NKDA.

Medications: Lithium, started 6 months ago.

PMH: Bipolar disorder, diagnosed 6 months ago.

SH: Two PPD for 10 years; stopped 3 months ago. No alcohol, no illicit drugs. Sexually active with husband only. Doesn't exercise.

Diet: Consists mainly of donuts, lots of coffee during the day, chicken, steak, Chinese food, and salad.

FH: Mother and sister are obese.

Physical Examination

Patient is in no acute distress.

VS: WNL.

HEENT: No conjunctival pallor, mouth and pharynx WNL.

Neck: No lymphadenopathy, thyroid normal.

Chest: Clear breath sounds bilaterally.

Heart: RRR; normal S1/S2; no murmurs, rubs, or gallops.

Abdomen: Soft, nontender, nondistended, ⊕BS, no hepatosplenomegaly.

Extremities: No edema, normal DTRs in lower extremities bilaterally.

Differential Diagnosis

1. Smoking cessation
2. Hypothyroidism
3. Lithium-related obesity
4. Familial obesity
5. Pregnancy
6. Cushing's syndrome

Diagnostic Workup

1. TSH
2. Urine hCG
3. Glucose, cholesterol, triglycerides
4. Dexamethasone suppression test
5. 24-hour urine free cortisol

CASE DISCUSSION

Differential Diagnosis

- **Smoking cessation:** Weight gain occurs in most patients following smoking cessation but usually averages only 2 kg (4.4 lbs). However, major weight gain such as that seen in this case may occur. Patients generally report increased appetite and calorie consumption.
- **Hypothyroidism:** The patient has classic symptoms of hypothyroidism, and it needs to be ruled out as a cause of her weight gain.
- **Lithium-related obesity:** Weight gain is a common side effect of lithium therapy and may contribute in this case.
- **Familial obesity:** There are probably strong genetic influences on the development of obesity, but a positive family history does not account for acute weight gain.
- **Pregnancy:** Regardless of the menstrual history given by the patient, suspect pregnancy in a woman of childbearing age who has unexplained weight gain.
- **Cushing's syndrome:** This is a cause of unexplained weight gain and can usually be diagnosed by physical exam (e.g., one can see hypertension, moon facies, plethora, supraclavicular fat pads, truncal obesity with thin limbs, and abdominal striae).

Diagnostic Workup

- **TSH:** To diagnose suspected hypothyroidism.
- **Urine hCG:** To rule out pregnancy.
- **Glucose, cholesterol, triglycerides:** To screen for medical complications of obesity.
- **Dexamethasone suppression test:** To screen for hypercortisolism. A suppressed morning cortisol following bedtime dexamethasone administration excludes Cushing's syndrome with 98% certainty.
- **24-hour urine free cortisol:** Performed if the dexamethasone suppression test is abnormal. Helps confirm hypercortisolism.

DOORWAY INFORMATION

Opening Scenario

Patricia Garrison, a 36-year-old female, comes to the office complaining of not having menstrual periods recently.

Vital Signs

BP: 120/85 mmHg
Temp: 98.0°F (36.7°C)
RR: 13/minute
HR: 65/minute, regular

Examinee Tasks

1. Take a focused history.
2. Perform a focused physical exam (do not perform rectal, genitourinary, or female breast exam).
3. Explain your clinical impression and workup plan to the patient.
4. Write the patient note after leaving the room.

Checklist/SP Sheet

PATIENT DESCRIPTION
Patient is a 36 yo F.

NOTES FOR THE SP
None.

CHALLENGING QUESTIONS TO ASK
"Am I going through menopause?"

SAMPLE EXAMINEE RESPONSE
"I doubt it. It would be extremely unusual at your age. I need to learn more by asking you about other symptoms and examining you, and then we can discuss possible reasons you are not having periods."

Examinee Checklist

ENTRANCE:

- [ ] Examinee knocked on the door before entering.
- [ ] Examinee introduced self by name.
- [ ] Examinee identified his/her role or position.
- [ ] Examine correctly used patient's name.
- [ ] Examinee made eye contact with the SP.

HISTORY:

- [ ] Examinee showed compassion for your illness.

☑ Question	Patient Response
☐ Chief complaint	I haven't had a period in three months.
☐ Menstrual history	I used to have regular periods every month lasting for 4–5 days, but over the last year I started having them less frequently— every 5–6 weeks lasting for seven days.
☐ Pads/tampons changed a day	It was 2–3 a day, but the blood flow is becoming less, and I use only one a day now.
☐ Age at menarche	Age 14.
☐ Weight changes	I have gained 15 pounds over the past year.
☐ Cold intolerance	No.
☐ Skin/hair changes	Actually, I noticed some facial hair recently that I am plucking.
☐ Voice change	No.
☐ Change in bowel habits	No.
☐ Appetite changes	I have a good appetite.
☐ Fad diet or diet pills	No, I've been a vegetarian for 10 years.
☐ Fatigue	No.
☐ Depression/anxiety/stress	No.
☐ Hot flashes	No.
☐ Vaginal dryness/itching	No.
☐ Sleeping problems (falling asleep, staying asleep, early waking, snoring)	No.
☐ Urinary frequency	No.
☐ Nipple discharge	Yes, just last week I noticed some milky discharge from my left breast.
☐ Visual changes	No.
☐ Headache	No.
☐ Abdominal pain	No.
☐ Sexual activity	Once a week on average with my husband.
☐ Contraceptives	The same pills for eight years.
☐ Pregnancies	I have one child; he is 10 years old.
☐ Problems during pregnancy/delivery	No, it was a normal delivery, and my child is healthy.
☐ Miscarriages/abortions	No.
☐ Last Pap smear	Ten months ago. It was normal.
☐ History of abnormal Pap smears	No.
☐ Current medications	None.
☐ Past medical history	None.
☐ Past surgical history	None.

☑ *Question*	*Patient Response*
☐ Family history	My father and mother are healthy; my mother began menopause at age 55.
☐ Occupation	Nurse.
☐ Alcohol use	None.
☐ Illicit drug use	Never.
☐ Tobacco	No.
☐ Exercise	I run two miles three times a week.
☐ Drug allergies	No.

Physical Examination:

☐ Examinee washed his/her hands.
☐ Examinee asked permission to start the exam.
☐ Examinee used respectful draping.
☐ Examinee did not repeat painful maneuvers.

☑ *Exam Component*	*Maneuver*
☐ Neck exam	Examined thyroid gland
☐ CV exam	Auscultation
☐ Pulmonary exam	Auscultation
☐ Abdominal exam	Auscultation, palpation, percussion
☐ Extremities	Inspection
☐ Neurologic exam	Visual fields, extraocular movements, checked DTRs

Closure:

☐ Examinee discussed initial diagnostic impressions.
☐ Examinee discussed initial management plans:
    ☐ Diagnostic tests.
    ☐ Follow-up tests: Examinee mentioned the need for a pelvic and breast exam.
☐ Examinee asked if the patient has any other questions or concerns.

Sample Closure:

Ms. Garrison, there are a few reasons you may not be having regular periods. The first thing we need to do is determine whether you are pregnant. We can do that with a simple urine test. The other thing we need to do is conduct a breast and pelvic exam, especially since you have had some nipple discharge, and look for any signs of menopause. Menopause is highly unlikely in your age group, but on rare occasions it may occur. A blood test to measure your hormone levels will also help us determine if you are menopausal or have a hormonal imbalance. This will give us a good start in figuring out why you haven't had your period, and we will go from there if we don't find anything. Do you have any questions for me?

PATIENT NOTE

History

Physical Examination

Differential Diagnosis

1.

2.

3.

4.

5.

Diagnostic Workup

1.

2.

3.

4.

5.

History

HPI: 36 yo F c/o amenorrhea for 3 months. She recently noticed some milky discharge from her left breast as well as abnormal facial hair but denies visual changes or headache. She also describes oligomenorrhea, hypomenorrhea, and a 15-pound weight gain over the past year but denies dry skin, cold intolerance, voice change, constipation, depression, fatigue, or sleep problems. She also denies hot flashes and vaginal dryness or itching.

OB/GYN: Menarche at age 14. For the last year, menses have cycled every 5–6 weeks and lasted for 7 days, with decreased blood flow. Before that, menses cycled every 4 weeks. G1P1; 1 uncomplicated vaginal delivery 10 years ago. Last Pap smear 10 months ago; no history of abnormal Pap smears. Sexually active with husband once a week on average; uses OCPs for contraception.

ROS: Negative except as above.

Allergies: NKDA.

Medications: None.

PMH/PSH: None.

SH: Denies tobacco, alcohol, or illicit drug use. Exercises regularly. Vegetarian; hasn't changed her diet recently.

FH: Mother had menopause at age 55.

Physical Examination

Patient is in no acute distress.

VS: WNL.

HEENT: EOMI without diplopia or lid lag; visual fields full to confrontation.

Neck: No thyromegaly.

Chest: Clear breath sounds bilaterally.

Heart: RRR; normal S1/S2; no murmurs, rubs, or gallops.

Abdomen: Soft, nontender, nondistended, ⊕BS, no hepatosplenomegaly.

Extremities: No edema, no tremor.

Neuro: See HEENT. Normal DTRs in lower extremities bilaterally.

Differential Diagnosis

1. Pregnancy
2. Hyperprolactinemia
3. Polycystic ovary syndrome
4. Thyroid disease
5. Premature ovarian failure
6. Asherman's syndrome

Diagnostic Workup

1. Pelvic and breast exam
2. Urine hCG
3. LH/FSH
4. Prolactin, TSH
5. Electrolytes, glucose, BUN/Cr, AST/ALT/ bilirubin/alkaline phosphatase
6. Testosterone, DHEAS
7. MRI—brain
8. Hysteroscopy

CASE DISCUSSION

Differential Diagnosis

- **Pregnancy:** This is the most common cause of secondary amenorrhea in women of childbearing age and should be ruled out during the initial evaluation.
- **Hyperprolactinemia:** This causes menstrual cycle disturbances, galactorrhea, and infertility. It may result from a variety of conditions, including pregnancy, hypothyroidism, renal failure, and cirrhosis, or it can be a side effect of medications. Roughly 70% of women with secondary amenorrhea and galactorrhea will have hyperprolactinemia.
- **Polycystic ovary syndrome (PCOS):** This manifests variably as hirsutism, obesity, virilization, infertility, and glucose intolerance. Half of patients have amenorrhea (due to chronic anovulation). The patient's oligomenorrhea and hirsutism in the context of recent weight gain suggest this diagnosis.
- **Thyroid disease:** Hyper- and hypothyroidism can both cause menstrual irregularities, although amenorrhea is more commonly due to hypothyroidism. Except for galactorrhea and weight gain, the patient does not have other signs or symptoms of thyroid disease.
- **Premature ovarian failure:** This refers to primary hypogonadism that occurs before age 40. Causes include autoimmunity against the ovary, pelvic radiation therapy, chemotherapy, surgical bilateral oophorectomy, and familial factors. The patient's lack of menopausal symptoms (e.g., fatigue, insomnia, headache, diminished libido, depression, and hot flashes) makes this diagnosis unlikely.
- **Asherman's syndrome:** This describes amenorrhea due to endometrial scarring, which can occur following uterine infections. The vaginal estrogen effect is normal.

Diagnostic Workup

- **Pelvic and breast exam:** Required to check for genital virilization (i.e., clitoromegaly), uterine or adnexal enlargement, and estrogen effect (via inspection of vaginal mucosa and Pap smear) and to elicit breast discharge.
- **Urine hCG:** To rule out pregnancy.
- **LH/FSH:** PCOS is a clinical diagnosis; an increased LH/FSH ratio is often seen but is neither necessary nor sufficient to make the diagnosis. Physiologically, increased levels of estrone (derived from obesity) are believed to suppress pituitary FSH, leading to a relative increase in LH. Constant LH stimulation of the ovary then results in anovulation (and often amenorrhea). An elevated FSH (> 40) is diagnostic for premature ovarian failure.
- **Prolactin, TSH:** To screen for hyperprolactinemia and thyroid disease. Free T_4 is also useful if hyperthyroidism (or central hypothyroidism) is suspected.
- **Electrolytes, glucose, BUN/Cr, AST/ALT/bilirubin/alkaline phosphatase:** To check renal and hepatic function and to screen for evidence of hypercortisolism (e.g., high sodium and low potassium).
- **Testosterone, DHEAS:** To screen for hyperandrogenism when amenorrhea is accompanied by hirsutism and virilization. Mild elevations are often due to PCOS, but high levels may be due to ovarian or adrenal tumors.
- **MRI—brain:** Required to evaluate the pituitary region in patients suspected of having amenorrhea due to a hypothalamic or pituitary etiology (e.g., hyperprolactinemia).
- **Hysteroscopy:** To look for endometrial adhesions that are diagnostic for Asherman's syndrome.

Opening Scenario

Stephanie McCall, a 28-year-old female, comes to the office complaining of pain during sex.

Vital Signs

BP: 120/85 mmHg
Temp: 98.0°F (36.7°C)
RR: 13/minute
HR: 65/minute, regular

Examinee Tasks

1. Take a focused history.
2. Perform a focused physical exam (do not perform rectal, genitourinary, or female breast exam).
3. Explain your clinical impression and workup plan to the patient.
4. Write the patient note after leaving the room.

Checklist/SP Sheet

PATIENT DESCRIPTION
Patient is a 28 yo F.

NOTES FOR THE SP
None.

CHALLENGING QUESTIONS TO ASK
When asked about vaginal discharge, ask, "Do you think I have a sexually transmitted disease?"

SAMPLE EXAMINEE RESPONSE
"There are many causes of vaginal discharge, only some of which are due to sexually transmitted infections. I will try to look for clues by asking you more questions and examining you, and we will definitely send a sample of the discharge to the lab to check for infection."

Examinee Checklist

ENTRANCE:

☐ Examinee knocked on the door before entering.
☐ Examinee introduced self by name.
☐ Examinee identified his/her role or position.
☐ Examinee correctly used patient's name.
☐ Examinee made eye contact with the SP.

HISTORY:

☐ Examinee showed compassion for your pain.

☑ Question	Patient Response
☐ Chief complaint	I have been experiencing pain during sex.
☐ Onset	Three months ago.
☐ Describe pain	Aching and burning.
☐ Timing	It happens every time I try to have sex.
☐ Location	In the vaginal area. It starts on the outside, and I feel it on the inside with deep thrusting.
☐ Vaginal discharge	Yes, recently.
☐ Color/amount/smell	White, small amount every day (I don't have to wear a pad); it smells like fish.
☐ Itching	Yes, a little bit.
☐ Douching	No.
☐ Last menstrual period	Two weeks ago.
☐ Frequency of menstrual periods	Regular, every month; lasts for three days.
☐ Pads/tampons changed a day	Three.
☐ Painful periods	Yes, they have started to be painful over the past year.
☐ Postcoital or intermenstrual bleeding	No.
☐ Sexual partner	I have had the same boyfriend for the last year; before that I had a relationship with my ex-boyfriend for five years.
☐ Contraception	I am using the patch.
☐ Sexual desire	Good.
☐ Conflicts with partner	No, we are pretty close.
☐ Feeling safe at home	Yes, I have my own apartment.
☐ History of physical, sexual, or emotional abuse	I don't usually talk about it, but I was raped in college, and that was when I contracted gonorrhea.
☐ History of vaginal infections or STDs	I had gonorrhea 10 years ago in college.
☐ Last Pap smear	Six months ago; it was normal.
☐ History of abnormal Pap smears	No.
☐ Depression/anxiety	No.
☐ Hot flashes	No.
☐ Vaginal dryness during intercourse	No.
☐ Sleeping problems	No.
☐ Urinary frequency/pain with urination	No.

✓ *Question*	*Patient Response*
☐ Pregnancies	I have never been pregnant.
☐ Current medications	None.
☐ Past medical history	None.
☐ Past surgical history	None.
☐ Family history	Both parents are healthy.
☐ Occupation	Editor for a fashion magazine.
☐ Alcohol use	A couple of beers on the weekends; sometimes a glass of wine on a romantic dinner.
☐ CAGE questions	No (to all four).
☐ Illicit drug use	Marijuana in college.
☐ Tobacco	No.
☐ Exercise	I swim and run regularly.
☐ Drug allergies	No.

Physical Examination:

- ☐ Examinee washed his/her hands.
- ☐ Examinee asked permission to start the exam.
- ☐ Examinee used respectful draping.
- ☐ Examinee did not repeat painful maneuvers.

✓ *Exam Component*	*Maneuver*
☐ CV exam	Auscultation
☐ Pulmonary exam	Auscultation
☐ Abdominal exam	Auscultation, palpation, percussion

Closure:

- ☐ Examinee discussed initial diagnostic impressions.
- ☐ Examinee discussed initial management plans:
  - ☐ Diagnostic tests.
  - ☐ Follow-up tests: Examinee mentioned the need for a pelvic exam.
- ☐ Examinee asked if the patient has any other questions or concerns.

Sample Closure:

Ms. McCall, your most likely diagnosis is an infection in the vagina or cervix. However, there are other, less common causes for your problem. I can't make a diagnosis until I do a pelvic exam and take a look at what I find under a microscope. I will also take a cervical swab and send it for gonorrhea and chlamydia testing. Do you have any questions for me?

PATIENT NOTE

History

Physical Examination

Differential Diagnosis

1.

2.

3.

4.

5.

Diagnostic Workup

1.

2.

3.

4.

5.

History

HPI: 28 yo F c/o pain during intercourse for 3 months, located both superficially and with deep thrusting. She also noticed a small white vaginal discharge with a fishy odor, accompanied by mild vaginal pruritus. Denies postcoital or intermenstrual vaginal bleeding. She is sexually active with her boyfriend (only) for the past year, and her sexual desire is good. She feels safe at home and denies any conflicts with her partner. She also denies vaginal dryness, hot flashes, hirsutism, depression, fatigue, sleep problems, dysuria, and urinary frequency.

OB/GYN: G0P0. Last menstrual period 2 weeks ago; has regular menses but started to be painful over the past year. No history of abnormal Pap smears; most recent was 6 months ago. Uses patch for contraception.

ROS: Negative except as above.

Allergies: NKDA.

Medications: None.

PMH: History of rape 10 years ago; subsequently contracted gonorrhea.

SH: No tobacco. Drinks a couple of beers on the weekends, occasional wine, CAGE 0/4; used marijuana in college. Exercises regularly.

FH: Noncontributory.

Physical Examination

Patient is in no acute distress.

VS: WNL.

Chest: Clear breath sounds bilaterally.

Heart: RRR; normal S1/S2; no murmurs, rubs, or gallops.

Abdomen: Soft, nontender, nondistended, ⊕BS, no hepatosplenomegaly.

Differential Diagnosis

1. Vulvovaginitis
2. Cervicitis
3. Endometriosis
4. Vulvodynia
5. Domestic violence
6. Pelvic tumor
7. Vaginismus

Diagnostic Workup

1. Pelvic exam
2. Wet mount, KOH prep, "whiff" test
3. Cervical cultures (chlamydia and gonorrhea DNA probes)
4. U/S—pelvis
5. MRI—pelvis
6. Laparoscopy

CASE DISCUSSION

Differential Diagnosis

- **Vulvovaginitis:** This describes infection or inflammation of the vagina. Etiologies include pathogens, allergic or contact reactions, or friction from intercourse. The presence of vaginal discharge (accompanied by a fishy odor and pruritus) makes this a likely diagnosis.
- **Cervicitis:** The presence of vaginal discharge and pain with deep thrusting suggests infection or inflammation of the cervix.
- **Endometriosis:** This describes abnormal ectopic endometrial tissue, which can cause inflammation and scarring in the lower pelvis. Endometriosis may account for the patient's dysmenorrhea over the past year and, if so, could also cause dyspareunia with deep thrusting. Her history of gonorrhea infection (if it caused PID) also puts her at risk for pelvic scarring and subsequent dyspareunia (due to impaired mobility of pelvic organs).
- **Vulvodynia:** This is the leading cause of dyspareunia in premenopausal women but is not well understood. Pain may be constant or intermittent, focal or diffuse, and superficial or deep. Physical findings are often absent, making it a diagnosis of exclusion. However, vulvar erythema can be seen in a subset of vulvodynia termed *vulvar vestibulitis.*
- **Domestic violence:** Physicians must screen for this in any woman presenting with dyspareunia. Serial screening is required, as victims may not disclose this history initially.
- **Pelvic tumor:** This could account for the patient's pain with deep thrusting and possibly for her history of dysmenorrhea. However, pelvic tumors are not associated with vaginal discharge and pruritus.
- **Vaginismus:** This describes severe involuntary spasm of muscles around the introitus and often results from fear, pain, or sexual or psychological trauma. The muscle contractions generally preclude penetration. Although this patient was raped in the past, she does not describe the muscle contractions characteristic of vaginismus.

Diagnostic Workup

- **Pelvic exam:** To localize and reproduce the pain or discomfort and to determine if any pathology is present. A complete exam includes external genital inspection and palpation, a speculum exam, and bimanual and rectal exams.
- **Wet mount, KOH prep, "whiff" test:** The vaginal discharge is examined microscopically. The presence of epithelial cells covered with bacteria (clue cells) suggests bacterial vaginosis, and the presence of hyphae and spores indicates candidal infection. Motile organisms are seen in trichomonal infection. A "fishy" odor after exposure of the discharge to a drop of potassium hydroxide is characteristic of bacterial vaginosis.
- **Cervical cultures:** To diagnose chlamydia, gonorrhea, and occasionally HSV infection (the latter is characterized by the presence of vesicles or ulcers on the cervix).
- **Imaging studies:** Ultrasound and MRI are useful to assess the size and positioning of pelvic organs and to help rule out masses or other pathology.
- **Laparoscopy:** This is the gold standard test used to confirm a clinical diagnosis of endometriosis.

CASE 27

Opening Scenario

Rick Meyer, a 51-year-old male construction worker, comes to the office complaining of back pain.

Vital Signs

BP: 120/85 mmHg
Temp: 98.2°F (36.8°C)
RR: 20/minute
HR: 80/minute, regular

Examinee Tasks

1. Take a focused history.
2. Perform a focused physical exam (do not perform rectal, genitourinary, or female breast exam).
3. Explain your clinical impression and workup plan to the patient.
4. Write the patient note after leaving the room.

Checklist/SP Sheet

PATIENT DESCRIPTION

Patient is a 51 yo M who lives with his girlfriend.

NOTES FOR THE SP

- Pretend that you have paraspinal lower back tenderness when examined.
- Show normal reflexes, sensation, and strength in both lower extremities.
- Lean forward slightly when walking.

CHALLENGING QUESTIONS TO ASK

"I don't think I can go to work, doctor. Can you write a letter to my boss so that I can have some days off?"

SAMPLE EXAMINEE RESPONSE

"You're right; heavy construction work can worsen your back pain or cause it to heal more slowly. I will ask your boss to reassign you to light duty for a while."

Examinee Checklist

ENTRANCE:

- ☐ Examinee knocked on the door before entering.
- ☐ Examinee introduced self by name.
- ☐ Examinee identified his/her role or position.
- ☐ Examinee correctly used patient's name.
- ☐ Examinee made eye contact with the SP.

HISTORY:

☐ Examinee showed compassion for your pain.

☑	Question	Patient Response
☐	Chief complaint	Pain in my back.
☐	Onset	One week ago.
☐	Associated/precipitating events	I was lifting some heavy boxes; then my back started hurting right away.
☐	Progression	It has been the same.
☐	Severity on a scale	8/10.
☐	Location	The middle of my lower back.
☐	Radiation	It radiates to my left thigh and sometimes reaches my left foot.
☐	Quality	Sharp.
☐	Alleviating factors	Lying still in bed.
☐	Exacerbating factors	Walking, sitting for a long time, coughing.
☐	Weakness/numbness	None.
☐	Difficulty urinating	I noticed that over the past six months I have had to strain in order to urinate. Sometimes I feel as if I haven't emptied my bladder fully.
☐	Urinary or fecal incontinence	No.
☐	Fever, night sweats, weight loss	No.
☐	History of back pain in the past	Well, for the past year I have been having back pain on and off, mainly when I walk. It is usually accompanied by pain in my legs. That pain goes away when I stop walking and sit down.
☐	Current medications	I take ibuprofen. It helps, but the pain is still there.
☐	Past medical history	None.
☐	Past surgical history	None.
☐	Family history	My father died of a heart attack at age 65, and my mother is healthy.
☐	Occupation	Construction worker.
☐	Alcohol use	Yes, a couple of beers on the weekends.
☐	CAGE questions	No (to all four).
☐	Illicit drug use	Never.
☐	Tobacco	Yes, one pack a day for the last 18 years.
☐	Drug allergies	Penicillin gives me a rash.

Physical Examination:

- [ ] Examinee washed his/her hands.
- [ ] Examinee asked permission to start the exam.
- [ ] Examinee used respectful draping.
- [ ] Examinee did not repeat painful maneuvers.

☑ Exam Component	Maneuver
[ ] Back exam	Inspection, palpation, range of motion
[ ] Extremities	Inspection, palpation of peripheral pulses, hip exam
[ ] Neurologic exam	Motor, DTRs, Babinski's sign, gait (including toe and heel walking), passive straight leg raising, sensory exam

Closure:

- [ ] Examinee discussed initial diagnostic impressions.
- [ ] Examinee discussed initial management plans:
  - [ ] Diagnostic tests.
  - [ ] Follow-up tests: Examinee mentioned the need for a rectal exam.
- [ ] Examinee asked if the patient has any other questions or concerns.

Sample Closure:

Mr. Meyer, I am concerned about your difficulty urinating, so I would like to do a rectal exam and assess your prostate for benign growths or cancer. I would also like to run some blood tests and order an x-ray and possibly an MRI of your back so that I can better determine the cause of your pain. In the meantime, as we discussed previously, I will write a note to your employer requesting that you be given only light duties while you are at work. Do you have any questions for me?

PATIENT NOTE

History

Physical Examination

Differential Diagnosis

1.

2.

3.

4.

5.

Diagnostic Workup

1.

2.

3.

4.

5.

History

HPI: *51 yo M construction worker c/o lower back pain that started after he lifted heavy boxes 1 week ago. The pain is 8/10, is sharp, and radiates to the left thigh and sometimes to the left foot. Pain worsens with movement, cough, and sitting for a long time. Pain is relieved by lying still and partially by ibuprofen. He denies urinary/stool incontinence or weakness/loss of sensation in lower extremities. No fever, night sweats, or weight loss. He does report difficulty urinating and incomplete emptying of the bladder for 6 months as well as a 1-year history of intermittent lower back pain and leg pain with ambulation that resolves with sitting.*
ROS: *Negative except as above.*
Allergies: *Penicillin, causes rash.*
Medications: *Ibuprofen.*
PMH: *None.*
PSH: *None.*
SH: *One PPD for 18 years, 1–2 beers on weekends, CAGE 0/4.*
FH: *Noncontributory.*

Physical Examination

Patient is in mild distress due to back pain.
Back: *Mild paraspinal muscle tenderness bilaterally, normal range of motion, no warmth or erythema.*
Extremities: *2+ popliteal, dorsalis pedis, and posterior tibial pulses bilaterally. Hips normal, nontender range of motion bilaterally.*
Neuro: *Motor: Strength 5/5 throughout, including left great toe dorsiflexion. DTRs: 2+ symmetric, ⊖Babinski bilaterally. Gait: Normal (including toe and heel walking), although he walks with back slightly bent forward. Straight leg raising ⊖bilaterally. Sensation: Intact.*

Differential Diagnosis

1. Disk herniation
2. Lumbar muscle strain
3. Degenerative arthritis
4. Lumbar spinal stenosis
5. Metastatic prostate cancer
6. Multiple myeloma
7. Malingering

Diagnostic Workup

1. Rectal exam
2. XR—L-spine
3. MRI—L-spine
4. PSA
5. CBC, calcium, BUN/Cr
6. Serum and urine protein electrophoresis

CASE DISCUSSION

Differential Diagnosis

- **Disk herniation:** Low back pain radiating down the buttock and below the knee suggests nerve root irritation due to disk herniation. However, this pattern is nonspecific and can also be caused by sacroiliitis, facet joint degenerative arthritis, spinal stenosis, or other causes of sciatica. Most disk herniations occur at the L4–L5 or L5–S1 vertebral levels. These nerve roots are quickly assessed by checking the knee-jerk reflex (L4), great toe dorsiflexion (L5), and ankle-jerk reflex (S1). Ipsilateral straight leg raising that produces radicular symptoms (with the leg raised < 60 degrees) is highly sensitive but nonspecific in herniations at these levels. This patient may have disk herniation but has no objective evidence of neurologic compromise at this point.
- **Lumbar muscle strain:** This often follows strenuous or unusual exertion, but pain usually does not radiate to the extremities. Paraspinal muscle tenderness is often present.
- **Degenerative arthritis:** Degenerative back diseases are common, and classically pain is exacerbated by activity and alleviated by rest. Radicular symptoms may be present.
- **Lumbar spinal stenosis:** This is most often seen in patients > 60 years of age. They present with gradual onset of back pain that radiates to the buttocks and legs with or without leg numbness and weakness. Pain usually occurs with walking or prolonged standing and subsides by sitting or leaning forward (as in this case).
- **Metastatic prostate cancer:** The most common cancers leading to vertebral body metastasis are prostate, breast, lung, multiple myeloma, and lymphoma. In metastatic disease, patients complain of gradual-onset back pain (or occasionally acute pain in the case of pathologic fracture) with or without neurologic symptoms. Pain may be worse at night and unrelieved by rest. This patient's urinary symptoms may be a sign of prostatic disease.
- **Multiple myeloma:** Typically, patients are > 50 years of age. Back and bone pain may be the only presenting complaint. Anemia, neuropathy, hypercalcemia, and renal failure are also common.
- **Malingering:** This is defined as intentional faking of symptoms for secondary gain (e.g., getting out of work).

Diagnostic Workup

The history and physical exam are often all that is required, as the majority of patients with low back pain will improve within four weeks. Patients who require more extensive or urgent evaluation are those suspected of having pain caused by infection, cancer, abdominal aortic aneurysm, or neurologic emergency (e.g., cauda equina syndrome).

- **Rectal exam (including "saddle area" sensory exam):** To evaluate the prostate, rectal sphincter tone, and integrity of sacral nerve roots.
- **XR–L-spine:** Can show evidence of vertebral osteomyelitis, cancer, or fractures. Degenerative changes are expected in older patients and correlate poorly with clinical symptoms.
- **MRI–L-spine:** Provides the best anatomic detail and is the test of choice for suspected herniation, infection, or malignancy. Remember that asymptomatic disk herniation is common, so its presence does not necessarily correlate with clinical disease.
- **PSA:** Screening test for prostate cancer.
- **CBC, calcium, BUN/Cr:** To detect anemia, hypercalcemia, and renal failure, which may be clues to underlying multiple myeloma.
- **Serum and urine protein electrophoresis:** To detect a monoclonal paraprotein in myeloma.

Opening Scenario

The mother of Theresa Wheaton, a six-month-old female child, calls the office complaining that her child has diarrhea.

Examinee Tasks

1. Take a focused history.
2. Explain your clinical impression and workup plan to the mother.
3. Write the patient note after leaving the room.

Checklist/SP Sheet

PATIENT DESCRIPTION

The patient's mother offers the history.

NOTES FOR THE SP

Show concern about your child's health, but add that you don't want to come to the office unless you have to because you do not have transportation.

CHALLENGING QUESTIONS TO ASK

"How sick is my baby?"

SAMPLE EXAMINEE RESPONSE

"It is hard for me to give you an accurate answer over the phone. I would like you to bring your baby here so that I can examine her and perhaps run some tests. After that, I should be able to give you a more accurate assessment."

Examinee Checklist

ENTRANCE:

☐ Examinee introduced self by name.
☐ Examinee identified his/her role or position.
☐ Examinee correctly used patient's name and identified caller and relationship of caller to patient.

HISTORY:

☐ Examinee showed compassion for your child's illness.

☑ Question	Patient Response
☐ Chief complaint	My baby has diarrhea.
☐ Onset	It started yesterday at 2 P.M.
☐ Progression	It is getting worse.

☑ Question	Patient Response
☐ Frequency of bowel movements	She has about six bowel movements per day.
☐ Description of bowel movements	Light brown, watery, large amounts.
☐ Blood in stool	No.
☐ Relationship to oral intake	None.
☐ Previous regular bowel movements	Yes.
☐ Abdominal distention	No.
☐ Appetite changes	She is not as hungry as she used to be.
☐ Activities	Not as playful as she was earlier.
☐ Awake and responsive	She is less responsive and looks drowsy.
☐ Number of wet diapers	None since yesterday.
☐ Dry mouth or sunken soft spot over the head	Yes, her mouth is dry.
☐ Treatment tried	I tried some Tylenol, but it did not help.
☐ Vigorous cry	No, her cry is weak.
☐ Recent URI	No.
☐ Fever	Yes; I took her temperature, and it was 100.5.
☐ Breathing fast	No.
☐ Nausea/vomiting	No.
☐ Rash	No.
☐ Shaking (seizures)	No.
☐ Cough, pulling ear, or crying when urine is passed	No.
☐ Day care center	Yes.
☐ Ill contacts in day care center	Not to my knowledge.
☐ Vaccinations	Up to date.
☐ Last checkup	Two weeks ago, and everything was normal.
☐ Birth history	It was an uncomplicated spontaneous vaginal delivery.
☐ Eating habits	Formula with iron; rice cereal at night; occasionally juice.
☐ Current medications	None.
☐ Past medical history	Nothing of note.
☐ Past surgical history	None.
☐ Family history	None.
☐ Drug allergies	None.

Physical Examination:

None.

Closure:

- ☐ Examinee discussed initial diagnostic impressions.
- ☐ Examinee discussed initial management plans:
  - ☐ Follow-up tests.
- ☐ Examinee asked if the patient has any other questions or concerns.

Sample Closure:

Mrs. Wheaton, from the information you have given me, I am concerned that your child may be dehydrated. She hasn't urinated since yesterday, and she is weak and drowsy. It is very hard for me to assess her over the telephone, and I do not want to jeopardize her health in any way. For this reason, I am going to ask you to bring her in for a physical exam and a full assessment, and we will then proceed according to what we find on the exam. I understand that you may have problems with transportation, but we are fortunate to have a social worker here who can help you handle these issues. After we are done on the phone, I will transfer your call to him, and he can help you. Do you have any questions for me?

PATIENT NOTE

History

Physical Examination

Differential Diagnosis

1.

2.

3.

4.

5.

Diagnostic Workup

1.

2.

3.

4.

5.

History

HPI: *The source of information is the patient's mother. The mother of a 6-month-old F c/o her child having 1 day of diarrhea, weakness, and drowsiness. The child has had 6 watery brown bowel movements per day. There was no blood in her stool, but she has not urinated since yesterday. She received Tylenol without improvement. The mother reports the child's temperature as 100.5°F and adds that her mouth is dry. The child has no known sick contacts but is in day care. The mother denies any nausea/vomiting, lethargy, excessive sleeping, abnormal behavior, or recent URIs. The child had a normal checkup 2 weeks ago and is up to date on her immunizations. She has a diet of formula with iron and rice cereal at night with occasional juice.*
ROS: *Negative.*
Allergies: *NKDA.*
Medications: *None.*
PMH: *Uncomplicated spontaneous vaginal delivery.*
PSH: *None.*
FH: *Noncontributory.*

Physical Examination

None.

Differential Diagnosis

1. Rotavirus
2. Bacterial diarrhea
3. Malabsorption
4. UTI
5. Intussusception
6. Bacteremia

Diagnostic Workup

1. Rotavirus enzyme immunoassay
2. Electrolytes
3. Stool leukocytes, culture, ova and parasitology, and pH
4. UA
5. AXR
6. Blood cultures

CASE DISCUSSION

Differential Diagnosis

- **Rotavirus:** This is the cause of 60% of cases of acute pediatric infectious diarrhea.
- **Bacterial diarrhea:** The most common types of bacterial diarrhea, in order of frequency, are *Shigella, Salmonella, Campylobacter jejuni,* and *Yersinia enterocolitica.*
- **Malabsorption:** This condition may result from a baby's consumption of juice and may be the culprit in the current patient's case. It is important to counsel parents that juice should not be introduced into the diet of babies in this age group. Some children may have milk intolerance as well. However, milk intolerance would probably not present as acutely as is seen here.
- **UTI:** Diarrhea in infants may be a nonspecific response to an infection such as UTI or pyelonephritis.
- **Intussusception:** Given the severe nature of this disease, intussusception must be considered in the differential. The classic presentation includes abdominal pain, vomiting, and bloody stools. Some 75% of patients with intussusception have only two of these findings. Intussusception is also associated with recent viral illness and low-grade fever.
- **Bacteremia:** Bacteremia/sepsis should be ruled out in any child with high fever, drowsiness, and no urine output.

Diagnostic Workup

- **Rotavirus enzyme immunoassay:** This test is 97% sensitive and 97% specific for rotavirus infection.
- **Electrolytes:** Children with diarrhea frequently have metabolic acidosis or other electrolyte abnormalities, such as hyponatremia.
- **Stool leukocytes, culture, ova and parasitology, and pH:** WBCs in the stool would suggest an infectious etiology, and cultures may reveal a bacterial pathogen. Microscopy may reveal ova or parasites such as *Giardia,* an infection that is common among the day care population. Stool pH can distinguish a secretory from an osmotic cause of diarrhea by revealing a pH of > 6 or < 5, respectively.
- **UA:** To assess for pyelonephritis or UTI.
- **AXR:** A plain film abdominal radiograph should pick up characteristics of nonspecific bowel obstruction in intussusception.
- **Blood cultures:** To rule out bacteremia.

CASE 29
DOORWAY INFORMATION

Opening Scenario

Paul Stout, a 75-year-old male, comes to the office complaining of hearing loss.

Vital Signs

BP: 132/68 mmHg
Temp: 98.4°F (36.9°C)
RR: 18/minute
HR: 84/minute, regular

Examinee Tasks

1. Take a focused history.
2. Perform a focused physical exam (do not perform rectal, genitourinary, or female breast exam).
3. Explain your clinical impression and workup plan to the patient.
4. Write the patient note after leaving the room.

Checklist/SP sheet

PATIENT DESCRIPTION
Patient is a 75 yo M.

NOTES FOR THE SP

- Ask the examinee to speak up if he or she did not speak in a loud and clear manner.
- Pretend that you have difficulty hearing in both ears.
- On physical exam, demonstrate that you have no lateralization on the Weber test (i.e., show that your hearing is equal in both ears).
- Pretend that you cannot hear when spoken to from behind.

CHALLENGING QUESTIONS TO ASK
"Do you think I am going deaf?"

SAMPLE EXAMINEE RESPONSE
"It is obvious from your symptoms and from the results of my exam that you do have some kind of hearing deficit. We need to perform more complicated tests to figure out the cause of the problem, to determine whether it is going to get worse, and to ascertain whether we can halt its progression or improve your hearing. For the time being, I would like you to stop taking aspirin."

Examinee Checklist

ENTRANCE:

☐ Examinee knocked on the door before entering.
☐ Examinee introduced self by name.

☐ Examinee identified his/her role or position.
☐ Examinee correctly used patient's name.
☐ Examinee made eye contact with the SP.

HISTORY:

☐ Examinee showed compassion for your illness.

☑ Question	Patient Response
☐ Chief complaint	I can't hear as well as I used to.
☐ Description	My wife has told me that I can't hear well, and lately I have noticed that I have been reading lips.
☐ Onset	This has been going on for one year.
☐ Progression	It has been getting worse.
☐ Location	Both ears.
☐ Is hearing lost for all sounds or for anything specific?	Nothing specific.
☐ Do words sound jumbled or distorted?	Yes, especially in crowded places or when I watch television.
☐ Can you locate the source of sound?	Yes.
☐ Do you have any problems understanding speech?	No.
☐ Treatment tried	I saw my doctor one month ago, and he cleaned out some wax from my ears.
☐ Did that help you?	No.
☐ Ear pain	No.
☐ Ear discharge	No.
☐ Sensation of room spinning around you	No.
☐ Feeling of imbalance	No.
☐ Recent infections	I had a urinary infection about a year ago. It was treated with an antibiotic, but I don't remember its name.
☐ Ringing in the ears	Sometimes.
☐ Trauma to the ears	No.
☐ Exposure to loud noises	Yes.
☐ Headaches	Rarely.
☐ Insertion of foreign body	No.
☐ Nausea/vomiting	No.
☐ Neurologic problems, loss of sensation, muscle weakness, numbness or tingling anywhere in the body	No.
☐ Current medications	Hydrochlorothiazide. For the past 25 years, I have also taken aspirin daily to protect my heart.

☑ Question	Patient Response
☐ Past medical history	Hypertension.
☐ Past surgical history	None.
☐ Family history of hearing loss	No.
☐ Occupation	Retired military veteran.
☐ Alcohol use	Never.
☐ Illicit drug use	Never.
☐ Tobacco	Never.
☐ Sexual activity	Only with my wife.
☐ Drug allergies	I develop a rash when I take penicillin.

Physical Examination:

☐ Examinee washed his/her hands.
☐ Examinee asked permission to start the exam.
☐ Examinee used respectful draping.
☐ Examinee did not repeat painful maneuvers.

☑ Exam Component	Maneuver
HEENT exam	Tested hearing by speaking with back turned; inspected sinuses, nose, mouth, and throat; funduscopic exam and otoscopy; assessed hearing with Rinne and Weber tests and whisper test
CV/pulmonary exam	Auscultation
Neurologic exam	Cranial nerves, sensation, motor, reflexes, cerebellar

Closure:

☐ Examinee discussed initial diagnostic impressions.
☐ Examinee discussed initial management plans:
   ☐ Follow-up tests.
☐ Examinee asked if the patient has any other questions or concerns.

Sample Closure:

Mr. Stout, I know that you are concerned about your problem, and I can confirm that you do have some hearing loss. I would like to run several tests, including some blood tests, and would also like you to stop taking aspirin, because this may be causing your hearing loss or at least contributing to it. I will refer you to an audiometrist who will assess you for a hearing aid. Do you have any questions for me?

PATIENT NOTE

History

Physical Examination

Differential Diagnosis

1.

2.

3.

4.

5.

Diagnostic Workup

1.

2.

3.

4.

5.

History

HPI: 75 yo M c/o bilateral hearing loss for all sounds that started 1 year ago and is progressively worsening. He had cerumen removal 1 month ago with no improvement. He reports occasional tinnitus and rare headaches. He notes that words sound jumbled in crowded places or when he is watching TV. He denies inserting any foreign body in the ear canal. No ear pain, no ear discharge, no vertigo, no loss of balance. No history of trauma to the ears; no difficulty comprehending or locating the source of sounds.
ROS: Negative.
Allergies: Penicillin, causes rash.
Medications: HCTZ, aspirin (for 25 years).
PMH: Hypertension. UTI 1 year ago, treated with antibiotics.
PSH: None.
SH: No smoking, no EtOH, no illicit drugs. Retired veteran. Sexually active with wife only.
FH: No history of hearing loss.

Physical Examination

Patient is in no acute distress.
VS: WNL.
HEENT: NC/AT, PERRLA, EOMI, no nystagmus, no papilledema, no cerumen. TMs with light reflex, no stigmata of infection, no redness to ear canal, no tenderness of auricle or periauricle, no lymphadenopathy, oropharynx normal. Weber test revealed no lateralization; ⊕Rinne test (revealed air conduction > bone conduction).
Chest: Clear breath sounds bilaterally.
Heart: RRR; S1/S2; no murmurs, rubs, or gallops.
Neuro: Cranial nerves: 2–12 grossly intact except for decreased hearing. Motor: Strength 5/5 throughout. DTRs: 2+ throughout. Sensation: Intact. Gait: Normal; no past pointing and ⊖heel to shin.

Differential Diagnosis

1. Presbycusis
2. Cochlear nerve damage due to loud noise
3. Otosclerosis
4. Ménière's disease
5. Ototoxicity
6. Acoustic neuroma

Diagnostic Workup

1. Audiometry
2. Tympanography
3. Brain stem auditory evoked potentials
4. CT—head
5. VDRL/RPR

CASE DISCUSSION

Differential Diagnosis

- **Presbycusis:** This is a process of the inner ear in which bone loss is greater than air loss, leading to a gradual loss of hearing. Presbycusis is a common diagnosis as people age and can be detected by performing the Rinne test. This patient should be referred to an audiologist who works in conjunction with an ENT specialist. He will likely need a hearing aid.
- **Cochlear nerve damage:** The cochlear nerve can become damaged as a result of loud noise. This patient is a military veteran and may thus have a history of exposure to loud artillery fire. Cochlear nerve damage would present in a manner similar to presbycusis. As with presbycusis, patients with suspected damage should be referred to an audiologist working in conjunction with an ENT specialist. Such patients will likely need hearing aids as well.
- **Otosclerosis:** This is a disease of the elderly that presents as gradual hearing loss. It is a conductive hearing loss, so air loss exceeds bone loss.
- **Ménière's disease:** This condition usually presents with hearing loss, tinnitus, and episodic vertigo. It is caused by endolymphatic disruption in the inner ear. Causes include head trauma and syphilis.
- **Ototoxicity:** Hearing loss caused by antibiotics will become more pronounced and may even continue to worsen for a time after the drug is discontinued. Any sensorineural hearing loss associated with these drugs is permanent. Aspirin can also cause hearing loss, but such loss is reversible with discontinuation of the drug.
- **Acoustic neuroma:** It is unlikely that the patient has an intracranial lesion such as a brain tumor in the absence of any other signs; however, this diagnosis should be considered if new evidence of focal neurologic deficits is found.

Diagnostic Workup

- **Audiometry:** To assess hearing function and deafness to specific frequencies.
- **Tympanography:** A graphic display that represents the conduction of sound in the middle ear. It may help distinguish middle ear from inner ear dysfunction.
- **Brain stem auditory evoked potentials:** Used to diagnose auditory neuropathy.
- **CT—head:** Used to rule out any intracranial process, tumor, bleed, or CVA. An MRI of the brain would be better for an acoustic neuroma or a schwannoma.
- **VDRL/RPR:** To rule out syphilis associated with Ménière's disease.

Opening Scenario

The mother of Adam Davidson, an eight-year-old male child, comes to the office concerned that her son continues to wet the bed.

Examinee Tasks

1. Take a focused history.
2. Explain your clinical impression and workup plan to the mother.
3. Write the patient note after leaving the room.

Checklist/SP Sheet

PATIENT DESCRIPTION

The patient's mother offers the history; her son is in the waiting room.

NOTES FOR THE SP

None.

CHALLENGING QUESTIONS TO ASK

- "Did I do something wrong to cause this problem?"
- "Is my child going to get better?"

SAMPLE EXAMINEE RESPONSE

"There are a few medical problems that can lead to your child's condition, but it's just as likely to be an isolated symptom. Bed-wetting is much more common than most people believe, and there is no reason for you or your child to feel embarrassed or guilty. There are a number of treatment options available for this condition, and after we have run a few tests to rule out any physiologic abnormalities, I will discuss them with you."

Examinee Checklist

ENTRANCE:

☐ Examinee knocked on the door before entering.
☐ Examinee introduced self by name.
☐ Examinee identified his/her role or position.
☐ Examinee correctly used patient's name.
☐ Examinee made eye contact with the SP.

HISTORY:

☐ Examinee showed compassion for your child's illness.

☑	Question	Patient Response
☐	Chief complaint	My child wets his bed.
☐	Frequency	Two or three times a week.
☐	Time of day	Only at night.
☐	Onset	I guess he has always had trouble at night. I don't think he has ever gone more than a few nights without an accident.
☐	Have you tried any interventions or drugs in the past?	We ordered one of those nighttime alarms, but everyone in the house could hear it, so we didn't use it for long.
☐	How has the behavior affected the child?	He is ashamed of himself. He avoids school trips because of it.
☐	How has the behavior affected you?	It bothers me. I'm afraid he has some underlying disease or abnormality.
☐	Have you ever punished or rewarded him?	I feel irritated sometimes, but I've never punished him. I try to encourage him by rewarding him on dry nights.
☐	Alleviating/exacerbating factors	None that I can think of.
☐	Does the problem increase in times of stress?	I'm not sure, but it probably does.
☐	Late-night eating or drinking	No.
☐	Volume of urine	He washes his own sheets, but I don't think it's ever a large amount.
☐	Dysuria	No.
☐	Urinary urgency	No.
☐	Fever	No.
☐	Urine color	Yellow.
☐	Hematuria	No.
☐	Abdominal pain	No.
☐	Constipation	No.
☐	Snoring	No.
☐	Nighttime awakening	No.
☐	Environmental changes related to wetting	No, I can't think of anything. We haven't moved or had any family problems.
☐	Any major stresses?	No, he does well in school and has great friends. I think the only hard thing for him is not being able to attend sleepovers.
☐	Family history of enuresis	Actually, his father had the same trouble as a kid. From my understanding, his father didn't gain full control until he was about 10 years old.
☐	Neurologic history	As far as I know, he has never had any problems of this kind.
☐	Birth history	Normal.
☐	Child weight, height, and language development	He was always on time with his development. He walked early, talked on time, and is reading at a third-grade level.
☐	Current medications	None.

✓ Question	Patient Response
☐ Past medical history	None.
☐ Past surgical history	None.
☐ Drug allergies	No.

Physical Examination:

None.

Closure:

☐ Examinee discussed initial diagnostic impressions.
☐ Examinee discussed initial management plans:
    ☐ Further examination.
    ☐ Follow-up tests.
☐ Examinee asked if the patient has any other questions or concerns.

Sample Closure:

Mrs. Davidson, your son's condition is probably an isolated symptom, but I would still like to run some tests to make sure he does not have an underlying infection or a more serious medical problem. We can then discuss his treatment options. Do you have any questions for me?

PATIENT NOTE

History

Physical Examination

Differential Diagnosis

1.

2.

3.

4.

5.

Diagnostic Workup

1.

2.

3.

4.

5.

History

HPI: *The source of the information is the patient's mother. The mother of an 8 yo M c/o her child continuing to wet the bed several times a week. The child has never had a significant period of continence. He has no dysuria, hematuria, fever, or urgency. The mother denies that the child c/o abdominal pain or constipation. The child does not snore or wake up multiple times during the night. There are no exacerbating factors, and there have been no major lifestyle changes or stresses in the family. The problem is causing distress for the child, who has been avoiding school trips, as well as for the mother, who is worried about the possibility of an underlying medical condition.*
ROS: *Negative.*
Allergies: *NKDA.*
Medications: *None.*
PMH: *None.*
PSH: *None.*
Birth history: *Normal.*
Developmental history: *Normal.*
FH: *Positive family history of male nocturnal enuresis.*

Physical Examination

None.

Differential Diagnosis

1. Monosymptomatic primary nocturnal enuresis
2. Secondary enuresis
3. Urinary tract infection
4. Constipation
5. Sleep apnea
6. Functional bladder disorder

Diagnostic Workup

1. Genital exam
2. UA
3. Urine culture
4. First-morning urine specific gravity
5. U/S—renal

CASE DISCUSSION

Differential Diagnosis

- **Monosymptomatic primary nocturnal enuresis:** This is a diagnosis of exclusion. This patient's lifetime history indicates a primary problem as opposed to a secondary one. The history and physical exam do not provide any related signs or symptoms, suggesting a monosymptomatic pathology. A urine sample must be taken to rule out infection, and old records should be evaluated to ensure that the presentation is not part of a global delay.
- **Secondary enuresis:** The patient's mother does not report a major trauma or life or environmental change such as the divorce of parents, a major illness, or an abuse that might result in regression to incontinence. This diagnosis is further unlikely because the child has not been continent for any significant period.
- **Urinary tract infection (UTI):** Asymptomatic UTIs are common in children and should be screened for at annual visits. This patient does not have dysuria, frequency, or urgency, but incontinence alone should trigger an evaluation. A positive UA is diagnostic, and culturing can direct treatment.
- **Constipation:** Infrequent or hard stools may indicate chronic constipation, which can put pressure on the bladder and decrease capacity. This may delay continence and look like a primary disorder. Physical examination can reveal impacted stool on the left side.
- **Sleep apnea:** Wetting occurs in all stages of sleep but is associated with particular disorders, such as sleep apnea and narcolepsy. This patient does not present with snoring or upper airway obstruction, and thus there is no indication of apnea that might warrant further evaluation.
- **Functional bladder disorder:** Children with functional disorders void several times a day, hold urine until the last moment, and wet small volumes almost every night, sometimes multiple times a night. This patient has normal voiding patterns during the day and remains continent a majority of nights.

Diagnostic Workup

- **Genital exam:** To evaluate for disorders such as abnormalities of the meatus, epispadias, and phimosis.
- **UA:** Clear urine, a negative dipstick, and a negative microscopic examination combined have a negative predictive value between 95% and 98%.
- **Urine culture:** The only 100% specific test for infection.
- **First-morning urine specific gravity:** An early-morning urine concentration of < 1.015 may indicate a lack of nighttime and early-morning ADH surges, which may predict a positive response to pharmacologic therapy with DDAVP.
- **U/S–renal:** Should be pursued if wetting continues with multiple treatments, abnormal voiding patterns, or recurrent UTIs confirmed by UA.

Opening Scenario

John Matthews, a 25-year-old male, comes to the ER following a motor vehicle accident.

Vital Signs

BP: 123/88 mmHg
Temp: 100°F (38°C)
RR: 22/minute
HR: 85/minute, regular

Examinee Tasks

1. Take a focused history.
2. Perform a focused physical exam (do not perform rectal, genitourinary, or female breast exam).
3. Explain your clinical impression and workup plan to the patient.
4. Write the patient note after leaving the room.

Checklist/SP Sheet

PATIENT DESCRIPTION

Patient is a 25 yo M.

NOTES FOR THE SP

- Exhibit pain in the left chest that worsens during inspiration and movement (i.e., when you breathe in, hold your side, and stop your breathing with a short gasp).
- Exhibit pain when your left chest is being palpated.
- Exhibit pain when your left upper abdomen is being palpated.
- Take fast, shallow breaths.
- Occasionally cough hard into a tissue.
- Moan occasionally and answer questions in short sentences.

CHALLENGING QUESTIONS TO ASK

"Do you think I am going to die?"

SAMPLE EXAMINEE RESPONSE

"Your condition raises concern and is obviously urgent. We will start by taking some images of your chest. Then, once we have a better idea of what might be wrong with you, we can give you some medication to help you with your pain. If there is air or blood around your lungs, there is a procedure we can perform that may release the pressure. We will be monitoring you very closely from this point on, and if you have any significant problems, we will be available to make sure you keep breathing."

Examinee Checklist

- ☐ Examinee knocked on the door before entering.
- ☐ Examinee introduced self by name.
- ☐ Examinee identified his/her role or position.
- ☐ Examinee correctly used patient's name.
- ☐ Examinee made eye contact with the SP.

HISTORY:

- ☐ Examinee showed compassion for your pain.

☑ Question	Patient Response
☐ Chief complaint	I'm having trouble breathing and have this excruciating pain (holds left side).
☐ Onset	It started last night.
☐ Severity on a scale	It's some of the worst pain I've ever had; I guess I would say 8/10.
☐ Context	I was driving my car and was trying to answer my cell phone. When I looked up, I found that I had veered off the road. I immediately tried to slow down but hit a tree. I wasn't going very fast, and my car was basically okay. I was embarrassed, so I didn't call the police. I was wearing my seat belt and felt okay at first, so I didn't think I needed to come to the hospital.
☐ Alleviating factors	Nothing I do makes it better.
☐ Exacerbating factors	It gets even worse when I try to take a deep breath or try to move.
☐ Cough	I have been coughing for a couple of days, I guess.
☐ Sputum production	I have to use a tissue because I keep bringing up all this yellow junk.
☐ Fever/chills	I have been feeling a little warm and have noticed that my muscles ache, but I don't think I've had any shaking or chills.
☐ Other injuries	I have a few abrasions on my limbs.
☐ Head trauma	No.
☐ Discharge from the ears, mouth, or nose (clear or bloody)	No.
☐ Loss of consciousness	No.
☐ Convulsions	No.
☐ Headache	No.
☐ Change in vision	No.
☐ Confusion, memory loss, or change in personality	No.
☐ Weakness or numbness in the extremities	No.

☑ **Question**	**Patient Response**
☐ Heart symptoms (left chest pain, palpitations)	No.
☐ Abdominal pain	Yes, I have sharp pain right here (point to the LUQ).
☐ Nausea/vomiting or stiff neck	No.
☐ Last meal/drink	I had breakfast this morning, about five hours ago.
☐ Were you under the influence of alcohol or recreational drugs?	No.
☐ Pain on urination	No.
☐ Current medications	None.
☐ Past medical history	I had a sore throat, mild fever, and fatigue two weeks ago, and my doctor diagnosed me with infectious mononucleosis, but it is resolved now.
☐ Past surgical history	None.
☐ Family history	My mother and father are both healthy and living.
☐ Occupation	I'm a banker.
☐ Alcohol use	Occasionally, on the weekends.
☐ Illicit drug use	No.
☐ Tobacco	No.
☐ Drug allergies	No.

Physical Exam:

☐ Examinee washed his/her hands.
☐ Examinee asked permission to start the exam.
☐ Examinee used respectful draping.
☐ Examinee did not repeat painful maneuvers.

☑ **Exam Component**	**Maneuver**
☐ Head and neck exam	Inspection
☐ CV exam	Auscultation
☐ Pulmonary exam	Inspection, auscultation, palpation, percussion
☐ Abdominal exam	Inspection, auscultation, palpation (examined specifically for organomegaly)
☐ Neurologic exam	Mental status, cranial nerves, gross motor
☐ Skin exam	Inspection

Closure:

- ☐ Examinee discussed initial diagnostic impressions.
- ☐ Examinee discussed initial management plans:
    - ☐ Diagnostic exams.
- ☐ Examinee asked if the patient has any other questions or concerns.

Sample Closure:

Mr. Matthews, you should always seek medical treatment after an accident like this. We must now observe you closely until we can determine what is causing your pain. We are going to run a few tests and take some x-rays of your chest. We will also give you something for your pain and will observe your breathing to make sure you are getting enough oxygen.

PATIENT NOTE

History

Physical Examination

Differential Diagnosis

1.

2.

3.

4.

5.

Diagnostic Workup

1.

2.

3.

4.

5.

PATIENT NOTE

History

HPI: *25 yo M c/o left chest pain and LUQ pain following an MVA. The patient struck a tree with his car at a slow speed. The pain is 8/10. It is exacerbated when he takes a deep breath, and nothing relieves it. He reports dyspnea and a productive cough with a low-grade fever but denies LOC, headache, change in mental status, or change in vision. No cardiovascular or neurologic symptoms. No nausea, vomiting, neck stiffness, or unusual fluid from mouth or nose. No dysuria. Last meal was 5 hours ago. Denies being under the influence of alcohol or drugs.*
ROS: *As per HPI.*
Allergies: *NKDA.*
Medications: *None.*
PMH: *Infectious mononucleosis.*
PSH: *None.*
SH: *No smoking, occasional EtOH, no illicit drugs.*
FH: *Noncontributory.*

Physical Examination

Patient is in acute distress, dyspneic.
VS: *Temp 100°F, RR 22.*
HEENT: *No JVD, no bruises, PERRLA, EOMI, no pharyngeal edema or exudates.*
Chest: *Two large bruises on left chest, left rib tenderness, decreased breath sounds over all of left lung field, right lung fields clear.*
Heart: *RRR; normal S1/S2; no murmurs, rubs, or gallops.*
Abdomen: *Soft, nondistended, ⊕BS, LUQ tenderness, no rebound or guarding, no organomegaly.*
Skin: *No bruises or lacerations.*
Neuro: Mental status: *Alert and oriented × 3.* Cranial nerves: *2–12 grossly intact.* Motor: *Strength 5/5 in all muscle groups.* Sensation: *Intact to pinprick and soft touch.*

Differential Diagnosis

1. Pneumothorax
2. Hemothorax
3. Pneumonia
4. Rib fracture
5. Splenic rupture
6. Pleuritis

Diagnostic Workup

1. CXR
2. XR/CT—abdomen
3. Pulse oximetry
4. Urine toxicology
5. Blood alcohol level
6. Sputum Gram stain and culture

CASE DISCUSSION

Differential Diagnosis

The most important steps in any trauma are to assess the ABCDEs: airway, breathing, circulation, disability (neurologic), and exposure. In this case, the exam is separated from the trauma by several hours and the patient is able to walk and talk, somewhat negating the urgency of a typical ER evaluation. At the same time, chest pain and dyspnea are serious symptoms that require swift evaluation and intervention.

- **Pneumothorax:** A pneumothorax forms when air collects between the pleural and visceral layers of the thorax. Physical findings include a unilateral loss of breath sounds with hyperresonance, shift of the trachea away from the injured side, and JVD. This patient's acute onset and distress suggest pneumothorax. CXR is the fastest diagnostic tool available.
- **Hemothorax:** This is defined by the presence of blood in the pleural space and is most commonly due to trauma. It presents with chest pain, shortness of breath, cough, and occasionally signs and symptoms of hypovolemic shock. A CXR will identify a pleural effusion. The final diagnosis can be made by pleurocentesis or chest tube placement.
- **Pneumonia:** Most commonly caused by *Streptococcus pneumoniae*, bacterial pneumonia can present with acute respiratory distress, fever, cough, pleuritic pain, and shaking chills. This patient has a cough, low-grade fever, and unilateral chest pain suggestive of pneumonia, but traumatic causes should be ruled out first. Physical signs include tachypnea, crackles, and dullness to percussion. The CXR will show a lobar infiltrate, and sputum cultures may help identify the bacterial pathogen.
- **Rib fracture:** Rib fractures are the most common chest injury and can result from almost any insult to the chest wall. A simple fracture could cause this patient's pain on inspiration and cough.
- **Splenic rupture:** Splenic injuries are always of great concern following a trauma because they can cause significant blood loss very quickly. If this patient was exposed to infectious mononucleosis, his chances of splenic injury or bleeding are greater. As this patient's pain is primarily left-sided, the spleen should be evaluated with an AXR.
- **Pleuritis:** Inflammation of the pleural membrane can cause severe pain that increases with inspiration or movement. The physical exam is generally negative with the exception of the chest pain. This patient may have a simple viral pleuritis, but more emergent causes should be ruled out first.

Diagnostic Workup

- **CXR:** On CXR, lobar consolidation may indicate pneumonia; hemothorax may cause linear consolidation; and tension pneumothorax will show mediastinal shift.
- **XR/CT—abdomen:** Although a CT scan may offer a better evaluation for internal abdominal injury, an AXR is a quick and cost-effective way to rule out free air in the abdomen.
- **Pulse oximetry:** Although not as sensitive as ABG analysis, pulse oximetry is a fast, noninvasive measure of respiratory distress. Remember that a patient with long-standing lung disease may have chronically suppressed oxygenation, which is necessary to maintain respiratory drive.
- **Urine toxicology and blood alcohol level:** Should be considered for any driver following a motor vehicle accident.
- **Sputum Gram stain and culture:** Used to screen sputum samples for sufficient bacterial content and to diagnose *S. pneumoniae*. Other stains, such as acid-fast stains and monoclonal antibodies, can identify tuberculosis and *Pneumocystis jiroveci* (formerly *P. carinii*).

DOORWAY INFORMATION

Opening Scenario

Julia Melton, a 25-year-old female, comes to the ER after having been assaulted.

Vital Signs

BP: 120/85 mmHg
Temp: 98.0°F (36.7°C)
RR: 17/minute
HR: 90/minute, regular

Examinee Tasks

1. Take a focused history.
2. Perform a focused physical exam (do not perform rectal, genitourinary, or female breast exam).
3. Explain your clinical impression and workup plan to the patient.
4. Write the patient note after leaving the room.

Checklist/SP Sheet

PATIENT DESCRIPTION

Patient is a 25 yo F.

NOTES FOR THE SP

- Look depressed and tearful.
- Start weeping when asked about physical and/or sexual assaults.
- Pretend to have right chest pain with deep inspiration, cough, and palpation.

CHALLENGING QUESTIONS TO ASK

"This is all my fault, doctor. Do you think my friends will ever accept me again?"

SAMPLE EXAMINEE RESPONSE

"I am so sorry for what happened to you; it is horrific and must be very difficult for you to handle. However, it is not your fault by any means. Whoever did this to you should be held accountable."

Examinee Checklist

ENTRANCE:

- [ ] Examinee knocked on the door before entering.
- [ ] Examinee introduced self by name.
- [ ] Examinee identified his/her role or position.
- [ ] Examinee correctly used patient's name.
- [ ] Examinee made eye contact with the SP.

HISTORY:

☐ Examinee showed compassion for your pain.

☑ Question	Patient Response
☐ Chief complaint	I was attacked by two men.
☐ Onset	About three hours ago.
☐ Incident location	It happened outside the bar that I usually go to.
☐ Did you recognize the assailants?	I have seen them in the bar but never talked to them.
☐ Did you report the incident?	No.
☐ Description of the assault	I was walking toward my car, and then all of a sudden I was pulled into a storage room. I started screaming, but the men started to slap me and beat me up with their fists.
☐ Assault objects	They used their fists and their bodies to hold me down.
☐ Sexual assault	Yes.
☐ Did they use condoms?	No.
☐ Did ejaculation occur?	I don't know.
☐ Type of intercourse (oral, vaginal, anal)	Vaginal.
☐ Foreign objects used	None.
☐ Last menstrual period	Three weeks ago.
☐ Contraceptives	None.
☐ Pain	Yes, I feel sore all over, especially on the right side of my chest.
☐ Location of the worst pain	The right chest.
☐ Radiation	No.
☐ Severity on a scale	About 8/10.
☐ Alleviating factors	It improves when I sit still.
☐ Exacerbating factors	It gets worse whenever I move or take a deep breath.
☐ Bleeding or bruises	No.
☐ Loss of consciousness	No.
☐ Headache	No.
☐ Change in vision	No.
☐ Dizziness	No.
☐ Weakness	No, I am just tired.
☐ Numbness	No.
☐ Shortness of breath	Yes, I feel that I can't get enough air.
☐ Palpitations	Yes.
☐ Blood in stool/urine	No, but I haven't gone to the bathroom since the incident.

☑ Question	Patient Response
☐ Vaginal bleeding	No.
☐ Nausea/vomiting	No.
☐ Abdominal pain	Yes, it hurts everywhere.
☐ Joint pain	No.
☐ Current medications	None.
☐ Past medical history	None.
☐ Past surgical history	None.
☐ Family history	None.
☐ Occupation	Student.
☐ Alcohol use	Occasionally.
☐ Illicit drug use	Never.
☐ Tobacco	No.
☐ Drug allergies	None.

Physical Examination:

- ☐ Examinee washed his/her hands.
- ☐ Examinee asked permission to start the exam.
- ☐ Examinee used respectful draping.
- ☐ Examinee did not repeat painful maneuvers.

☑ Exam Component	Maneuver
☐ Head and neck exam	Inspection, palpation
☐ Mouth exam	Inspection
☐ CV exam	Auscultation
☐ Pulmonary exam	Inspection, auscultation, palpation, percussion
☐ Abdominal exam	Inspection, auscultation, palpation
☐ Neurologic exam	Mental status, cranial nerves, gross motor
☐ Musculoskeletal exam	Inspection, palpation

Closure:

- ☐ Examinee discussed initial diagnostic impressions.
- ☐ Examinee discussed initial management plans:
    - ☐ Follow-up tests: Examinee mentioned the need for a pelvic exam.
- ☐ Examinee asked if the patient has any other questions or concerns.

Sample Closure:

Ms. Melton, I am really sorry for what happened to you. I want to emphasize, however, that it is not your fault, and you should not feel guilty about it. I recommend that you report the incident to the police. In the meantime, I will need to do a pelvic examination to make sure that you have no injuries in the genital area. I will also need to collect some specimens and swabs from your body and genital area so that they can be used as evidence if you choose to file charges, and also to look for STDs. We will run some blood tests for potential STDs, a pregnancy test, and some x-rays. If your pregnancy test is negative, we will offer you different options for emergency contraception. It would also be prudent to give you some antibiotics to protect you from infections. Finally, I can have our social worker come talk to you and provide you with phone numbers for support groups and other resources. Do you have any questions for me?"

PATIENT NOTE

History

Physical Examination

Differential Diagnosis

1.

2.

3.

4.

5.

Diagnostic Workup

1.

2.

3.

4.

5.

History

HPI: *25 yo F comes to the ER after having been sexually and physically assaulted. The event happened about 3 hours ago, as she was leaving a bar. She was beaten and raped by two unknown men. They had vaginal intercourse with her without using condoms, and she is unsure if ejaculation occurred. She also c/o shortness of breath, palpitations, and right chest pain that is nonradiating. The chest pain is exacerbated by movement and deep breaths and is relieved by sitting still. No nausea or vomiting; no dizziness or headache. No weakness or numbness in her extremities; no vaginal, rectal, or urinary bleeding.*
ROS: *Negative except as above.*
Allergies: *NKDA.*
Medications: *None.*
PMH: *None.*
PSH: *None.*
SH: *No smoking, occasional EtOH, no illicit drugs.*
FH: *Noncontributory.*

Physical Examination

Patient is anxious and in acute distress.
VS: *WNL.*
HEENT: *No JVD, PERRLA, EOMI.*
Chest: *Clear breath sounds bilaterally; tenderness on palpation of right chest wall.*
Heart: *Normal S1/S2; no murmurs, rubs, or gallops.*
Abdomen: *Soft, nontender, nondistended, ⊕BS, no rebound or organomegaly.*
Neuro: Mental status: *Alert and oriented × 3.* Cranial nerves: *2–12 grossly intact.* Motor: *Strength 5/5 in all muscle groups.*

Differential Diagnosis

1. Rib/bone fracture
2. Pneumothorax/hemothorax
3. STDs
4. Pregnancy

Diagnostic Workup

1. Pelvic exam
2. Urine hCG
3. Wet mount, KOH prep, cervical culture
4. XR—skeletal survey
5. HIV antibody, VDRL, HBV antigen
6. CXR
7. Evidence collection using rape kit

CASE DISCUSSION

Differential Diagnosis

- **Rib fracture:** Can result from any insult to the chest wall. A simple fracture could cause pain on inspiration and cough.
- **Pneumothorax/hemothorax:** Defined as the presence of air or blood in the pleural space between the visceral and parietal pleura. Physical findings include unilateral loss of breath sounds with hyperresonance, shifting of the trachea away from the injured side, and JVD. Because she has been beaten, this patient may have traumatic pneumothorax. A CXR is a fast and easy tool with which to evaluate patients for a pneumothorax.
- **STDs:** Sexual assault victims may acquire a variety of pathogens during the incident, including trichomoniasis, chlamydia, gonorrhea, HIV, and hepatitis B.
- **Pregnancy:** All sexual assault victims should be evaluated for possible existing pregnancy and should be offered emergency contraception.

Diagnostic Workup

- **Pelvic exam:** To evaluate for any possible physical injury of the genital or anal area and to collect specimens for medical and forensic purposes.
- **Urine hCG:** To rule out pregnancy.
- **Wet mount, KOH prep, cervical culture:** The vaginal discharge is examined microscopically to evaluate for previous or newly acquired infection. The presence of epithelial cells covered with bacteria (clue cells) suggests bacterial vaginosis, and the presence of hyphae and spores points to candidal infection. Motile organisms are seen in trichomonal infection. A "fishy" odor after the addition of KOH to the discharge is indicative of bacterial vaginosis. If sperm are detected in the victim, testing of sperm DNA may aid in the identification of the assailants.
- **XR—skeletal survey:** To detect possible bone or rib fractures.
- **HIV antibody, VDRL, HBV antigen:** To rule out HIV, syphilis, and hepatitis B infection.
- **CXR:** To detect pneumothorax, pleural effusions, and rib fractures.
- **Evidence collection using rape kit:** Rape kits are available to facilitate and guide the evidence collection process.

Opening Scenario

Tanya Parker, a 28-year-old female, comes to the clinic with a positive pregnancy test.

Vital Signs

BP: 120/70 mmHg
Temp: 98.6°F (37°C)
RR: 14/minute
HR: 76/minute

Examinee Tasks

1. Take a focused history.
2. Perform a focused physical exam (do not perform rectal, genitourinary, or female breast exam).
3. Explain your clinical impression and workup plan to the patient.
4. Write the patient note after leaving the room.

Checklist/SP Sheet

PATIENT DESCRIPTION

Patient is a 28 yo female, married with no children.

NOTES FOR THE SP

If asked, tell the doctor that you feel tired all the time.

CHALLENGING QUESTIONS TO ASK

"We had not planned to have a baby so soon after marriage. What should I do, doctor?"

SAMPLE EXAMINEE RESPONSE

"I understand your anxiety about this unplanned pregnancy. I suggest that you discuss this with your husband. As your physician, I want to assure you that I am here to support and advise you regardless of the decision you make. If you wish, I would be happy to discuss your options with both of you."

Examinee Checklist

ENTRANCE:

☐ Examinee knocked on the door before entering.
☐ Examinee introduced self by name.
☐ Examinee identified his/her role or position.
☐ Examinee correctly used patient's name.
☐ Examinee made eye contact with the SP.

HISTORY:

☐ Examinee showed compassion for your concerns.

☑ Question	Patient Response
☐ Chief complaint	Positive pregnancy test.
☐ Onset/duration	My periods have always been regular, but last month it was very light, and this month I haven't had one yet. So I checked a pregnancy test, and it was positive.
☐ Last menstrual period	Six weeks ago.
☐ Menarche	At the age of 14.
☐ Menstrual history	My periods last 3–4 days and occur at the same time every month. Last month I had some spotting for only a day or two. Usually I have moderate flow and use 4–5 pads per day.
☐ Pain with periods	No.
☐ Spotting between periods	No.
☐ Contraception	My husband withdraws before ejaculation.
☐ Pregnancy/miscarriages	None.
☐ Sexual activity/partners	I am sexually active only with my husband.
☐ History of STDs	None.
☐ Nausea/vomiting	I do feel nauseated lately, but I have not been vomiting.
☐ Postcoital bleeding	No.
☐ Abdominal pain	No.
☐ Appetite changes	I don't feel like eating anything because of the nausea.
☐ Weight changes	I haven't checked my weight recently, but I do feel bloated lately.
☐ Fatigue	Yes.
☐ Breast discharge/tenderness	My breasts are a little heavier than before.
☐ Last Pap smear	Eight months ago, and it was normal.
☐ Fever	No.
☐ Bowel habits	Once a day.
☐ Urinary habits	I feel I have to use the bathroom frequently now. I have no burning or itching.
☐ Shortness of breath	No.
☐ Skin changes	I have not noticed anything.
☐ Exercise	I run five miles a day.
☐ Current medications	Multivitamins.
☐ Past medical history	None.

☑ Question	Patient Response
☐ Past surgical history	My appendix was removed when I was 20.
☐ Family history	My father is a diabetic. My mom has thyroid and obesity problems.
☐ Occupation	Graduate student.
☐ Alcohol use	Occasionally a beer or two a week.
☐ Illicit drug use	None.
☐ Tobacco	None.
☐ Drug allergies	None.
☐ Planned pregnancy	No.
☐ Desired pregnancy	Unsure.
☐ Domestic abuse	No.

Physical Examination:

☐ Examinee washed his/her hands.
☐ Examinee asked permission to start the exam.
☐ Examinee used respectful draping.
☐ Examinee did not repeat painful maneuvers.

☑ Exam Component	Maneuver
☐ HEENT exam	Inspection/palpation of thyroid
☐ CV exam	Auscultation
☐ Pulmonary exam	Auscultation
☐ Abdominal exam	Inspection, auscultation, palpation
☐ Skin exam	Inspected for pigmentation or pallor

Closure:

☐ Examinee discussed initial diagnostic impressions.
☐ Examinee discussed initial management plans:
    ☐ Follow-up tests: Examinee mentioned the need for a pelvic/breast exam.
☐ Examinee asked if the patient has any other questions or concerns.

Sample Closure:

Ms. Parker, on the basis of my observations and what you have told me, it would appear that you are pregnant. I will have to repeat a urine pregnancy test to confirm the diagnosis. Your last period may not have been a real menstrual period, as spotting can frequently occur in the first trimester. Unfortunately, natural methods of contraception are the least effective. We will perform a pelvic ultrasound to more accurately estimate the duration of your pregnancy and the expected date of delivery. If you are pregnant, we will check some more blood tests, a Pap smear, and some vaginal cultures that we routinely perform in every pregnancy. For now, I would recommend stopping alcohol consumption and avoiding intense exercises and excess caffeine. I will be giving you some supplements to take orally, and we will schedule your future prenatal visits. I will be able to advise you further as soon as we receive these tests. Do you have any questions or concerns?

PATIENT NOTE

History

Physical Examination

Differential Diagnosis

1.

2.

3.

4.

5.

Diagnostic Workup

1.

2.

3.

4.

5.

History

HPI: *28 yo G0 presents with a positive pregnancy test. Her LMP was 6 weeks ago and was unusually scant. She reports bilateral breast engorgement, poor appetite, nausea with no vomiting, urinary frequency, and feeling bloated and fatigued. She is sexually active with her husband only, with coitus interruptus as the only method of contraception. This is an unplanned pregnancy, and she is unsure whether she will continue.*
OB/GYN: *G0, menarche at age 14, has regular periods 4–5/30. No history of STDs; last Pap smear was taken 8 months ago and was normal.*
ROS: *Denies abnormal bleeding, abdominal pain, fever, shortness of breath, or change in bowel habits.*
Allergies: *NKDA.*
Medications: *Multivitamins.*
PMH: *None.*
PSH: *Appendectomy at age 20.*
SH: *No smoking, 1–2 beers/week, no illicit drugs. Married graduate student; feels safe at home.*
FH: *Father is a diabetic. Mother has thyroid problems and obesity.*

Physical Examination

Patient appears comfortable.
VS: *WNL.*
HEENT: *NC/AT, PERRLA, no icterus, no pallor, mouth and oropharynx normal.*
Neck: *No thyroid enlargement.*
Chest: *Clear breath sounds bilaterally.*
Heart: *RRR; normal S1/S2; no murmurs, rubs, or gallops.*
Abdomen: *Soft, nontender, nondistended, ⊕BS, no evidence of guarding or hepatosplenomegaly.*

Differential Diagnosis

1. Normal pregnancy
2. Ectopic pregnancy
3. Molar pregnancy

Diagnostic Workup

1. Breast/pelvic exam
2. Urine hCG
3. U/S—pelvis
4. CBC, serum glucose
5. TSH
6. RPR, rubella IgG, HBsAg, HIV antibody
7. Blood type, Rh, antibody screen
8. Pap smear
9. Cervical GC DNA testing
10. UA, urine culture

CASE DISCUSSION

Differential Diagnosis

- **Normal pregnancy:** Any history of delayed periods or amenorrhea in a reproductive-age woman who is sexually active should prompt the diagnosis of pregnancy unless otherwise ruled out. This patient has symptoms of nausea, weight gain, and breast engorgement, all signs of early pregnancy.
- **Ectopic pregnancy:** Extrauterine implantation resulting in ectopic pregnancy should always be in the differential diagnosis of women with a positive pregnancy test until intrauterine pregnancy is identified.
- **Molar pregnancy:** Molar pregnancies are uncommon. Very high serum β-hCG levels, severe nausea and vomiting, new-onset hyperthyroidism, and a uterus that is larger than expected for gestational age should raise suspicion for molar pregnancy. The diagnosis is usually confirmed by pelvic ultrasound.

Diagnostic Workup

- **Breast/pelvic exam:** Breast engorgement and galactorrhea are some of the physiologic changes that occur in pregnancy. A pelvic examination should be performed to evaluate the cervix (lesions, length, dilation, consistency), the uterus (size, fibroids), and the adnexa (masses) and to collect necessary specimens for cytology, cultures, and PCR studies.
- **Urine hCG:** A urine hCG test can confirm pregnancy. Alternatively, a quantitative serum β-hCG can be ordered if an abnormal pregnancy (e.g., abortion, ectopic pregnancy, molar pregnancy) is suspected.
- **U/S—pelvis:** It is important to confirm the location of the pregnancy (intrauterine vs. extrauterine) and the gestational age in patients with an uncertain LMP or irregular periods. This can also aid in the diagnosis of molar pregnancies, uterine fibroids, and adnexal masses.
- **CBC, serum glucose:** Given her family history of diabetes, assessing blood glucose is mandatory for this patient. If it is confirmed that she is pregnant, it also serves as a baseline value if the patient does develop gestational diabetes mellitus in advanced pregnancy. A CBC is done to rule out anemia.
- **TSH:** Neurologic development may be adversely affected in children born to mothers with hypothyroidism, while maternal hyperthyroidism can lead to fetal and maternal complications.
- **RPR, rubella IgG, HBsAg, HIV antibody:** These infections can be transmitted perinatally, and early detection would allow for measures that could decrease the possibility of transmission to the fetus. HIV screening should be discussed separately, and the patient's consent is required.
- **Blood type, Rh, antibody screen:** To detect antibodies that could potentially cause hemolytic disease of the newborn. Rh(D)-negative women should receive anti-D immune globulin as indicated.
- **Pap smear:** To screen for cervical dysplasia and cervical cancer. However, since this patient had a normal Pap smear eight months ago, a repeat Pap smear is not necessarily indicated at this visit and could be postponed for another four months.
- **Cervical gonorrhea and chlamydia DNA testing:** Early diagnosis and treatment of these STDs can prevent serious neonatal infections.
- **UA, urine culture:** Pregnant women with untreated asymptomatic bacteriuria are at high risk of developing pyelonephritis.

Opening Scenario

Gwen Potter, a 20-year-old female, comes to the clinic complaining of sleeping problems.

Vital Signs

BP: 120/80 mmHg
Temp: 98.6°F (37°C)
RR: 18/minute
HR: 102/minute

Examinee Tasks

1. Take a focused history.
2. Perform a focused physical exam (do not perform rectal, genitourinary, or female breast exam).
3. Explain your clinical impression and workup plan to the patient.
4. Write the patient note after leaving the room.

Checklist/SP Sheet

PATIENT DESCRIPTION

Patient is a 20 yo F.

NOTES FOR THE SP

- Look anxious and irritable.
- Pretend that you are worried about performing well in graduate school.
- Exhibit a fine tremor on outstretched fingertips and brisk reflexes.

CHALLENGING QUESTIONS TO ASK

"Will I ever be able to sleep well again, doctor?"

SAMPLE EXAMINEE RESPONSE

"I think so, but first we need to run some tests to rule out underlying medical problems. In the meantime, I would recommend that you proceed with some lifestyle changes. If you drink coffee, I would strongly recommend that you cut down on it. You could also benefit from exercising, preferably during the day. Finally, you should get into the habit of going to bed early—for example, at 10 P.M. each night. You might try listening to some soothing music before you go to sleep."

Examinee Checklist

ENTRANCE:

☐ Examinee knocked on the door before entering.
☐ Examinee introduced self by name.
☐ Examinee identified his/her role or position.

☐ Examinee correctly used patient's name.
☐ Examinee made eye contact with the SP.

HISTORY:

☐ Examinee showed compassion for your pain.

☑ Question	Patient Response
☐ Chief complaint	Inability to fall asleep.
☐ Duration	It has been going on for about a month now.
☐ Total hours of sleep per night	I sleep around four hours a night, but I usually need eight hours of sleep to feel refreshed.
☐ Time you fall asleep	Around 2 A.M.
☐ Activities prior to sleep	I watch TV.
☐ Sleep interruptions	Yes, I wake up a couple of times during the night.
☐ Early spontaneous awakening	No, the alarm goes off and wakes me up at 6 A.M.
☐ Snoring	I do snore. My boyfriend told me about my snoring a few months ago, but he said that he is fine with it.
☐ Daytime sleepiness	I feel very sleepy during class and while driving to school at 7 A.M.
☐ Daytime naps	I feel the need to take naps but have no time for them. My final exams are coming up soon, and I am concerned about them.
☐ Recent stressful events/illnesses	Well, I am stressed out about getting good grades in grad school. I have been working hard to get an A+ in all of my classes.
☐ Relationship	My boyfriend is very understanding but has a hard time waking me up in the mornings for class.
☐ Sadness, depression, loss of interest in hobbies	No.
☐ Exercise	Before I started graduate school, I worked out one hour a day every evening, but lately it has become harder and harder for me to find the time to hit the gym.
☐ Caffeine intake	I drink at least 5–6 cups of coffee every day to stay awake.
☐ Tremors	None.
☐ Shortness of breath	No.
☐ Palpitations	Yes, I feel my heart racing most of the time, especially after I drink coffee.
☐ Sweating	Not really, but lately I have noticed that my palms are wet most of the time.
☐ Irritability	Yes.
☐ Intolerance to heat/cold	No.
☐ Weight changes	I have lost six pounds over the past month despite having a good appetite and eating more than usual.

✓	Question	Patient Response
☐	Frequency of menstrual period	Regular. I have been on oral contraceptive pills for the past two years.
☐	Contraceptives	Condoms and oral contraceptive pills.
☐	Fever	No.
☐	Change in bowel habits or in stool color or consistency	I used to go once a day, but lately I've been going two or three times each day. I have no loose stools or blood in my stool.
☐	Urinary habits	Normal.
☐	Neck pain	No.
☐	Skin changes	No.
☐	Any pain in joints/muscle	No.
☐	Hair loss/thinning	No.
☐	Current medications (antidepressants, antihistamines, pain medication)	All I take are multivitamins and oral contraceptive pills.
☐	Past medical history	None.
☐	Past surgical history	I had a tonsillectomy when I was 12.
☐	Family history	None.
☐	Occupation	Graduate student.
☐	Alcohol use	Occasionally a beer or two a week.
☐	Illicit drug use	None.
☐	Tobacco	None.
☐	Drug allergies	None.

Physical Examination:

☐ Examinee washed his/her hands.
☐ Examinee asked permission to start the exam.
☐ Examinee used respectful draping.
☐ Examinee did not repeat painful maneuvers.

✓	Exam Component	Maneuver
☐	HEENT exam	Inspection, palpation, auscultation of thyroid for lymphadenopathy
☐	CV exam	Auscultation
☐	Pulmonary exam	Auscultation
☐	Abdominal exam	Inspection, auscultation, palpation
☐	Extremities	Checked for tremor on outstretched fingertips; looked for edema

✓ *Exam Component*	*Maneuver*
☐ Skin exam	Inspection
☐ Neurologic exam	Looked for brisk reflexes

Closure:

☐ Examinee discussed initial diagnostic impressions.
☐ Examinee discussed initial management plans:
    ☐ Follow-up tests.
☐ Examinee asked if the patient has any other questions or concerns.

Sample Closure:

Ms. Potter, on the basis of your history and my examination, I think there are a few factors that might be contributing to your sleeping problems. The first is the anxiety and stress you've been experiencing over performing well in grad school. Although this is perfectly understandable, you may not be able to perform at your best if you don't get a good night's sleep. On the other hand, your problems could stem from your caffeine use, which I would urge you to reduce or stop completely. Another possibility has to do with your thyroid function. Sometimes hyperactivity of the thyroid gland can cause some of the symptoms you describe, and the only way to rule this out is through a blood test. I will also check a urine drug screen, and in light of your history of snoring, we may need to do a sleep study to rule out sleep apnea. At this point, I would encourage you to proceed with the lifestyle changes I have recommended, and I will see you for follow-up. Do you have any questions or concerns?

PATIENT NOTE

History

Physical Examination

Differential Diagnosis	Diagnostic Workup
1.	1.
2.	2.
3.	3.
4.	4.
5.	5.

History

HPI: 20 yo F graduate student c/o inability to sleep. She has difficulty falling asleep until 2 A.M. and also has difficulty staying asleep. She used to get 8 hours of sleep, but for the past month she has been getting a total of only 4 hours per night. She has difficulty getting up after hearing the alarm and feels tired while at school. She notes inability to concentrate during classes and while driving. The patient appears to be stressed about her coursework and about her performance at school. She has also been snoring for the past few months and has had palpitations, especially after drinking caffeine. She has a history of drinking 4–5 cups of coffee per day. She has lost weight (6 lbs in 1 month) and has sweaty palms. There is an increase in frequency of bowel movements. She lives with her boyfriend, and they use condoms and OCPs for contraception. There is no history of sexual abuse, recent infection, or recent tragic events in her life.

ROS: Negative except as above.
Allergies: NKDA.
Medications: Multivitamins, OCPs.
PMH: None.
PSH: Tonsillectomy at age 12.
SH: No smoking, 1–2 beers/week, no illicit drugs.
FH: Not significant.

Physical Examination

Patient appears anxious and restless.
Chest: Clear breath sounds bilaterally.
Heart: Tachycardic; normal S1/S2; no murmurs, rubs, or gallops.
Abdomen: Soft, nontender, nondistended, ⊕BS, no guarding, no hepatosplenomegaly.
Skin: Normal, no rashes, palms moist.
Neuro: Brisk reflexes.
Extremities: Tremor on outstretched fingertips.

Differential Diagnosis

1. Anxiety
2. Caffeine-induced insomnia
3. Hyperthyroidism
4. Insomnia related to depression
5. Adjustment insomnia
6. Illicit drug abuse
7. Obstructive sleep apnea

Diagnostic Workup

1. TSH, free T_4
2. CBC with differential, chem 8
3. Urine toxicology
4. Polysomnography
5. ECG

CASE DISCUSSION

Differential Diagnosis

- **Anxiety:** Fatigue and sleep disturbances are common in anxiety states. The clinical manifestations of anxiety are both psychological (e.g., tension, fears, difficulty concentrating) and somatic (e.g., tachycardia, sweating, hyperventilation, palpitations, tremor).
- **Caffeine-induced insomnia:** The most common pharmacologic cause of insomnia, caffeine use produces increased latency to sleep onset, more frequent arousals during sleep, and a reduction in total sleep time several hours after ingestion. Even small amounts of caffeine can significantly disturb sleep in some patients.
- **Hyperthyroidism:** Clinical hyperthyroidism is associated with anxiety, tremor, palpitations, sweating, frequent bowel movements, fatigue, menstrual irregularities, and heat intolerance. The patient presented in this case has some of these symptoms, suggesting the need to rule out hyperthyroidism.
- **Insomnia due to depression:** Several mood disorders are associated with insomnia. Depression can be associated with sleep onset insomnia, sleep maintenance insomnia, or early-morning wakefulness. Hypersomnia occurs in some depressed patients, especially adolescents and those with either bipolar or seasonal (fall/winter) depression.
- **Adjustment insomnia:** Any significant life event, such as a change of occupation, loss of a loved one, illness, or anxiety over a deadline or an examination, can cause adjustment insomnia. Increased sleep latency, frequent awakenings from sleep, and early-morning awakening can all result. Recovery is rapid, usually occurring within a few weeks.
- **Illicit drug use:** Drugs such as cocaine and amphetamine increase sympathetic activity and can thus cause insomnia.
- **Obstructive sleep apnea (OSA):** More than 50% of patients evaluated for OSA complain of symptoms of insomnia, including difficulty in initiating and maintaining sleep and early-morning awakening.

Diagnostic Workup

- **TSH, free T_4:** The patient gives a history of weight loss, increased frequency of bowel movements, palpitations, and sweaty palms, all of which are suggestive of hyperthyroidism. An elevated free T_4 with suppressed TSH is diagnostic.
- **CBC:** Can help detect anemia, hidden infection, or malignancy, all of which can cause the fatigue and weight loss seen in this patient.
- **Urine toxicology:** Although this patient denies illicit drug use, a toxicology screen will help rule out the use of CNS stimulants that can cause insomnia (e.g., cocaine, amphetamine).
- **Polysomnography:** A diagnostic test for OSA syndrome that can also help assess the severity of the disease as well as any comorbidities with which it might be associated.
- **ECG:** Nonspecific changes can be seen with hyperthyroidism and anxiety disorders.

Opening Scenario

Jack Edwards, a 27-year-old male, comes to the ER complaining of seeing strange writing on the wall.

Vital Signs

BP: 140/80 mmHg
Temp: 98.3° F (36.8°C)
RR: 15/minute
HR: 98/minute, regular

Examinee Tasks

1. Take a focused history.
2. Perform a focused physical exam (do not perform rectal, genitourinary, or female breast exam).
3. Explain your clinical impression and workup plan to the patient.
4. Write the patient note after leaving the room.

Checklist/SP Sheet

PATIENT DESCRIPTION
Patient is a 27 yo M.

NOTES FOR THE SP
- Sit up on the bed.
- Give the impression that you are staring at the wall.

CHALLENGING QUESTIONS TO ASK
"Do you think someone is trying to give me instructions through the writing I see on the wall?"

SAMPLE EXAMINEE RESPONSE
"I don't think anyone is trying to give you instructions. If you have been taking illicit drugs, it may be that the drugs are causing you to see this writing. In any case, we are going to do some tests to try to figure out what's going on."

Examinee Checklist

ENTRANCE:
☐ Examinee knocked on the door before entering.
☐ Examinee introduced self by name.
☐ Examinee identified his/her role or position.
☐ Examinee correctly used patient's name.
☐ Examinee made eye contact with the SP.

HISTORY:

☐ Examinee showed compassion for your pain.

☑ Question	Patient Response
☐ Chief complaint	I have been seeing strange writing on the wall.
☐ Onset	It started yesterday.
☐ Content	It is not clear, and I can't read it most of the time.
☐ Duration	It lasts less than a minute.
☐ Constant/intermittent	It comes and goes.
☐ Frequency	It has happened 3–4 times since yesterday.
☐ Do you see the writing while your eyes are closed?	Sometimes.
☐ Alleviating factors	None.
☐ Exacerbating factors	None.
☐ Major life changes or stressors	Not really.
☐ Headache	None.
☐ Visual changes or vision loss	None.
☐ Hearing changes	I feel as though I hear strange voices when I see the writing.
☐ Hearing loss	No.
☐ Content of the voices	I can't understand them; the voices seem distant.
☐ Feeling of being controlled	No.
☐ Do the voices/writing order you to harm yourself or others?	No.
☐ Do you think about harming yourself or others?	No.
☐ Enjoyment of daily activities	Yes.
☐ Mental illness in family	No.
☐ Sleeping problems	No, but sometimes I find it difficult to wake up in the morning.
☐ Do you fall asleep suddenly during the day?	No, but sometimes I feel very sleepy during the day.
☐ Fever	No.
☐ Weight changes	None.
☐ Current medications	None.
☐ Past medical history	None.
☐ Head trauma	No.
☐ Past surgical history	None.
☐ Family history	My father had high blood pressure.

☑ Question	Patient Response
☐ Occupation	I work as a bartender.
☐ Alcohol use	No.
☐ Illicit drug use	Occasionally.
☐ Which illicit drugs do you use?	Angel dust; sometimes Ecstasy.
☐ Last use of illicit drugs	Two days ago at a party at my friend's house.
☐ Tobacco	Yes, I have smoked one pack a day for six years.
☐ Exercise	No.
☐ Sexual activity	Yes, with my girlfriend.
☐ Use of condoms	Yes, I use them.
☐ Drug allergies	None.

Physical Examination:

☐ Examinee washed his/her hands.
☐ Examinee asked permission to start the exam.
☐ Examinee used respectful draping.
☐ Examinee did not repeat painful maneuvers.

☑ Exam Component	Maneuver
☐ Eye exam	Inspected pupils; checked for reactivity
☐ CV exam	Auscultation, vital signs
☐ Pulmonary exam	Auscultation
☐ Abdominal exam	Palpation
☐ Neurologic exam	Mini-mental status exam, cranial nerves, motor exam, DTRs, gait, sensory exam

Closure:

☐ Examinee discussed initial diagnostic impressions.
☐ Examinee discussed initial management plans:
    ☐ Follow-up tests: Examinee mentioned the need for a rectal exam.
☐ Examinee asked if the patient has any other questions or concerns.

Sample Closure:

Mr. Edwards, your symptoms could be caused by your illicit drug use or they may be the result of a mental problem or even a medical condition. We will run some tests to try to clarify your condition. In addition, I would recommend that you stop using illicit drugs and quit smoking.

PATIENT NOTE

History

Physical Examination

Differential Diagnosis

1.

2.

3.

4.

5.

Diagnostic Workup

1.

2.

3.

4.

5.

History

HPI: *27 yo M c/o episodes of seeing strange writing on the wall since yesterday. These episodes last less than a minute and have happened 3–4 times. The patient states that the writing is not clear and he cannot read the messages, but he thinks he might be getting instructions from them. He denies any other visual changes or visual loss. The patient also mentions hearing strange voices associated with the writing, adding that he cannot understand them either. He admits to having used illicit drugs 2 days prior to these events. He denies any headache, seizures, head trauma, or previous similar episodes. No appetite or weight changes, fever, or sleep problems.*
ROS: *Negative except as above.*
Allergies: *NKDA.*
Medications: *None.*
PMH: *None.*
PSH: *None.*
SH: *One PPD for 6 years; uses PCP ("angel dust") and MDMA (Ecstasy) occasionally; no EtOH. Works as a bartender.*
FH: *Noncontributory.*

Physical Examination

Patient seems anxious and in mild distress.
VS: *WNL.*
HEENT: *Pupils reactive to light.*
Chest: *Clear breath sounds bilaterally.*
Heart: *RRR; normal S1/S2; no murmurs, rubs, or gallops.*
Abdomen: *Soft, nontender, nondistended, no hepatosplenomegaly.*
Neuro: Mental status: *Alert and oriented × 3, spells backward and recalls 3 objects.* Cranial nerves: *2–12 intact.*
Motor: *Strength 5/5 in all muscle groups.* DTRs: *Symmetric.* Gait: *Normal.*

Differential Diagnosis

1. Substance-induced psychosis
2. Brief psychotic disorder
3. Psychosis secondary to a medical condition
4. Narcolepsy
5. Seizure

Diagnostic Workup

1. Urine toxicology
2. Mental status exam
3. Electrolytes, BUN/Cr
4. AST/ALT
5. TSH, free T_4
6. EEG

CASE DISCUSSION

Differential Diagnosis

- **Substance-induced psychosis:** Psychosis may result from the ingestion of medications, alcohol, or illicit drugs, or it may stem from the withdrawal of alcohol or sedative drugs such as benzodiazepines. The presence of offending substances is usually detectable and points to the diagnosis.
- **Brief psychotic disorder:** Symptoms of psychosis may be induced by stressful events and may resolve with removal of the stressor. Auditory hallucinations are more common and typically accompany visual hallucinations. The content of the hallucinations is usually disturbing and antagonistic. The duration and frequency of hallucinations are highly variable.
- **Psychosis secondary to a medical condition:** A variety of medical conditions can lead to hallucination. These include neurologic problems such as CNS infections and neoplasms; endocrine conditions such as thyroid, parathyroid, or adrenal abnormalities; and hepatic and renal disorders.
- **Narcolepsy:** The visual hallucinations of narcolepsy are complex, generally occurring immediately before falling asleep (hypnagogic) or just after waking up (hypnopompic). Auditory or tactile sensations can be associated with visual hallucinations as well. The duration and frequency are variable. Associated symptoms of narcolepsy include excessive daytime sleepiness, sleep paralysis, and cataplexy.
- **Seizure:** Visual hallucinations of epileptic origin can be simple or complex. They are variable in frequency and usually last for a few seconds. An example would be idiopathic occipital epilepsy.

Diagnostic Workup

- **Urine toxicology:** To detect commonly used illicit drugs, such as amphetamines, barbiturates, benzodiazepines, cannabinoids, cocaine, opioids, and phencyclidine (PCP).
- **Mental status exam:** To evaluate for any possible neurologic disorder.
- **Electrolytes, BUN/Cr, AST/ALT, TSH, free T_4:** To detect any medical condition that may cause neurologic or mental changes.
- **EEG:** To detect any seizure activity.

Opening Scenario

The mother of Louise Johnson, a 10-year-old female child, comes to the office because she is concerned that her daughter was recently diagnosed with diabetes.

Examinee Tasks

1. Take a focused history.
2. Explain your clinical impression and workup plan to the mother.
3. Write the patient note after leaving the room.

Checklist/SP Sheet

PATIENT DESCRIPTION

The patient's mother offers the history; her daughter is in the waiting room.

NOTES FOR THE SP

None.

CHALLENGING QUESTIONS TO ASK

- "Doctor, I have no history of diabetes in my family. Why is this happening to my daughter?"
- "Will my child ever be able to eat sweets again?"

SAMPLE EXAMINEE RESPONSE

"Your daughter probably had a genetic tendency to develop diabetes. Then certain unknown environmental factors led her to get full-blown diabetes. Your daughter may have either type 1 or type 2 diabetes. In type 1 diabetes, the immune system attacks the pancreas and destroys the cells that are responsible for making insulin. Since insulin regulates and maintains blood sugar, a deficiency of insulin will lead to high levels of blood sugar. On the other hand, if your child is overweight and is not physically active, she may have type 2 diabetes, which is a combination of insulin deficiency and resistance to the action of insulin resulting from being overweight. In either case, it is not essential to have a positive family history. As far as sweets are concerned, this is a myth. Your daughter can still eat sweets, but in moderation. She will need to see a dietitian to develop healthy meal plans and to learn to recognize which foods contain carbohydrates."

Examinee Checklist

ENTRANCE:

- [ ] Examinee knocked on the door before entering.
- [ ] Examinee introduced self by name.
- [ ] Examinee identified his/her role or position.
- [ ] Examinee correctly used patient's name.
- [ ] Examinee made eye contact with the SP.

HISTORY:

- [ ] Examinee showed compassion for your child's illness.

☑	Question	Patient Response
☐	Chief complaint	My child was recently diagnosed with diabetes.
☐	Type of diabetes	I am not sure.
☐	Onset	A month ago.
☐	Presenting symptoms at the time of diagnosis	Excessive thirst and urination.
☐	Effect on child	She is concerned about the effect this will have on her normal activities, such as playing tennis and attending school.
☐	Depression	I'm not sure, but she seems more concerned than depressed.
☐	Irritability	No.
☐	Effect on parents	We were shocked.
☐	Medication	Insulin injections.
☐	Site of injection	In the tummy.
☐	Insulin injector	I do it when she is at home, but when she is away from me, she does the injections herself.
☐	Compliance with insulin	Yes.
☐	Schedule of insulin	Two types: one with meals and one at bedtime.
☐	Measuring glucose at home	Yes, before each meal and at bedtime.
☐	Ranges of blood glucose readings	Her blood sugar levels are normally in the low 100s in the morning and in the high 100s before meals.
☐	Recent level of glucose	Today her morning glucose was 96 in the fasting state.
☐	Hypoglycemia	Not really; the lowest blood glucose reading was 80 in the morning.
☐	Urination	Normal.
☐	Abnormal thirst or extreme hunger	No, but she was excessively thirsty earlier.
☐	Weakness or fatigue	No.
☐	Vision problems (blurring of vision)	No.
☐	Weight changes	She has lost about nine pounds within the past three months, but now her weight is stable.
☐	Patient's weight and height	She weighs 180 pounds and has been on the heavy side for a long time. She is 5 feet, 1 inch tall.
☐	Tingling or numbness in limbs	No.
☐	Infections of skin or gums	No.
☐	Itchy skin	No.
☐	Any specific diet	We are trying to give her a balanced diet as suggested previously by a dietitian.
☐	Exercise and playful activities	Yes, she is active and plays tennis.
☐	When does she play?	Evenings.

☑ Question	Patient Response
☐ Loss of consciousness while playing	No.
☐ Last menstrual period	She has not yet started menstruating.
☐ Sleeping problems	No.
☐ Birth history	Normal.
☐ Child weight, height, and language development	She was always on time with her development. She walked early, talked on time, and is doing well in school.
☐ Past medical history	None.
☐ Past surgical history	None.
☐ Drug allergies	No.

Physical Examination:

None.

Closure:

☐ Examinee discussed initial diagnostic impressions.
☐ Examinee discussed initial management plans:
    ☐ Further examination.
    ☐ Follow-up tests.
    ☐ Examinee asked if the patient has any other questions or concerns.

Sample Closure:

Mrs. Johnson, I can understand how you have felt since your daughter was diagnosed with diabetes. Diabetes may alter the dynamics of the entire family and affects everyone, so your life is going to be a little different now. But believe me, we can manage this disease very well through a combination of insulin, a balanced diet, and regular exercise. First of all, you should understand the disease and know how to manage it. You will need to attend diabetes classes with your daughter. Second, everyone in your family, including your daughter, should learn to recognize signs of low glucose levels, such as confusion, disorientation, or fainting, and should be in a position to provide appropriate care. Your daughter should always carry glucose tablets or juices as an "emergency kit." Her teachers and friends should also be aware of her disease. I hope you understood what we discussed today. Do you have any additional questions or concerns?

PATIENT NOTE

History

Physical Examination

Differential Diagnosis

1.

2.

3.

4.

5.

Diagnostic Workup

1.

2.

3.

4.

5.

History

HPI: *The source of the information is the patient's mother. The mother of a 10 yo F states that her child was diagnosed with DM one month ago, when she presented with excessive thirst and frequent urination. The parents were shocked after the diagnosis was made. The child seems concerned but not irritable or depressed. She is active, plays tennis, and is currently on a diet prescribed by a dietitian. She is on insulin injections and regularly monitors her blood glucose levels at home. Her compliance is good; she checks her blood glucose before each meal and at bedtime. Fasting glucose levels are usually 80 to the low 100s and in the high 100s before meals. She has not had any episodes of hypoglycemia. She has lost 9 pounds in the past 3 months, but her weight is stable now. She denies any weakness, fatigue, tingling over limbs, visual symptoms, or rash/itch at the injection sites. She has not yet started menstruating.*

ROS: *Negative.*
Allergies: *NKDA.*
Medications: *Insulin.*
PMH: *None.*
PSH: *None.*
Birth history: *Normal.*
Developmental history: *Normal.*
FH: *No family history of diabetes.*

Physical Examination

None.

Differential Diagnosis

1. Type 1 diabetes mellitus
2. Type 2 diabetes mellitus
3. Secondary causes of diabetes (such as Cushing's)

Diagnostic Workup

1. Basal metabolic profile
2. Glycosylated hemoglobin/HbA$_{1c}$
3. UA, urine microalbumin
4. Insulin and C-peptide levels
5. Islet cell antibodies
6. 24-hour urine free cortisol

CASE DISCUSSION

Differential Diagnosis

- **Diabetes mellitus:** Although most cases of diabetes in the pediatric population are type 1, the increasing prevalence of obesity and physical inactivity in the urban population has led to a growing incidence of type 2 diabetes among children. In every suspected case of diabetes mellitus, it is mandatory to rule out other causes of diabetes.
- **Secondary causes of diabetes (hyperglycemia):** Diabetes can be secondary to other factors or medical conditions, such as drugs (e.g., thiazide diuretics, glucocorticoids), Cushing's syndrome, pancreatitis, cystic fibrosis, hemochromatosis, and acromegaly.

Diagnostic Workup

- **Basal metabolic profile:** To evaluate serum electrolytes and glucose levels.
- **Glycosylated hemoglobin/HbA$_{1c}$:** Not a test to diagnose DM, but conducted to estimate blood glucose control during the preceding 2–3 months. Elevated levels suggest existing diabetes as well as lack of control of blood glucose levels within the past 2–3 months.
- **UA, urine microalbumin:** To screen for diabetic nephropathy.
- **Insulin and C-peptide levels:** When combined, can be a useful tool in identifying type 1 diabetes.
- **Islet cell antibodies:** This finding will support the diagnosis of type 1 diabetes mellitus.
- **24-hour urine free cortisol:** To rule out coexisting Cushing's syndrome.

Opening Scenario

Riva George, a 35-year-old female, comes to the hospital complaining of pain in her right calf.

Vital Signs

BP: 130/70 mmHg
Temp: 98.2°F (36.8°C)
RR: 13/minute
HR: 74/minute

Examinee Tasks

1. Take a focused history.
2. Perform a focused physical exam (do not perform rectal, genitourinary, or female breast exam).
3. Explain your clinical impression and workup plan to the patient.
4. Write the patient note after leaving the room.

Checklist/SP Sheet

PATIENT DESCRIPTION

Patient is a 35 yo F, married with two children.

NOTES FOR THE SP

- Exhibit pain in your calf when the doctor dorsiflexes your right ankle.
- Place a bandage on your right leg to cover the cuts that you got after a fall.

CHALLENGING QUESTIONS TO ASK

"My father had a clot in his leg. What do you think I should do to make sure I don't get one too?"

SAMPLE EXAMINEE RESPONSE

"There are several measures you can take that may prevent you from having a clot. Above all, you should avoid immobilization for long periods of time—for example, while sitting at your computer desk or on long-distance plane trips. Try to move in place and perhaps take a short walk. If you are on oral contraceptive pills, I would strongly recommend that you stop taking them, as they are known to precipitate clotting. Studies have also shown that obesity increases your risk of having a clot, so I suggest that you exercise regularly and manage your diet."

Examinee Checklist

ENTRANCE:

☐ Examinee knocked on the door before entering.
☐ Examinee introduced self by name.
☐ Examinee identified his/her role or position.

☐ Examinee correctly used patient's name.
☐ Examinee made eye contact with the SP.

HISTORY:

☐ Examinee showed compassion for your pain.

✓ Question	Patient Response
☐ Chief complaint	Pain in my right calf muscle.
☐ Onset	The pain started a few days ago and has gotten worse.
☐ Frequency	It is present all the time.
☐ Progression	The pain was mild in the beginning, but now it hurts even when I take just one step.
☐ Severity on a scale	8/10.
☐ Radiation	No.
☐ Quality	Pressure, spasms.
☐ Alleviating factors	Pain medication (ibuprofen). It also helps if I prop up my leg with a pillow.
☐ Exacerbating factors	Walking and extending my knee.
☐ Swelling	At the end of the day, my legs feel heavy and pit on pressure.
☐ Injury	Yes, I fell down and scratched my right leg (points to bandage).
☐ Redness	Yes.
☐ Warmth	My right leg feels warmer than my left.
☐ Varicose veins	No.
☐ Shortness of breath	No.
☐ Chest pain	No.
☐ Recent immobilization	I travel frequently as part of my consulting business, and a week ago I took a 15-hour flight to meet an important client.
☐ Fever	No.
☐ Last menstrual period	Two weeks ago.
☐ Contraceptives	I have been taking oral contraceptives for two years.
☐ Frequency of menstrual periods	Regular. My periods last three days, and I use 3–4 pads. They are not accompanied by pain.
☐ Obstetric history	I have had two kids, both with a normal delivery.
☐ Last Pap smear	One year ago; it was normal.
☐ Weight changes	I gained 50 pounds after having my last child three years ago.
☐ Past medical history	None.

☑ Question	Patient Response
☐ Past surgical history	None.
☐ Family history	My dad had a clot in his leg.
☐ Occupation	Executive consultant.
☐ Alcohol use	No.
☐ Illicit drug use	No.
☐ Tobacco	No.
☐ Sexual activity	With my husband.
☐ Drug allergies/herbal medication	None.

Physical Examination:

- ☐ Examinee washed his/her hands.
- ☐ Examinee asked permission to start the exam.
- ☐ Examinee used respectful draping.
- ☐ Examinee did not repeat painful maneuvers.

☑ Exam Component	Maneuver
☐ CV/pulmonary exam	Inspection, auscultation, palpation; compared pulses (femoral, popliteal, dorsalis pedis) on both sides
☐ Joint exam	Inspection, palpation, range of motion (knee, ankle, hip joint on both sides)
☐ Extremities	Inspection, palpation; checked for Homans' sign
☐ Neurologic exam	Sensory and motor reflexes (knee, ankle)

Closure:

- ☐ Examinee discussed initial diagnostic impressions.
- ☐ Examinee discussed initial management plans.
- ☐ Examinee asked if the patient has any other questions or concerns.

Sample Closure:

Mrs. George, on the basis of your history and my physical examination, I believe it is possible that you had a venous clot. First, however, we will have to look for other possible causes of your symptoms, such as an infection or a ruptured cyst. We will be running a few blood tests as well as some imaging studies that should help us make a final diagnosis. If your test results show a clot, we will start you on blood thinners, which should prevent further complications such as the possibility of a clot traveling to your lungs.

PATIENT NOTE

History

Physical Examination

Differential Diagnosis

1.

2.

3.

4.

5.

6.

Diagnostic Workup

1.

2.

3.

4.

5.

History

HPI: 35 yo F c/o calf pain of a few days' duration. The pain is constant, 8/10 in intensity, not radiating, aggravated on walking and extending the knee, and associated with swelling, redness, and warmth. It is alleviated on elevation of the foot and with ibuprofen. The patient took a 15-hour flight 1 week ago. She has a history of trauma to the right leg and weight gain postpartum. She has 2 children, both normal deliveries. LMP was 2 weeks ago. The patient says she has gained 50 lbs in the last 3 years. She has been on OCPs for 2 years. No history of chest pain or shortness of breath.

ROS: Negative except as above.

Allergies: NKDA.

Medications: OCPs, ibuprofen.

PMH: None.

PSH: None.

SH: No smoking, no EtOH, no illicit drugs.

FH: Father had DVT. No history of sudden deaths in the family.

Physical Examination

Patient is in severe pain.

VS: WNL.

Chest: Clear breath sounds bilaterally; no rales or rhonchi.

Heart: RRR; normal S1/S2; no murmurs, rubs, or gallops.

Abdomen: Soft, nontender, nondistended, ⊕BS.

Extremities: Inspection: Right calf appears red and swollen compared to left; contours of the muscles appear normal; no ulcers or pigmentation. Palpation: Right leg is warmer compared to left; pitting pedal edema ⊕ on right side; dorsalis pedis pulse felt and equal on both sides; mobility normal at ankle joint, knee, and hip joint; ⊕Homans' sign on right side.

Neuro: Mental status: Alert and oriented. DTRs: Symmetric 2+. Motor/sensation: Normal. Cranial nerves: 2–12 intact. Gait: Normal.

Differential Diagnosis

1. Deep venous thrombosis
2. Cellulitis/myositis
3. Rupture of Baker's cyst
4. Hematoma
5. Rupture of the medial head of the gastrocnemius
6. Spasm due to injury or sprain

Diagnostic Workup

1. Doppler U/S
2. D-dimer
3. Hypercoagulability testing
4. CBC with differential
5. CPK and myoglobin level
6. CT venography
7. MRI

CASE DISCUSSION

Differential Diagnosis

- **Deep venous thrombosis (DVT):** DVT is common in the lower limbs and may arise under conditions of stasis, hypercoagulability, and venous endothelial injury. Conditions that result in prolonged immobilization (e.g., post-surgery, trauma, sedentary jobs, long hours of travel) are predisposing factors. DVT may produce pain and edema of the affected limb or may be asymptomatic. A positive Homans' sign (pain on dorsiflexion of the ankle) is indicative of DVT.
- **Cellulitis/myositis:** Trauma can lead to cellulitis of the skin and subcutaneous tissue or to myositis of the calf muscle. All the classic signs of inflammation associated with fever may point to the diagnosis. Myositis ossificans may occur as a complication of this disorder, causing hardening of the muscle and pain on contraction. Radiographs may show ossification in the muscle.
- **Rupture of Baker's cyst:** Baker's cysts (also known as popliteal cysts) are seen in the popliteal fossa. Arthritis or a cartilage tear of the knee joint may cause excess fluid to be accumulated, forming a cyst. Ruptures can present with tightness and swelling behind the knee, pain on knee extension, and stiffness of the calf muscle.
- **Hematoma:** Injuries can cause bleeding intramuscularly (in which no bruising occurs) or intermuscularly (in which bruising is usually present). Patients present with pain, swelling, and restricted movement. The condition may lead to posterior compartment syndrome.
- **Rupture of the gastrocnemius muscle:** Presents with sudden pain associated with rupture at the musculotendinous junction of the gastrocnemius muscle, halfway between the knee and the heel. There may be bruising and pain on standing on the tips of the toes. Patients also present with pain on dorsiflexion of the ankle against resistance.
- **Spasm/sprain:** Undue strain may cause physical tearing of muscles or tendons, inducing spasm and pain. Ligaments can be ruptured or torn due to overstretching or injuries.

Diagnostic Workup

- **Doppler U/S:** An initial diagnostic test that is noninvasive and can visualize clots in the veins of the leg.
- **D-dimer:** A cross-linked fibrin degradation product that may be increased in DVT. The negative predictive value of this test is sufficiently high to rule out DVT.
- **Hypercoagulability testing:** Several autoantibodies are implicated in thrombophilic states. Protein C and S deficiency, partial antithrombin deficiency, hyperhomocysteinemia, antiphospholipid antibody syndrome, and paroxysmal nocturnal hemoglobinuria may all lead to increased coagulability.
- **CBC with differential:** To detect infections such as cellulitis.
- **CPK and myoglobin:** Both can be elevated in muscle injury (myositis).
- **CT/MRI:** CT venography is used to diagnose DVT in conjunction with contrast-enhanced spiral CT to rule out pulmonary embolism. MRI is noninvasive and can detect acute, symptomatic proximal DVTs as well as muscle or tendon rupture.

Opening Scenario

Will Foreman, a 31-year-old male, comes to his primary care physician complaining of heel pain.

Vital Signs

BP: 125/80 mmHg
Temp: 99.5°F (37.5°C)
RR: 14/minute
HR: 69/minute, regular

Examinee Tasks

1. Take a focused history.
2. Perform a focused physical exam (do not perform rectal, genitourinary, or female breast exam).
3. Explain your clinical impression and workup plan to the patient.
4. Write the patient note after leaving the room.

Checklist/SP Sheet

PATIENT DESCRIPTION

Patient is a 31 yo M.

NOTES FOR THE SP

- Pretend to have pain on the bottom of your right heel and into the arch of your right foot when the examinee extends your toes (moves them up).
- Exhibit pain when the examinee palpates the arch of your right foot and the bottom of your right heel.
- Give the appearance of pain with the first few steps you take after sitting.

CHALLENGING QUESTIONS TO ASK

"Doctor, can you just give me some powerful pain meds so that I can keep running? I am training for a marathon."

SAMPLE EXAMINEE RESPONSE

"First we need to do a complete evaluation to determine the cause of your pain, and from that point we can discuss the nature of your treatment."

Examinee Checklist

ENTRANCE:

☐ Examinee knocked on the door before entering.
☐ Examinee introduced self by name.
☐ Examinee identified his/her role or position.

☐ Examinee correctly used patient's name.
☐ Examinee made eye contact with the SP.

HISTORY:

☐ Examinee showed compassion for your pain.

☑ Question	Patient Response
☐ Chief complaint	Right heel pain.
☐ Location	It hurts the most on the bottom of my heel.
☐ Onset	It came on gradually over the past two weeks.
☐ Precipitating events	Not really, but I have been training for a marathon.
☐ Constant/intermittent	Intermittent.
☐ Frequency	It usually hurts every day. It seems to be the worst in the morning.
☐ When does it hurt in the morning?	It hurts the most with the first few steps I take after I get out of bed.
☐ Progression	It has stayed about the same.
☐ Severity on a scale	When it hurts, it can get up to a 7/10.
☐ Radiation	It occasionally radiates into the arch of my foot.
☐ Radiation proximally (up the leg or down from the back)	No.
☐ Quality	Stretching/tearing pain.
☐ Burning, tingling, numbness	No.
☐ Alleviating factors	Massaging the arch of my foot and applying ice.
☐ Exacerbating factors	Walking barefoot or walking after sitting for a prolonged period of time.
☐ Other joint pain	No.
☐ Previous episodes of similar pain	No.
☐ Previous injury to your feet or ankles.	No.
☐ Constitutional symptoms (nausea/ vomiting, weight/appetite changes, fever/ chills, diarrhea/constipation, fatigue)	No.
☐ Current medications	Occasionally I take ibuprofen for the pain.
☐ Past medical history (be sure to address diabetes, rheumatologic disorders, and cancer)	No.
☐ Past surgical history	None.
☐ Family history (be sure to address diabetes, rheumatologic disorders, and cancer)	My father has arthritis.
☐ Occupation	I work as an accountant.

☑ Question	Patient Response
☐ Avocation	Runner.
☐ Alcohol use	I have approximately 1–2 beers a week.
☐ Illicit drug use	No.
☐ Tobacco	No.
☐ Sexual activity	I am sexually active with my wife of 10 years.
☐ Drug allergies	No.

Physical Examination:

☐ Examinee washed his/her hands.
☐ Examinee asked permission to start the exam.
☐ Examinee used respectful draping.
☐ Examinee did not repeat painful maneuvers.

☑ Exam Component	Maneuver
☐ CV exam	Auscultation, distal pulses (posterior tibialis, dorsalis pedis), capillary refill of the toes
☐ Pulmonary exam	Auscultation
☐ Abdominal exam	Auscultation, palpation
☐ Extremities	• Inspection of both feet and ankles—non–weight bearing, weight bearing, and with ambulation • Palpation of medial calcaneal tuberosity, Achilles tendon, plantar fascia, retrocalcaneal bursae • Passive range of motion and general strength of ipsilateral knee and hip • Ankle dorsiflexion and great toe extension and passive range of motion; strength testing of ankle dorsiflexion and plantarflexion
☐ Neurologic exam	Checked sensation to light touch for dermatomes of foot and ankle; assessed Achilles tendon reflex

Closure:

☐ Examinee discussed initial diagnostic impressions.
☐ Examinee discussed initial management plans:
    ☐ Diagnostic tests: X-ray of right ankle.
☐ Examinee asked if the patient has any other questions or concerns.

Sample Closure:

Mr. Foreman, the most likely cause of your heel pain is plantar fasciitis, which is the most common cause of pain on the bottom of the heel. It typically resolves over a few months, with conservative treatment consisting of stretching, massage, NSAIDs, and avoidance of painful activities. We will get an x-ray today to help confirm that there is no obvious fracture or foreign body and to look for possible bone spurs. If you would like, I can send you to physical therapy to help you get started on these exercises. If your symptoms are not responsive to this treatment over the next two months, we may consider a bone scan to rule out a stress fracture.

PATIENT NOTE

History

Physical Examination

Differential Diagnosis	Diagnostic Workup
1.	1.
2.	2.
3.	3.
4.	4.
5.	5.

History

HPI: *31 yo M c/o pain on the plantar surface of his right heel. The pain started insidiously about 2 weeks ago and has not progressed. The patient denies trauma or a specific inciting event but does admit to training for a marathon. He states that the pain is worse with the first few steps after getting out of bed in the morning and after prolonged sitting. He reports that the pain has a tearing/stretching quality and that it can get as high as 7/10. He has used ice and massage with minor relief. The patient denies any tingling, burning, or numbness. He denies proximally radiating symptoms but does report occasional pain radiating into his arch.*

ROS: *Denies nausea/vomiting, weight/appetite changes, fever/chills, diarrhea/constipation, or fatigue.*

Allergies: *NKDA.*

Medications: *Occasional ibuprofen.*

PMH: *None. Denies cancer, rheumatologic disorders, diabetes.*

PSH: *None.*

SH: *No smoking, 1–2 beers/week, no illicit drugs. Works as an accountant; sexually active only with wife of 10 years. Marathon runner.*

FH: *Father with arthritis, probable osteoarthritis. Denies FH of cancer, rheumatologic disorders, or diabetes.*

Physical Examination

Patient is pleasant and in no acute distress.

VS: *WNL.*

Chest: *Clear to auscultation bilaterally.*

Heart: *RRR; normal S1/S2; no murmurs, rubs, or gallops.*

Abdomen: *Soft, nontender, nondistended, ⊕BS.*

Extremities: *Posterior tibialis and dorsalis pedis pulses 2+ bilaterally; mild bilateral rear/midfoot pronation; range of motion WNL for hip/knee/ankle and foot. Tender to palpation over medial calcaneal tuberosity and plantar fascia; plantar heel and arch pain with passive extension of toes.*

Neuro: *Motor: Strength 5/5 in hip/knee/ankle/foot. Sensation: Intact to light touch in saphenous, sural, and deep/superficial peroneal nerve distribution (dermatomes L4–S1). DTRs: 1+ in Achilles tendon. Gait: Nonantalgic gait pattern.*

Differential Diagnosis

1. Plantar fasciitis
2. Calcaneal stress fracture
3. Achilles tendinitis
4. Retrocalcaneal bursitis
5. Tarsal tunnel syndrome
6. Foreign body
7. Ankle sprain

Diagnostic Workup

1. XR—right ankle
2. Bone scan
3. MRI

CASE DISCUSSION

Differential Diagnosis

Heel pain in adults can be caused by several distinct entities. For this reason, it is essential that the examiner ascertain the precise location of the symptoms, as this is the first step in determining the most likely diagnosis.

- **Plantar fasciitis:** The most common cause of plantar heel pain in adults, plantar fasciitis typically results from repetitive use or excessive loading (e.g., training for a marathon). Pes planus, pes cavus, decreased subtalar joint mobility, and a tight Achilles tendon can all predispose to plantar fasciitis. The pain is typically gradual in onset and worse with the first few steps in the morning and after prolonged sitting. Examination reveals marked tenderness over the medial calcaneal tuberosity and increased pain with passive dorsiflexion of the toes. Conservative management includes analgesics, stretching, exercise, orthotics, and night splinting.
- **Calcaneal stress fracture:** The calcaneus is second only to the metatarsals in terms of stress fractures of the foot. Stress fractures are common in athletes who are involved in running or jumping sports, as well as in patients who have risk factors for osteopenia. Patients typically have diffuse heel pain that is made worse by medial and lateral compression. A calcaneal stress fracture may be considered in this patient if his symptoms prove refractory to conservative management. Follow-up diagnostic testing (e.g., x-ray, bone scan) may then be warranted.
- **Achilles tendinitis:** Patients with Achilles tendinitis typically complain of posterior heel pain either on the Achilles tendon insertion site or on the tendon itself during running, jumping, and harsh activities. Tenderness to palpation and swelling along the Achilles tendon are common. Pain may also increase with passive dorsiflexion of the ankle. Again, this is commonly due to overuse or to poor biomechanics. Conservative management includes rest, analgesics, and stretching/strengthening exercises.
- **Retrocalcaneal bursitis:** Patients with this condition usually complain of posterior heel pain secondary to chronic irritation of the underlying bursae. The bursae are located between the posterior calcaneus and the Achilles tendon, and between the Achilles tendon and the skin. The condition is commonly be caused by ill-fitting footwear that has a poorly fitting, rigid heel cup. It can also be associated with Haglund's deformity (a bony spur on the posterosuperior aspect of the calcaneus), which may exacerbate the condition. Conservative management includes analgesics, proper shoe wear, and heel padding.
- **Tarsal tunnel syndrome:** The tarsal tunnel is on the medial aspect of the heel and is formed by the flexor retinaculum traversing over the talus and calcaneus. Compression of the tibial nerve in the tunnel can lead to pain, burning, tingling, or numbness that can radiate to the plantar heel and even to the distal sole and toes. Symptoms may be exacerbated by percussion of the tarsal tunnel or with dorsiflexion and eversion of the foot. Conservative management includes analgesics and correction of foot mechanics with orthotics.
- **Foreign body:** If a foreign body is suspected, the foot should be inspected for signs of an entrance wound. The patient may or may not describe a mechanism of injury. Signs of local infection such as warmth, erythema, pain, induration, or a fluctuant mass should also be sought. Conservative management includes foreign body removal, topical antimicrobials, and appropriate dressing.
- **Ankle sprain:** Ankle ligament injuries are the most common musculoskeletal injury, with the lateral collateral ligament complex most commonly involved. Patients typically describe an injury pattern consistent with "rolling" the ankle, often in the plantarflexed and inverted position. Examination reveals tenderness to palpation over the involved ligaments and increased laxity on stress testing. Significant edema and ecchymosis are often present in the acute/subacute stages. Conservative treatment involves rest, ice, compression, elevation, NSAIDs, and bracing.

Diagnostic Workup

- **XR—right ankle:** X-rays in this region may demonstrate calcaneal spur formation (calcification) at the proximal plantar fascia (as in this patient) or at the Achilles tendon insertion. Care must be taken to correlate these findings with symptoms and with the physical examination, as such calcification can also be seen in asymptomatic patients. Increased prominence of the posterosuperior calcaneus (Haglund's deformity) may also be demonstrated.
- **Bone scan:** If conservative treatment fails in this patient, follow-up with a bone scan would be recommended in two months to rule out calcaneal stress fracture, as would be demonstrated by an increased area of uptake.
- **MRI:** Reserved for suspected soft tissue involvement, which could include the degree of Achilles tendon degeneration, rupture of the Achilles tendon, or articular cartilage defects.

Opening Scenario

The mother of David Whitestone, a five-day-old male child, calls the office complaining that her child has yellow skin and eyes.

Examinee Tasks

1. Take a focused history.
2. Explain your clinical impression and workup plan to the mother.
3. Write the patient note after leaving the room.

Checklist/SP Sheet

PATIENT DESCRIPTION

The patient's mother offers the history.

NOTES FOR THE SP

Show concern about your child's health, but add that you do not want to come to the office unless you have to because you do not have transportation.

CHALLENGING QUESTIONS TO ASK

"Can this jaundice hurt my baby?"

SAMPLE EXAMINEE RESPONSE

"Newborns often develop a mild case of natural jaundice after birth. This type of jaundice will resolve and rarely poses a threat to the baby. However, if your newborn has a more severe type of jaundice, his pigment levels may rise too high and cause damage to his brain. In order to give you a better idea of the severity of your child's illness, I must examine him in the office and then obtain some blood tests. After seeing him, I should be able to give you a more accurate assessment of his condition."

Examinee Checklist

ENTRANCE:

☐ Examinee introduced self by name.
☐ Examinee identified his/her role or position.
☐ Examinee correctly used patient's name and identified caller and relationship of caller to patient.

HISTORY:

☐ Examinee showed compassion for your child's illness.

☑ Question	Patient Response
☐ Chief complaint	My baby has yellow skin and eyes.
☐ Onset	I noticed it yesterday.

☑ Question	Patient Response
☐ Progression	It is not getting worse, but I'm still concerned.
☐ Parts of body involved	It is mainly visible on his face and hands.
☐ Age of child	Five days old.
☐ Vomiting	None.
☐ Abdominal distention	No.
☐ Frequency of bowel movements	He has 2–3 bowel movements a day.
☐ Color of stool	Brown.
☐ Blood in stool	No.
☐ Urinary frequency	Every 3–4 hours.
☐ Number of wet diapers	About 7–8 diapers per day.
☐ Breast-feeding and frequency	Started soon after birth. Every 4–5 hours.
☐ Sucking well	Yes.
☐ Activities and cry	Yes, he is playful and active. He cries occasionally.
☐ Awake and responsive	Yes.
☐ Recent URI	No.
☐ Fever	No.
☐ Breathing fast	No.
☐ Dry mouth	No.
☐ Cough, pulling ear	No.
☐ Shaking (seizures)	No.
☐ Your own blood group and the blood groups of your husband and baby	I'm B Rh positive and my husband is A Rh positive. My baby is also B Rh positive.
☐ Ill contacts	Not to my knowledge.
☐ Other pregnancies and miscarriages	I have a three-year-old daughter and have had no miscarriages.
☐ Birth history	It was an uncomplicated vaginal delivery.
☐ Complications during pregnancy	Yes, I had a positive culture for some bacteria and received antibiotics before delivery.
☐ Delivery at term or premature	At term.
☐ Smoking, alcohol, or recreational drugs during pregnancy	No.
☐ First bowel movement of baby	Soon after delivery.
☐ Discharge from hospital	Uneventful.
☐ Current medications	None.
☐ Past medical history	None.
☐ Past surgical history	None.

✓ *Question*	*Patient Response*
☐ Family history	My daughter also had jaundice after the first week of birth. She was admitted to the hospital.
☐ Drug allergies	Not known.

Physical Examination:

None.

Closure:

☐ Examinee discussed initial diagnostic impressions.
☐ Examinee discussed initial management plans:
    ☐ Follow-up tests.
☐ Examinee asked if the patient has any other questions or concerns.

Sample Closure:

Mrs. Whitestone, given the information you have provided, I'm considering the possibility of physiologic or natural jaundice. This condition usually peaks on day 4 or 5 and then gradually disappears over 1–2 weeks. However, breast-feeding, some other pathologic conditions, and certain birth defects can also cause jaundice in infants, and these need to be ruled out. I would suggest that you bring your child to the medical center for further evaluation. I hope you understood what we discussed today. Do you have any concerns or questions?

PATIENT NOTE

History

Physical Examination

Differential Diagnosis

1.

2.

3.

4.

5.

Diagnostic Workup

1.

2.

3.

4.

5.

History

HPI: *The source of information is the patient's mother. The mother of a 5-day-old M c/o her child having yellow discoloration of the eyes and skin for 2 days. It has not worsened. The child is awake, responsive, playful, and active. He is breast-fed. His stomach is soft and he has 2–3 daily bowel movements. The color of the stools is brown. She denies any h/o recent fever, vomiting, seizure, URI, or breathlessness. There is no noticeable dryness of the mouth. He is wetting 7–8 diapers per day every 3–4 hours. He was delivered vaginally at full term. The mother did receive antibiotics for a positive culture before delivery. The blood group of both mother and neonate is B positive, while that of the father is A positive.*
ROS: *Negative.*
Allergies: *NKDA.*
Medications: *None.*
PMH: *None.*
PSH: *None.*
FH: *His elder sister was hospitalized after the first week of birth for jaundice.*

Physical Examination

None.

Differential Diagnosis

1. Physiologic jaundice
2. ABO or Rh incompatibility
3. Neonatal sepsis
4. Cephalohematoma
5. Breast-feeding jaundice
6. Polycythemia
7. Familial neonatal hyperbilirubinemia

Diagnostic Workup

1. Total and indirect bilirubin
2. Blood typing
3. Direct Coombs' test
4. C-reactive protein
5. CBC
6. Titers for CMV, toxoplasmosis, and rubella (if required)

CASE DISCUSSION

Differential Diagnosis

Early-onset neonatal jaundice (within one week):

- **Physiologic jaundice:** A condition that peaks between the third and seventh day of life. Underlying causes include accelerated destruction of erythrocytes, decreased excretory capacity, and decreased activity of the bilirubin-conjugating enzymes in hepatic cells. It is predominately seen in preterm infants.
- **ABO or Rh incompatibility:** The hemolysis that results from blood group incompatibility may also cause clinically significant jaundice in neonates.
- **Neonatal sepsis:** Signs of infection such as lethargy, vomiting, poor feeding, fever, and/or abnormally colored urine are often present in neonatal sepsis. A history of maternal infections, particularly TORCH and group B streptococcus, yields an additional clue to this diagnosis.
- **Cephalohematoma:** As this scalp hemorrhage reabsorbs, it can also serve as a source of increased bilirubin production.
- **Breast-feeding jaundice:** This is usually seen toward the end of the first week of life in an infant who is otherwise thriving.
- **Polycythemia:** A condition that may also lead to abnormal levels of bilirubin.
- **Familial neonatal hyperbilirubinemia:** Look for a positive history of a sibling who had neonatal jaundice requiring phototherapy.

Late-onset neonatal jaundice (after one week):

- **Breast milk jaundice.**
- **Biliary atresia.**
- **Metabolic disorders:** Hypothyroidism, galactosemia, or hereditary hemolytic disorders such as spherocytosis or G6PD deficiency.

Diagnostic Workup

- **Total and indirect bilirubin:** The first step in determining the severity and type of jaundice. Phototherapy is usually indicated when bilirubin levels exceed 15 mg/dL.
- **Blood typing and direct Coombs' testing:** To evaluate for jaundice stemming from blood group incompatibility. All infants who are born to mothers with type O blood should routinely receive direct Coombs' testing to check for maternal-fetal incompatibility. Such children should also be closely followed for evidence of jaundice from hemolysis.
- **C-reactive protein:** For early assessment and to monitor for signs of infection.
- **CBC:** To evaluate the status of blood parameters such as hematocrit and hemoglobin due to suspected underlying hemolysis. Differential counts may provide additional clues about infections causing sepsis.
- **Titers for CMV, toxoplasmosis, and rubella:** In suspected maternal TORCH infections.

Opening Scenario

The mother of Angelina Harvey, a two-year-old female child, calls the office complaining that her child has noisy and strange breathing.

Examinee Tasks

1. Take a focused history.
2. Explain your clinical impression and workup plan to the mother.
3. Write the patient note after leaving the room.

Checklist/SP Sheet

PATIENT DESCRIPTION

The patient's mother offers the history.

NOTES FOR THE SP

Show concern about your child's health, but add that you don't want to come to the office unless you have to because you do not have transportation.

CHALLENGING QUESTIONS TO ASK

"Can you explain to me exactly what is going on with my child and what can be done for it?"

SAMPLE EXAMINEE RESPONSE

"It is hard for me to give you an accurate answer over the phone. I would like you to bring your baby here so that I can examine her and perhaps run some tests. After that, I will be able to give you a more accurate assessment of her condition."

Examinee Checklist

ENTRANCE:

☐ Examinee introduced self by name.
☐ Examinee identified his/her role or position.
☐ Examinee correctly used patient's name and identified caller and relationship of caller to patient.

HISTORY:

☐ Examinee showed compassion for your child's illness.

☑ Question	Patient Response
☐ Chief complaint	My baby has noisy and strange breathing.
☐ Onset	It started suddenly about an hour ago.
☐ Progression	It is getting worse.

☑ Question	Patient Response
☐ Description of the activity that proceded the event	She was playing with toys.
☐ Description of the sound	It is a noisy sound, as if she swallowed a washing machine.
☐ Consistency	The sound is always the same.
☐ Best heard on inhalation or exhaling air	On inhalation.
☐ Can you identify anything that may have caused it?	None.
☐ Alleviating/exacerbating factors (feeding, crying, supine position, sleep)	None.
☐ Associated problems (cough, fever)	Yes, there is some coughing, but it was present earlier. She has no fever.
☐ Is the cough barking in nature?	No.
☐ Is it productive?	No.
☐ Any blood in cough?	No.
☐ Is she crying?	Yes.
☐ Is her crying muffled or weak?	Weak.
☐ Breathing fast	No.
☐ Nausea/vomiting	No.
☐ Drooling	No.
☐ Blueness of skin or fingers	No.
☐ Difficulty in swallowing food	No.
☐ Similar episodes in the past	No.
☐ Hoarseness of voice	No.
☐ Snoring at night	No.
☐ History of allergies in the family	No.
☐ Psychological or social stress in the recent past	No.
☐ Day care center	Yes.
☐ Ill contacts in day care center	Not to my knowledge.
☐ Vaccinations	Up to date.
☐ Last checkup	Two weeks ago, and everything was normal.
☐ Growth, development, and milestones	All were fine. She met all milestones in a timely manner.
☐ Birth history	It was an uncomplicated spontaneous vaginal delivery.
☐ Eating habits	Normal.
☐ Current medications	None.
☐ Past medical history	Nothing of note.

☑ *Question*	*Patient Response*
☐ Past surgical history	None.
☐ Family history	None.

Physical Examination:

None.

Closure:

☐ Examinee discussed initial diagnostic impressions.
☐ Examinee discussed initial management plans:
    ☐ Follow-up tests.
☐ Examinee asked if the patient has any other questions or concerns.

Sample Closure:

Mrs. Harvey, on the basis of the information I have gathered from you, I'm considering the possibility that your daughter might have aspirated a foreign body. However, the possibility that some infection might be causing her problem needs to be ruled out. Right now, however, I feel that your daughter needs emergency medical attention. Since you do not have access to transportation, I would strongly suggest that you call 911 immediately and bring her to the medical center. In the meantime, I would suggest that you avoid putting a finger in her mouth or performing any blind finger sweep, as doing so may cause the foreign body to become more deeply lodged if it is actually present. If you observe significant respiratory compromise or choking, please perform the Heimlich maneuver by thrusting you daughter's tummy with sudden pressure. I hope you understood what we have discussed today. Do you have any questions or concerns? All right, I will see you once you get to the hospital. Take care.

PATIENT NOTE

History

Physical Examination

Differential Diagnosis	**Diagnostic Workup**
1.	1.
2.	2.
3.	3.
4.	4.
5.	5.

PATIENT NOTE

History

HPI: *The source of information is the patient's mother. The mother of a 2 yo F c/o her child suddenly developing noisy breathing that is getting progressively worse. The child was playing with her toys when she developed the noisy breathing. The sound is consistent, best heard on inhalation, and similar to that of a washing machine. There is no relation to posture. It is associated with a nonproductive cough without any associated fever, hemoptysis, tachypnea, hoarseness of voice, drooling, or bluish discoloration of the skin. Her vaccinations are up to date.*
ROS: *Negative.*
Allergies: *NKDA.*
Medications: *None.*
PMH: *Uncomplicated spontaneous vaginal delivery.*
PSH: *None.*
FH: *Noncontributory.*

Physical Examination

None.

Differential Diagnosis

1. Foreign body aspiration
2. Croup
3. Laryngitis
4. Epiglottitis
5. Retropharyngeal abscess
6. Angioedema
7. Peritonsillar abscess
8. Laryngeal papilloma

Diagnostic Workup

1. ABG
2. CXR—PA and lateral
3. XR—neck, AP and lateral
4. CBC with differential
5. Direct laryngoscopy
6. Bronchoscopy

CASE DISCUSSION

Differential Diagnosis

There are three types of stridor:

- **Inspiratory stridor:** Indicates obstruction at the level of larynx or superior to it.
- **Expiratory stridor:** Points to obstruction inferior to the larynx.
- **Biphasic stridor:** Suggests obstruction in the trachea.

When associated hoarseness presents along with stridor, it suggests involvement of the vocal cords.

- **Aspiration of a foreign body:** The sudden and dramatic onset of symptoms, especially when a foreign body (usually a toy or peanuts) is in the vicinity before the patient develops symptoms, helps support this diagnosis.
- **Croup:** Common in children six months to three years of age; develops insidiously as an URI. A characteristic barking cough is often present.
- **Laryngitis:** Occurs in children older than five years of age. The absence of stridor and the presence of a hoarse voice is characteristic.
- **Epiglottitis:** Occurs more frequently in children 2–6 years of age and begins with a short prodrome. Significant drooling, with symptomatic relief while bending forward, is the hallmark feature. A history of incomplete vaccinations is often present.
- **Retropharyngeal abscess:** Patients are usually < 6 years of age. They lack stridor, their voice is muffled, and drooling is often present.
- **Angioedema:** Can occur at any age. Onset is sudden, and the clinical features of stridor and facial edema are found. Respiration is laborious.
- **Peritonsillar abscess:** Occurs in children > 10 years of age. Onset is gradual, with a history of a sore throat and tonsillitis. There is no stridor.
- **Laryngeal papilloma:** A chronic condition characterized by a hoarse voice; most commonly diagnosed in children three months to three years of age.

Diagnostic Workup

- **ABG:** It is essential to determine blood gas concentrations in order to indirectly assess ventilation and gaseous exchange in the lung.
- **CXR—PA and lateral:** It is noteworthy that the majority of foreign bodies are not visible on CXR PA plain films. Therefore, a normal radiograph cannot rule out an aspirated foreign body. However, when a foreign body obstructs the lower airway and causes air trapping, the expiratory film may sometimes reveal air trapping as a result of the ball-and-valve effect.
- **XR—neck, lateral:** May show narrowing of the trachea (steeple sign), extrinsic pressure, or a classic swollen glottis (thumbprint sign), which may assist with the specific diagnosis of croup or epiglottitis, respectively.
- **CBC with differential:** To rule out or rule in an underlying infective pathology.
- **Direct laryngoscopy:** Of use when differentials of laryngomalacia or laryngeal lesions such as papilloma are suspected.
- **Bronchoscopy:** Used as a diagnostic and therapeutic modality in cases of foreign body aspiration.

CASE 41
DOORWAY INFORMATION

Opening Scenario

Frank Emanuel, a 32-year-old male, comes to the office for a pre-employment medical checkup as requested by his prospective employer.

Vital Signs

BP: 130/85 mmHg
Temp: 98.3°F (36.8°C)
RR: 15/minute
HR: 70/minute, regular

Examinee Tasks

1. Take a focused history.
2. Perform a focused physical exam (do not perform rectal, genitourinary, or female breast exam).
3. Explain your clinical impression and workup plan to the patient.
4. Write the patient note after leaving the room.

Checklist/SP Sheet

PATIENT DESCRIPTION
Patient is a 32 yo M.

NOTES FOR THE SP

- Sit up on the bed.
- Hold the physical exam request form in your hand.

CHALLENGING QUESTIONS TO ASK
"Do you think they are going to give me the job?"

SAMPLE EXAMINEE RESPONSE

"Employers routinely request medical examinations to ensure that potential employees are fit for the job, as well as to determine if they have any medical conditions that may prove hazardous to others in the work environment. I will ask you few questions and perform a physical examination, and on the basis of what I find, I may or may not order further tests. Hopefully everything will be fine."

Examinee Checklist

ENTRANCE:

☐ Examinee knocked on the door before entering.
☐ Examinee introduced self by name.
☐ Examinee identified his/her role or position.

☐ Examinee correctly used patient's name.
☐ Examinee made eye contact with the SP.

HISTORY:

☐ Examinee showed compassion for your situation.

☑ Question	Patient Response
☐ Medical complaints or problems	No.
☐ Chest pain (current and past)	No.
☐ Shortness of breath (current and past)	No.
☐ Palpitations or slow heart rate	No.
☐ Swelling in legs	No.
☐ Loss of consciousness/seizures	No.
☐ Headache	No.
☐ Weakness/numbness	No.
☐ Cough	Yes.
☐ Onset of cough	I've had this cough for years.
☐ Changes in the cough during the day	None.
☐ Progression of the cough	It is the same.
☐ Wheezing	No.
☐ Do you cough at night?	No.
☐ Sputum production	Yes.
☐ Amount of sputum	I am not sure. Around half a teaspoonful; stable.
☐ Color	White mucus.
☐ Odor	None.
☐ Blood in sputum	No.
☐ Fever/chills	None.
☐ Night sweats	No.
☐ Exposure to TB	No.
☐ Recent travel	I emigrated from Africa one month ago.
☐ Last PPD	I have never had this test.
☐ Joint pain or swelling	No.
☐ Nausea/vomiting	No.
☐ Abdominal pain	No.
☐ Diarrhea/constipation	No.
☐ Weight changes	No.

☑ *Question*	*Patient Response*
☐ Appetite changes	No.
☐ Change in stool color	No.
☐ Current medications	None.
☐ Past medical history	None.
☐ Past surgical history	None.
☐ Medical problems or diseases in your family	None.
☐ Vaccinations	My immunizations are up to date. I have my papers at home; I can fax them to you.
☐ Occupation	I used to work in a coal mine back home. I am applying for a new job.
☐ Alcohol use	No.
☐ Illicit drug use	No.
☐ Tobacco	Yes, one pack a day for 10 years.
☐ Sexual activity	Yes, with my wife.
☐ Drug allergies	None.

Physical Examination:

☐ Examinee washed his/her hands.
☐ Examinee asked permission to start the exam.
☐ Examinee used respectful draping.
☐ Examinee did not repeat painful maneuvers.

☑ *Exam Component*	*Maneuver*
☐ Head and neck exam	Inspected mouth, throat; palpated lymph nodes
☐ CV exam	Auscultation
☐ Pulmonary exam	Auscultation, palpation, percussion
☐ Abdominal exam	Auscultation, palpation
☐ Extremities	Inspection
☐ Neurologic exam	Cranial nerves, motor exam, DTRs, gait.

Closure:

☐ Examinee discussed initial diagnostic impressions.
☐ Examinee discussed initial management plans:
    ☐ Follow-up tests: Examinee mentioned the need for a rectal exam.
☐ Examinee asked if the patient has any other questions or concerns.

Sample Closure:

Mr. Emanuel, your physical examination is normal, but your cough may raise concern for some possible medical problems. We need to order some tests to make sure you are free of any serious medical conditions, and if we find anything, we will treat it right away. Since you just came here from Africa and you have never been tested for TB, we should rule out pulmonary tuberculosis, not only because it is harmful to you but also because you may transmit it to your future coworkers. The other issue I want to talk to you about is your smoking. It puts you at increased risk of heart and lung disease, and I would strongly urge you to quit. Do you have any questions?

PATIENT NOTE

History

Physical Examination

Differential Diagnosis

1.

2.

3.

4.

5.

Diagnostic Workup

1.

2.

3.

4.

5.

History

HPI: 32 yo M with no PMH came in for a pre-employment medical examination. He has no medical complaints or problems. Nevertheless, he mentioned having a chronic cough for many years with no recent change in frequency or severity. The cough is productive of half a teaspoonful of white mucus with no blood. The patient denies any dyspnea, fever or chills, chest pain, or wheezing and has had no appetite or weight changes. The patient is an African immigrant who came to the United States 1 month ago and reports no TB exposure. He has never had a PPD test. However, he states that his immunizations are up to date, and he will be faxing us the report to review.
ROS: Negative except as above.
Allergies: NKDA.
Medications: None.
PMH: Per HPI.
PSH: None.
SH: One PPD for 10 years, no EtOH, no illicit drugs. Sexually active with wife only.
FH: Noncontributory.

Physical Examination

VS: WNL.
HEENT: Mouth and pharynx WNL.
Neck: No JVD, no lymphadenopathy.
Chest: Clear breath sounds bilaterally; no rhonchi, rales, or wheezing; tactile fremitus normal.
Heart: RRR; normal S1/S2; no murmurs, rubs, or gallops.
Abdomen: Soft, nontender, nondistended, ⊕BS, no hepatosplenomegaly.
Extremities: No clubbing, cyanosis, or edema.
Neuro: Cranial nerves: 2–12 intact. Motor: Strength 5/5 in all muscle groups. DTRs: Symmetric. Gait: Normal.

Differential Diagnosis

1. Pulmonary tuberculosis
2. COPD/chronic bronchitis
3. Pulmonary silicosis
4. Asthma
5. GERD

Diagnostic Workup

1. CXR—PA and lateral
2. PPD test
3. Sputum Gram stain, AFB smear, routine and mycobacterial sputum cultures
4. CBC

CASE DISCUSSION

Differential Diagnosis

- **Pulmonary tuberculosis:** TB should be ruled out in this patient before he starts a new job, since he is an immigrant and has never been tested for TB.
- **COPD/chronic bronchitis:** This patient's chronic cough and sputum production might be due to COPD/chronic bronchitis secondary to his smoking history.
- **Pulmonary silicosis:** Considering his occupational history as a coal miner, this patient is at increased risk of pulmonary silicosis, which might predispose him to pulmonary tuberculosis.
- **Other possible causes:** There are other possible causes of the patient's chronic cough that may be benign, such as GERD and asthma.

Diagnostic Workup

- **CXR—PA and lateral:** A good initial test in evaluating chronic cough. It may demonstrate cavitary lesions in TB or may show nodular calcification in silicosis. It is usually normal in benign causes of cough, such as asthma or GERD.
- **PPD (tuberculin skin test):** Used as a screening tool to identify individuals who have been infected with *Mycobacterium tuberculosis*, but does not distinguish between active and latent infection.
- **Sputum Gram stain, AFP smear, routine and mycobacterial sputum cultures:** To identify a causative agent of possible infection.
- **CBC:** To identify leukocytosis in infection (nonspecific).

Top-Rated Review Resources

This section is a database of recommended clinical science review books, sample examination books, and commercial review courses marketed to medical students studying for the USMLE Step 2 CS. For each book, we list the **Title** of the book, the **First Author** (or editor), the **Current Publisher**, the **Copyright Year**, the **Edition**, the **Number of Pages**, the **ISBN Code**, the **Approximate List Price**, the **Format** of the book, and the **Number of Test Questions**. Most entries also include Summary Comments that describe their style and utility for studying. Finally, each book receives a **Rating**.

A letter rating scale with six different grades reflects the detailed student evaluations. Each book receives a rating as follows:

A+	Excellent for boards review.
A	
A–	Very good for boards review; choose among the group.

B+	
B	Good, but use only after exhausting better sources.
B–	

The **Rating** is meant to reflect the overall usefulness of the book in preparing for the USMLE Step 2 CS examination. This is based on a number of factors, including:

- The cost of the book
- The readability of the text
- The appropriateness and accuracy of the book
- The quality and number of sample questions
- The quality of written answers to sample questions
- The quality and appropriateness of the illustrations (e.g., graphs, diagrams, photographs)
- The length of the text (longer is not necessarily better)
- The quality and number of other books available in the same discipline
- The importance of the discipline on the USMLE Step 2 CS examination

Please note that **the rating does not reflect the quality of the book for purposes other than reviewing for the USMLE Step 2 CS examination.** Many books with low ratings are well written and informative but are not ideal for boards preparation. We have also avoided listing or commenting on the wide variety of general textbooks available in the clinical sciences.

Evaluations are based on the cumulative results of formal and informal surveys of hundreds of medical students from medical schools across the country. The summary comments and overall ratings represent a consensus opinion, but there may have been a large range of opinions or limited student feedback on any particular book.

Please note that the data listed are subject to change because:

- Publishers' prices change frequently.
- Individual bookstores often charge an additional markup.
- New editions come out frequently, and the quality of updating varies.
- The same book may be reissued through another publisher.

We actively encourage medical students and faculty to submit their opinions and ratings of these clinical science review books so that we may update our database (see "How to Contribute," p. xv). In addition, we ask that publishers and authors submit review copies of clinical science review books, including new editions and books not included in our database, for evaluation. We also solicit reviews of new books or suggestions for alternate modes of study that may be useful in preparing for the examination, such as flash cards, computer-based tutorials, commercial review courses, and Internet Web sites.

DISCLAIMER/CONFLICT OF INTEREST STATEMENT

No material in this book, including the ratings, reflects the opinion or influence of the publisher. All errors and omissions will gladly be corrected if brought to the attention of the authors through the publisher.

A

USMLE Step 2 CS: Complex Cases—35 Cases You Are Likely to See on the Exam
BROTTMAN

$40.00   Review

Kaplan, 2007, 296 pages, 1st edition, ISBN 9781419595509

A thorough review book that is not presented in workbook format. **Pros:** Features a lengthy section on exam basics, including high-yield tips on the physical exam, as well as 35 cases providing doorway information, suggested checklists for the history and physical exam, and a note with a differential diagnosis and follow-up exam. A discussion of history taking, the physical exam, and the patient note is included with each case. Also includes 96 flash cards featuring the chief complaint/patient scenario on one side and the differential/workup on the other. Additional online clinical cases are available with purchase of the book. **Cons:** If you need a workbook-style text, this is not the one for you. **Summary:** A good text for examinees who are willing to put in the time but don't need the redundancy of a workbook-style text.

A

Mastering the USMLE Step 2 CS
RETEGUIZ

$42.95   Review

McGraw-Hill, 2005, 442 pages, 3rd edition, ISBN 9780071443340

A large workbook-style text. **Pros:** Easy to read, with a large font and a smattering of cartoon-like illustrations. Offers a detailed general discussion of the Step 2 CS exam. Also features 50 workbook-style cases covering a wide range of topics, with each case including doorway information, an SP checklist, a patient note, a differential diagnosis, and a diagnostic workup. Learning objectives with "pearls" on history taking, the physical exam, and the patient note are also provided. High-yield chapters cover the top 10 reasons for failure and a quick review with commonly tested scenarios. **Cons:** A large book with a lot of repetition, especially if examinees feel they don't need a workbook format. Limited information is provided on physical exam techniques. **Summary:** A highly comprehensive text that may be too detailed for quick review.

A

Blueprints USMLE Step 2 CS
WAHL

$24.95   Review

Lippincott Williams & Wilkins, 2005, 146 pages, 1st edition,
ISBN 9781405104388

A pocket-sized text presented in workbook format. **Pros:** A highly concise review book that still allows space for practice. Makes good use of standard mnemonics to guide the history. **Cons:** Printed in a small font. Provides sufficient but cursory information on the basics of the Step 2 CS exam. Includes only 20 cases, with no accompanying master list or categories. No clinical correlation is provided for the cases, and the discussion of physical exam techniques is limited. **Summary:** A high-yield text that is ideal for examinees who are comfortable with the Step 2 CS format and seek only a quick review. May not be suitable for IMGs or for those who are less familiar with the exam.

A⁻

CS Checklists: Portable Review for the USMLE Step 2 CS
ROONEY

$32.95   Review

McGraw-Hill, 2007, 348 pages, 2nd edition, ISBN 9780071488235

A pocket-sized text presented in workbook format. **Pros:** Provides detailed descriptions of the components of a complete health history, physical exam, and patient note write-up, presented in bullet-point format. Also features 55 cases organized by chief complaint along with a brief paragraph on history. A patient history checklist, a physical exam checklist, and physical exam findings are also provided. One-page "answers" listed at the end of the book include a differential diagnosis, an appropriate workup, and a brief paragraph on clinical correlation. Also features a case index with diagnoses and corresponding page numbers. **Cons:** Offers limited general information on the physical exam and on how to perform and interpret exam findings. **Summary:** A concise and high-yield text that contains all the information needed for Step 2 CS review. Cases are streamlined to allow for practice without taking up copious amounts of space. Overall, a high-yield book that may require additional texts if more in-depth information is needed on the physical exam.

B+

NMS Review for the USMLE Clinical Skills Exam
ARIAS

$41.95   Review

Lippincott Williams & Wilkins, 2008, 296 pages, 2nd edition,
ISBN 9780781766937

A sleek review book presented in non-workbook format. **Pros:** Provides extensive coverage of physical exam techniques and signs and symptoms, and includes a wealth of basic science information. Chapters devoted to the physical exam and note writing cover OB/GYN, neurology, psychology, pediatrics, and trauma medicine. Also features 91 review cases covering internal medicine and family practice, surgery and orthopedics, OB/GYN, the nervous system, pediatric and phone medicine, and trauma medicine. **Cons:** Some of the material may not be sufficiently high yield for the Step 2 CS. Cases are compressed into a one-page format with a written patient note, a differential diagnosis, a diagnostic workup plan, and a short paragraph on clinical correlation. **Summary:** A great book for both Step 2 CS and Step 2 CK preparation that provides a large number of very concise cases. However, no attention is paid to a step-by-step approach toward the patient exam or patient note.

B+

The Ultimate Guide and Review for the USMLE Step 2 Clinical Skills Exam
SWARTZ

$37.95   Review

Saunders, 2007, 402 pages, 1st edition, ISBN 9781416037279

A large workbook-style review text. **Pros:** Easy to read, and printed in a large font. Includes a detailed chapter outlining the basics of the exam. Approximately 20 pages are devoted to communication skills, and an additional 10 pages are devoted to a guide to U.S. culture. **Cons:** Because the workbook format takes up a significant amount of space, only 30 review cases are provided. **Summary:** A text that may be best suited to examinees who seek practice documenting checklists and patient notes. The lengthy sections on communication skills and U.S. culture make it more suitable for IMGs. Those who seek a quick review might be better served by a more concise text.

Acronyms and Abbreviations

Abbreviation	Meaning
AAMC	Association of American Medical Colleges
ABG	arterial blood gas
ACE	angiotensin-converting enzyme
ACh	acetylcholine
ACTH	adrenocorticotropic hormone
ADH	antidiuretic hormone
ADHD	attention-deficit hyperactivity disorder
ADLs	activities of daily living
AFB	acid-fast bacillus
AFP	α-fetoprotein
AIDS	acquired immunodeficiency syndrome
ALT	alanine aminotransferase
ANA	antinuclear antibody
AP	anteroposterior
AST	aspartate aminotransferase
AXR	abdominal x-ray
BP	blood pressure
BPH	benign prostatic hypertrophy
BPPV	benign paroxysmal positional vertigo
BS	bowel sounds
BUN	blood urea nitrogen
CABG	coronary artery bypass graft
C-ANCA	cytoplasmic antineutrophil cytoplasmic antibody
CBC	complete blood count
CC	chief complaint
CD	cluster of differentiation
CEA	carcinoembryonic antigen
CHF	congestive heart failure
CIS	communication/interpersonal skills [CSE score]
CMV	cytomegalovirus
CN	cranial nerve
CNS	central nervous system
c/o	complains of
COPD	chronic obstructive pulmonary disease
CPK	creatine phosphokinase
CPK-MB	creatine phosphokinase, MB fraction
Cr	creatinine

Abbreviation	Meaning
CREST	calcinosis, Raynaud's phenomenon, esophageal dysmotility, sclerodactyly, telangiectasia [syndrome]
CRP	C-reactive protein
CS	Clinical Skills
CSA	Clinical Skills Assessment
CSEC	Clinical Skills Evaluation Collaboration [center]
CSF	cerebrospinal fluid
CT	computed tomography
CV	cardiovascular
CVA	costovertebral angle, cerebrovascular accident
CXR	chest x-ray
D&C	dilatation and curettage
DDAVP	1-deamino (8-D-arginine) vasopressin
DEXA	dual-energy x-ray absorptiometry
DFA	direct fluorescent antibody [test]
DG	data gathering [CSE score]
DHEAS	dehydroepiandrosterone sulfate
DI	diabetes insipidus
DIC	disseminated intravascular coagulation
DM	diabetes mellitus
DNA	deoxyribonucleic acid
dsDNA	double-stranded deoxyribonucleic acid
DTR	deep tendon reflex
DVT	deep venous thrombosis
EBNA	Epstein-Barr nuclear antigen
EBV	Epstein-Barr virus
ECFMG	Educational Commission for Foreign Medical Graduates
ECG	electrocardiogram
ED	erectile dysfunction
EEG	electroencephalogram
EMG	electromyogram
ENT	ear, nose, and throat
EOMI	extraocular movements intact
ER	emergency room
ERCP	endoscopic retrograde cholangiopancreatography

Abbreviation	Meaning
ESR	erythrocyte sedimentation rate
ET	essential tremor
EtOH	ethyl alcohol
FH	family history
FSH	follicle-stimulating hormone
FT_4	free thyroxine
GBS	group B *Streptococcus*
GC	gonorrhea and *Chlamydia*
GERD	gastroesophageal reflux disease
GI	gastrointestinal
HbA_{1c}	hemoglobin A_{1c}
HBsAg	hepatitis B surface antigen
HBV	hepatitis B virus
hCG	human chorionic gonadotropin
HCTZ	hydrochlorothiazide
HEENT	head, eyes, ears, nose, and throat
5-HIAA	5-hydroxyindoleacetic acid
HIDA	hepatobiliary iminodiacetic acid [scan]
HIV	human immunodeficiency virus
HPI	history of present illness
HR	heart rate
HRT	hormone replacement therapy
HSV	herpes simplex virus
IADLs	instrumental activities of daily living
ICE	integrated clinical encounter [CSE score]
Ig	immunoglobulin
IMED	International Medical Education Directory
IMG	international medical graduate
IPS	interpersonal skills [CSE score]
IV	intravenous
IVDU	intravenous drug use
IVP	intravenous pyelography
IWA	Interactive Web Application
JVD	jugular venous distention
KOH	potassium hydroxide
LDH	lactose dehydrogenase
LH	luteinizing hormone
LLQ	left lower quadrant
LMP	last menstrual period
LOC	loss of consciousness
LP	lumbar puncture
LUQ	left upper quadrant
LVH	left ventricular hypertrophy
MCP	metacarpophalangeal [joint]
MDI	metered-dose inhaler
MDMA	methylenedioxymethamphetamine ("ecstasy")
MI	myocardial infarction
MRA	magnetic resonance angiography
MRCP	magnetic resonance cholangiopancreatography
MRI	magnetic resonance imaging
MS	multiple sclerosis

Abbreviation	Meaning
MTP	metatarsophalangeal [joint]
MVA	motor vehicle accident
NBME	National Board of Medical Examiners
NC/AT	normocephalic/atraumatic
NKDA	no known drug allergies
NOS	not otherwise specified
NSAID	nonsteroidal anti-inflammatory drug
N/V	nausea or vomiting
OASIS	Online Applicant Status and Information System
OCP	oral contraceptive pill
OSA	obstructive sleep apnea
OTC	over the counter
PA	posteroanterior
PCOS	polycystic ovary syndrome
PCP	*Pneumocystis carinii* pneumonia
PCR	polymerase chain reaction
PD	Parkinson's disease
PERRLA	pupils equal, round, and reactive to light and accommodation
PFT	pulmonary function test
PID	pelvic inflammatory disease
PMH	past medical history
PMI	point of maximal impulse
PN	patient note
PPD	pack per day; purified protein derivative [tuberculin skin test]
prn	pro re nata [as needed]
PSA	prostate-specific antigen
PSH	past surgical history
PT	prothrombin time
PTSD	post-traumatic stress disorder
PTT	partial thromboplastin time
RBC	red blood cell
RF	rheumatoid factor
RLQ	right lower quadrant
ROS	review of systems
RPR	rapid plasma reagin
RR	respiratory rate
RRR	regular rate and rhythm
RUQ	right upper quadrant
SEP	spoken English proficiency [CSE score]
SH	social history
SIADH	syndrome of inappropriate antidiuretic hormone
SLE	systemic lupus erythematosus
SP	standardized patient
SPECT	single-photon emission computed tomography
SPEP	serum protein electrophoresis
STD	sexually transmitted disease
T_3	triiodothyronine
T_4	thyroxine
TB	tuberculosis

Abbreviation	Meaning	Abbreviation	Meaning
TCA	tricyclic antidepressant	U/S	ultrasound
TEE	transesophageal echocardiography	USMLE	United States Medical Licensing Examination
TIA	transient ischemic attack	UTD	up to date [vaccinations]
TIBC	total iron-binding capacity	UTI	urinary tract infection
TM	tympanic membrane	VCA	virus capsid antigen
TMJ	temporomandibular joint	VDRL	Venereal Disease Research Laboratory
TOEFL	Test of English as a Foreign Language	V/Q	ventilation-perfusion [scan]
TSE	test of spoken English	VS	vital signs
TSH	thyroid-stimulating hormone	WBC	white blood cell
TTE	transthoracic echocardiography	WNL	within normal limits
UA	urinalysis	XR	x-ray
UPEP	urine protein electrophoresis	yo	year old
URI	upper respiratory infection		

Index

Fifth disease, 179
Flexible proctosigmoidoscopy, 161
Follicle-stimulating hormone (FSH), 259, 290
Foreign body aspiration, 386

G

Galactosemia, 380
Gastric cancer, 135
Gastritis, 110, 135
Gastrocnemius muscle, rupture of, 366
Gastroenteritis (infectious diarrhea), 109, 124, 142, 173
Gastroesophageal reflux disease (GERD), 99, 167, 192, 393
  atypical, 135
  and chronic cough, 393
Gastrointestinal bleeding
  blood in stool, 110–111, 156–161
    angiodysplasia, 161
    colorectal cancer, 111, 161
    diverticulosis, 111, 161
    hemorrhoids, 161
    ulcerative colitis, 111, 161
  upper, 110
    gastritis, 110
    peptic ulcer, bleeding, 110
Giant cell arteritis (temporal arteritis), 83, 246
Gilbert's syndrome, 199
Glomerulonephritis, 252
Glucocorticoids, 360
Glucose-6-phosphate dehydrogenase (G6PD) deficiency, 380
Glycosylated hemoglobin, 360
Gonococcal arthritis, 266
Gonorrhea, 121, 334, 341
  disseminated, 121
Gout, 266
Group A streptococcal pharyngitis, 155
Guillain-Barré syndrome, 92

H

Haglund's deformity, 373
Hallucinations, 349–354
  hypnagogic, 354
  hypnopompic, 354
Headache, 83–85, 241–246
  cluster, 83, 246
  depression, 246

intracranial mass lesion, 246
  meningitis, 84
  migraine, 83, 246
  pseudotumor cerebri, 84, 246
  sinusitis, 84, 246
  subarachnoid hemorrhage, 84
  temporal arteritis (giant cell arteritis), 83
  tension, 84, 246
  trigeminal neuralgia, 85
Hearing loss, 309–314
  acoustic neuroma, 314
  cochlear nerve damage, 314
  Ménière's disease, 314
  otosclerosis, 314
  ototoxicity, 314
  presbycusis, 314
Heel pain, 367–374
  Achilles tendinitis, 373
  ankle sprain, 373
  calcaneal stress fracture, 373
  foreign body, 373
  plantar fasciitis, 373
  retrocalcaneal bursitis, 373
  tarsal tunnel syndrome, 373
Helicobacter pylori, 135
Hematoma, 366
Hematuria, 111–112, 247–252
  benign prostatic hyperplasia (BPH), 252
  bladder cancer, 112, 252
  glomerulonephritis, 252
  polycystic kidney disease, 112
  prostate cancer, 252
  renal cell carcinoma, 112, 252
  urinary tract infection (UTI), 252
  urolithiasis, 252
Hemochromatosis, 360
Hemorrhoids, 161
Hemothorax, 327, 334
Hepatitis
  acute, 105
  alcoholic, 199
  B, 334
  viral, 199
HIDA (hepatobiliary) scan, 135
Hip
  dislocation, traumatic, 120
  fracture, 120
History, taking the, 42–53
  additional tips, 44–45
  common questions to ask the patient, 45–53

abuse, 53
  alcohol history, 50
  appetite, 48
  bowel symptoms, 48
  cough, 46
  daily activities (for dementia patients), 53
  diet, 48
  dizziness, 49
  family history, 49
  feeding history, 51
  fever, 47
  growth and development, 51
  gynecologic/obstetric history, 50–51
  headache, 46–47
  joint pain, 49
  nausea, 46
  opening of the encounter, 45
  pain, 45–46
  past medical history, 49
  pediatric history, 51
  psychiatric history, 52
  routine care, 51
  sexual history, 50
  shortness of breath, 47
  sleep, 48
  social history, 49–50
  travel history, 49
  urinary symptoms, 47–48
  vomiting, 46
  weight, 48
  guidelines, 43
  overview, 43
HIV, 96, 155, 185, 226, 334
  antibody, 185, 226, 334
Holter monitor, 278
Homans' sign, 366
Horner's syndrome, 246
Humeral fracture, 148
Hyperbilirubinemia, 199, 380
  familial neonatal, 380
Hypercalcemia, 206
Hypercoagulability testing, 366
Hypercortisolism, 284
Hyperglycemia, 206, 233, 360
Hyperhomocysteinemia, 366
Hypernatremia, 206, 233
Hyperprolactinemia, 290
Hypersomnia, 348
Hypertension, 253–259
  erectile dysfunction (ED)
    caused by vascular disease, 259
    drug-induced, 259

Tao Le, MD, MHS   Vikas Bhushan, MD   Mae Sheikh-Ali, MD   Fadi Abu Shahin, MD

Tao Le, MD, MHS

Tao has been a well-recognized figure in medical education for the past 16 years. As senior editor, he has led the expansion of *First Aid* into a global educational series. In addition, he is the founder of the *USMLERx* online test bank series as well as a cofounder of the *Underground Clinical Vignettes* series. As a medical student, he was editor-in-chief of the University of California, San Francisco *Synapse,* a university newspaper with a weekly circulation of 9000. Tao earned his medical degree from the University of California, San Francisco in 1996 and completed his residency training in internal medicine at Yale University and allergy and immunology fellowship training at Johns Hopkins University. At Yale, he was a regular guest lecturer on the USMLE review courses and an adviser to the Yale University School of Medicine curriculum committee. Tao subsequently went on to cofound Medsn and served as its chief medical officer. He is currently pursuing research in asthma education at the University of Louisville.

Vikas Bhushan, MD

Vikas is an author, editor, entrepreneur, and roaming teleradiologist who divides his days between Los Angeles, Maui, and balmy remote locales with abundant bandwidth. In 1992 he conceived and authored the original *First Aid for the USMLE Step 1*, and in 1998 he originated and coauthored the *Underground Clinical Vignettes* series. His entrepreneurial adventures include a successful software company; a medical publishing enterprise (S2S); an e-learning company (Medsn); and, most recently, an ER teleradiology venture (24/7 Radiology). His eclectic interests include medical informatics, independent film, humanism, Urdu poetry, world music, South Asian diasporic culture, and avoiding a day job. He has also coproduced a music documentary on qawwali; coproduced and edited *Shabash 2.0: The Hip Guide to All Things South Asian in North America;* and is now completing a CD/book project on Sufi poetry translated into four languages. Vikas completed a bachelor's degree in biochemistry from the University of California, Berkeley; an MD with thesis from the University of California, San Francisco; and a radiology residency from the University of California, Los Angeles.

Mae Sheikh–Ali, MD

Mae is currently an assistant professor of medicine, division of endocrinology at the University of Florida College of Medicine, Jacksonville. She earned her medical degree from Damascus University School of Medicine in Syria. She completed her residency training in internal medicine at Drexel University College of Medicine in Philadelphia and endocrinology fellowship training at Mayo Clinic College of Medicine, Jacksonville, Florida. She is an editor and contributing author of several editions of the *First Aid for the® USMLE* and the *Underground Clinical Vignettes series.* Mae is passionate about medical education. She is taking an active role in teaching and empowering medical students, residents, fellows and patients. Mae is currently pursuing an academic career in endocrinology, with a focus on vitamin D, obesity and diabetes research projects..

Fadi Abu Shahin, MD

Fadi is a distinguished graduate of Damascus University medical school in Syria. He subsequently moved to the United States and worked in the Department of Obstetrics and Gynecology at Yale University as a postdoctoral fellow. His research was focused on ovarian cancer and the effects of estrogen on the immune system. Currently, he is a chief resident in obstetrics and gynecology at Northwestern University in Chicago. He will soon be starting his fellowship in gynecologic oncology at the Cleveland Clinic. He has been a contributor, an editor, and an author of several editions of the *First Aid for the® USMLE* and the *Underground Clinical Vignettes* series.

ABOUT THE AUTHORS

usmle Rx™
From the Authors of FIRST AID®

STEP 2 CK Qmax
New!

▷ **2600+** high-yield Step 2 CK questions with detailed explanations

▷ Create highly custom tests

▷ Select questions by difficulty level

▷ Simulate a half-day or full-day exam

▷ Predictive of actual USMLE performance

▷ Pass guarantee – pass or we will double your subscription

www.usmlerx.com
Your Prescription for USMLE Success